THE WASHINGTON MANUAL®

Nephrology

FOURTH EDITION

Editors

Tarek Alhamad, MD, MS

Assistant Professor of Medicine
Department of Medicine
Division of Nephrology
Washington University School of Medicine
St. Louis, Missouri

Steven Cheng, MD

Associate Professor of Medicine
Department of Medicine
Division of Nephrology
Washington University School of Medicine
St. Louis, Missouri

Anitha Vijayan, MD

Professor of Medicine
Department of Medicine
Division of Nephrology
Washington University School of Medicine
St. Louis, Missouri

Series Editors

Thomas M. De Fer, MD, FACP

Executive Editor
Professor of Medicine
Associate Dean for Medical Student
    Education
Department of Medicine
Division of Medical Education
Washington University School of Medicine
St. Louis, Missouri

Thomas M. Ciesielski, MD

Assistant Professor of Medicine
Associate Program Director
Department of Medicine
Division of Medical Education
Washington University School of Medicine
St. Louis, Missouri

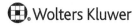. Wolters Kluwer

Philadelphia • Baltimore • New York • London
Buenos Aires • Hong Kong • Sydney • Tokyo

Acquisitions Editor: Sharon Zinner
Development Editor: Ariel S. Winter
Editorial Coordinator: Anthony Gonzalez
Marketing Manager: Phyllis Hitner
Design Coordinator: Teresa Mallon
Production Project Manager: Barton Dudlick
Manufacturing Coordinator: Beth Welsh
Prepress Vendor: Aptara, Inc.

9 8 7 6 5 4

Printed in The United States of America

978-1-9751-1345-2
Library of Congress Cataloging-in-Publication Data
available upon request

Library of Congress Control Number: 2019916472

shop.lww.com

Contributing Authors

Fizza Abbas, MD
Fellow
Department of Medicine
Division of Nephrology
Washington University School of Medicine
St. Louis, Missouri

Nurelign Abebe, MD
Fellow
Department of Medicine
Division of Nephrology
Washington University School of Medicine
St. Louis, Missouri

Tarek Alhamad, MD, MS
Assistant Professor of Medicine
Department of Medicine
Division of Nephrology
Washington University School of
    Medicine
St. Louis, Missouri

Deepa Amberker, MD
Fellow
Department of Medicine
Division of Nephrology
Washington University School of
    Medicine
St. Louis, Missouri

Owais Bhatti, MD
Fellow
Department of Medicine
Division of Nephrology
Washington University School of Medicine
St. Louis, Missouri

Clarice E. Carthon, PharmD, BCBS
Clinical Pharmacy Specialist
Department of Pharmacy
Barnes-Jewish Hospital
St. Louis, Missouri

Monica Chang-Panesso, MD
Assistant Professor of Nephrology
Department of Medicine
Division of Nephrology
Washington University School of Medicine
St. Louis, Missouri

Ying Chen, MD
Assistant Professor of Medicine
Department of Medicine
Division of Nephrology
Washington University School of
    Medicine
St. Louis, Missouri

Steven Cheng, MD
Associate Professor of Medicine
Department of Medicine
Division of Nephrology
Washington University School of Medicine
St. Louis, Missouri

Daniel Coyne, MD
Professor of Medicine
Department of Medicine
Division of Nephrology
Washington University School of Medicine
St. Louis, Missouri

Reem Daloul, MD
Transplant Fellow
Department of Medicine
Division of Nephrology
Washington University School of Medicine
St. Louis, Missouri

Fahad Edrees, MD
Fellow
Department of Medicine
Division of Nephrology
Washington University School of Medicine
St. Louis, Missouri

Seth Goldberg, MD
Associate Professor of Medicine
Department of Medicine
Division of Nephrology
Washington University School of Medicine
St. Louis, Missouri

Sagar Gupta, MD
Transplant Fellow
Department of Medicine
Division of Nephrology
Washington University School of Medicine
St. Louis, Missouri

Jennifer Hagopian, BS, PharmD, BCPS
Transplant Clinical Pharmacist
Department of Pharmacy
Barnes Jewish Hospital
St. Louis, Missouri

Brittany Heady, PA-C
Physician Assistant
Division of Nephrology
Washington University School of Medicine
St. Louis, Missouri

Andreas Herrlich, MD
Associate Professor of Medicine
Department of Medicine
Division of Nephrology
Washington University School of Medicine
St. Louis, Missouri

Timothy A. Horwedel, PharmD
Clinical Pharmacy Specialist
Department of Pharmacy
Barnes-Jewish Hospital
St. Louis, Missouri

Benjamin D. Humphreys, MD, PhD
Joseph Friedman Professor of Renal Diseases
Department of Medicine
Division of Nephrology
Washington University School of Medicine
St. Louis, Missouri

George Jarad, MD
Associate Professor of Medicine
Department of Medicine
Division of Nephrology
Washington University School of Medicine
St. Louis, Missouri

Anuja Java, MD
Assistant Professor of Medicine
Department of Medicine
Division of Nephrology
Washington University School of Medicine
St. Louis, Missouri

Patricia F. Kao, MD, MS
Associate Professor of Medicine
Department of Medicine
Division of Nephrology
Washington University School of Medicine
St. Louis, Missouri

Sreelatha Katari, MD
Transplant Fellow
Department of Medicine
Division of Nephrology
Washington University School of Medicine
St. Louis, Missouri

Lisa Koester, ANP, CNN-NP
Nurse Practitioner
Department of Medicine
Division of Nephrology
Washington University School of
  Medicine
St. Louis, Missouri

Pooja Koolwal, MD
Fellow
Department of Medicine
Division of Nephrology
Washington University School of
  Medicine
St. Louis, Missouri

Ryan Kunjal, MD
Fellow
Department of Medicine
Division of Nephrology
Washington University School of
  Medicine
St. Louis, Missouri

Randy Laine, MD
Resident
Department of Medicine
Division of Medical Education
Washington University School of
  Medicine
St. Louis, Missouri

Tingting Li, MD, MSCI
Associate Professor of Medicine
Department of Medicine
Division of Nephrology
Washington University School of Medicine
St. Louis, Missouri

Andrew Malone, MB, BCh
Assistant Professor of Medicine
Department of Medicine
Division of Nephrology
Washington University School of Medicine
St. Louis, Missouri

Brent Miller, MD
Professor of Medicine
Department of Medicine
Division of Nephrology
Washington University School of Medicine
St. Louis, Missouri

Aubrey Morrison, MBBS, MACP, FASN
Professor of Medicine
Department of Medicine
Division of Nephrology
Washington University School of Medicine
St. Louis, Missouri

Frank O'Brien, MD
Assistant Professor of Medicine
Department of Medicine
Division of Nephrology
Washington University School of
  Medicine
St. Louis, Missouri

Rungwasee Rattanavich, MD
Transplant Fellow
Department of Medicine
Division of Nephrology
Washington University School of Medicine
St. Louis, Missouri

Will Ross, MD
Associate Dean for Diversity
Department of Medical School Diversity
  Programs
Washington University School of Medicine
St. Louis, Missouri

Marcos Rothstein, MD
Professor of Medicine
Department of Medicine
Division of Nephrology
Washington University School of Medicine
St. Louis, Missouri

Rowena Delos Santos, MD
Assistant Professor of Medicine
Department of Medicine
Division of Nephrology
Transplant Nephrology
Washington University School of Medicine
St. Louis, Missouri

Bethany Tellor, PharmD, BCPS
Clinical Pharmacy Specialist
Department of Pharmacy
Barnes-Jewish Hospital
St. Louis, Missouri

Fadi Tohme, MD
Adjunct Assistant Professor of Medicine
Department of Medicine
Division of Nephrology
Washington University in St. Louis
St. Louis, Missouri

Karthikeyan Venkatachalam, MD
Fellow
Department of Medicine
Division of Nephrology
Washington University School of Medicine
St. Louis, Missouri

Anitha Vijayan, MD
Professor of Medicine
Department of Medicine
Division of Nephrology
Washington University School of
  Medicine
St. Louis, Missouri

Miraie Wardi, MD
Fellow
Department of Medicine
Division of Nephrology
Washington University School of Medicine
St. Louis, Missouri

Timothy Yau, MD
Assistant Professor of Medicine
Department of Medicine
Division of Nephrology
Washington University in St. Louis
St. Louis, Missouri

Usman Younus, MD
Fellow
Department of Medicine
Division of Nephrology
Washington University School of Medicine
St. Louis, Missouri

Chairman's Note

It is a pleasure to present the new edition of *The Washington Manual*® Subspecialty Consult Series: *Nephrology Subspecialty Consult*. This pocket-size book continues to be a primary reference for medical students, interns, residents, and other practitioners who need ready access to practical information to diagnose and treat patients with a variety of kidney disorders. Medical knowledge continues to increase at an astounding rate, which creates a challenge for physicians who need to keep up-to-date with new diagnostics, biomarkers, and therapeutics. Rapid access to updated information positively impacts patient care. The *Washington Manual* Subspecialty Consult Series addresses this challenge by providing concise, practical information to aid clinicians in the diagnosis, investigation, and treatment of kidney diseases.

I want to personally thank the authors, which include house officers, fellows, and attendings at the Washington University School of Medicine and Barnes-Jewish Hospital. Their commitment to patient care and education is unsurpassed. Their efforts and skill in compiling this manual are evident in the quality of the final product. In particular, I would like to acknowledge our editors, Drs. Tarek Alhamad, Steven Cheng, and Anitha Vijayan, and the series editors, Drs. Tom De Fer and Thomas Ciesielski, who have worked tirelessly to produce another outstanding edition of this manual. I would also like to thank Dr. Melvin Blanchard, Chief of the Division of Medical Education in the Department of Medicine at the Washington University School of Medicine, for his advice and guidance. This Subspecialty Manual provides practical knowledge that can be directly applied at the bedside and in outpatient settings to improve patient care.

Victoria J. Fraser, MD
Adolphus Busch Professor
Chairman of Medicine
Washington School University of Medicine

Preface

Online medical education and social media are rapidly changing the availability of information in health care. However, easy access to high-quality medical literature during day-to-day hospital rounds and clinics is essential. A manual, written by experts, that stays in the white coat pocket as a quick, handy reference remains a necessity. In the fourth edition of *The Washington Manual Nephrology Subspecialty Consult*, we maintained the original high standards and reformatted the text into a "bullet-style" layout, transforming pages of text into easily accessible tables and figures.

The unique aspect of this fourth edition is the completely renovated transplant section, which includes seven new chapters. With ongoing innovation in the areas of HLA typing and cross-match testing, living donation, immunosuppression medications, and posttransplant care, kidney transplantation remains the treatment of choice for patients with advanced chronic kidney disease. We have carefully incorporated the relevant aspects of kidney transplantation into this edition to serve as a handy reference at the bedside.

The field of nephrology remains a fascinating, challenging, and exciting area of medicine. In addition to the section on kidney transplantation, we have added new chapters on onconephrology and complement-mediated diseases and revamped the other chapters with up-to-date information. Electrolyte and acid-base problems will always pose an interesting thought-provoking dilemma to the trainee and the attending alike. The thrill of working up a patient with hyponatremia or narrowing down the differential diagnoses to get to the underlying etiology of hypokalemia never changes with time. We hope to transfer our passion for nephrology to medical students and trainees and inspire them to pursue a career in nephrology. We hope the readers find this publication to be a relevant, informative, and useful tool in their clinical day-to-day practice.

We would like to acknowledge and thank the authors for all the time and effort vested in this publication. We sincerely thank Dr. Benjamin Humphreys for his support and mentorship. Last, but not least, we would like to thank our parents and families for their love and support: Abdulsalam, Fawzieh, and Basma (TA); Abby and Isaac (SC); and Vichu, Maya, and Dev (AV).

Contents

Contributing Authors   *iii*
Chairman's Note   *vii*
Preface   *viii*

PART I. GENERAL APPROACH TO KIDNEY DISEASE

1. Assessment of Kidney Function   **1**
   Fizza Abbas and Steven Cheng

2. Approach to Proteinuria and Hematuria   **10**
   Ryan Kunjal and Timothy Yau

PART II. ELECTROLYTES AND ACID–BASE DISORDERS

3. Disorders of Water Balance   **20**
   Usman Younus and Steven Cheng

4. Disorders of Potassium Balance   **28**
   Pooja Koolwal and Andreas Herrlich

5. Disorders of Calcium and Phosphorus Balance   **38**
   Miraie Wardi and Daniel Coyne

6. Acid–Base Disorders   **51**
   Owais Bhatti and Steven Cheng

PART III. ACUTE KIDNEY INJURY

7. Approach to the Patient with Acute Kidney Injury   **62**
   Fadi Tohme

8. Intrinsic Causes of Acute Kidney Injury   **79**
   Anitha Vijayan

PART IV. GLOMERULAR DISEASES

9. Primary Glomerulopathies **101**
Ying Chen

10. Secondary Glomerular Disease **115**
Tingting Li

11. Thrombotic Microangiopathy **127**
Anuja Java

PART V. CHRONIC KIDNEY DISEASE

12. Management of Chronic Kidney Disease **130**
Nurelign Abebe and Marcos Rothstein

13. Diabetic Nephropathy **141**
George Jarad

14. Cystic Disease of the Kidney **149**
Seth Goldberg

PART VI. MISCELLANEOUS RENAL DISORDERS

15. Renal Diseases in Pregnancy **162**
Deepa Amberker and Will Ross

16. Nephrolithiasis **173**
Seth Goldberg

17. Renal Artery Stenosis and Renovascular Hypertension **184**
Reem Daloul and Aubrey Morrison

18. Secondary Causes of Hypertension **194**
Randy Laine and Patricia F. Kao

19. Onconephrology **207**
Monica Chang-Panesso and Benjamin D. Humphreys

PART VII. RENAL REPLACEMENT THERAPIES AND THERAPEUTIC PLASMA EXCHANGE

20. Hemodialysis **217**
Frank O'Brien

21. Peritoneal Dialysis and Home Hemodialysis **228**
    Lisa Koester and Brent Miller

22. Continuous and Prolonged Intermittent
    Renal Replacement Therapies **246**
    Fahad Edrees and Anitha Vijayan

23. Therapeutic Plasma Exchange **254**
    Brittany Heady and Tingting Li

PART VIII. DRUG DOSING

24. Principles of Drug Dosing in Renal Impairment **261**
    Bethany Tellor and Jennifer Hagopian

PART IX. TRANSPLANT NEPHROLOGY

25. Overview of Kidney Transplantation **280**
    Rowena Delos Santos

26. Evaluation of the Kidney Transplant Candidate **293**
    Sreelatha Katari

27. Evaluation of the Living Kidney Donor Candidate **302**
    Rungwasee Rattanavich

28. Management of the Kidney Transplant Patient **314**
    Clarice E. Carthon and Timothy A. Horwedel

29. Immunologic Complications After Kidney Transplantation **324**
    Karthikeyan Venkatachalam and Tarek Alhamad

30. Nonimmunologic Complications After Kidney Transplantation **331**
    Sagar Gupta and Tarek Alhamad

31. Combined Organ Transplantation **340**
    Andrew Malone

Index **349**

Assessment of Kidney Function

Fizza Abbas and Steven Cheng

1

GENERAL PRINCIPLES

- Assessing kidney function is a critical step in the recognition and monitoring of acute and chronic kidney disease (CKD).
- Kidney function is most commonly approximated by the **glomerular filtration rate (GFR).** This provides a quantitative measurement of the kidney's ability to filter and clear solute from the body.
- Equally important is the quality of the filtrate that is produced by the kidneys. This can be assessed by examining the content of the urinary filtrate, which reflects renal tubular function and the integrity of the filtration barrier.
- Clinicians need to understand the assumptions and pitfalls regarding the various measurements of kidney function in order to use and interpret them appropriately.
- The amount of fluid that is processed by the kidney is reflected by the **GFR.**
  - GFR is defined as the sum of the filtration rates of all functional nephrons.
  - The normal GFR is ~125 mL/min/1.73 m^2 in men and 100 mL/min/1.73 m^2 in women.
  - Changes in the *overall* filtering capacity of the kidney will result in parallel changes in GFR. For example, diseased kidneys with significantly impaired filtering capacity will have a reduced GFR.
- The content or composition of the urinary filtrate is also highly regulated. An intact nephron has an effective filtration barrier and tight control over solute concentration in the urine.
  - Abnormal urinary findings can suggest damage to specific sites in the nephron.
  - Proteinuria and hematuria, for example, may reflect impaired glomerular architecture, thus compromising the filtration barrier.

DIAGNOSIS

Differential Diagnosis

- Renal dysfunction, identified by a reduction in GFR, an abnormality in urine content, and/or direct tissue evaluation with biopsy, can be categorized in the following ways:
  - **Acute kidney disease versus CKD:** The acuity of the renal disease is important for both diagnostic and prognostic purposes. Establishing a time course for the loss of renal function helps the clinician to narrow the differential diagnosis to processes that acutely injure the kidney or those that cause a more gradual, insidious loss of function. It also provides important information about the likelihood of renal recovery, since most CKD processes cause irreversible damage.
  - **Localization of renal injury:** With intrinsic renal injury, the underlying process should be localized to vascular, glomerular, tubular, or interstitial compartments. This can be done using the clinical context, serologic tests, and urinary findings, as discussed later in this textbook. Localization of the injury helps the clinician to narrow the differential diagnosis and provide treatment targeted to specific lesions.

○ **Stage of disease:** In both acute and chronic renal diseases, it is important to identify the severity or stage of the disease process. The rise in creatinine and fall in urine output can be used to stratify the stage of acute kidney injury, while the estimated GFR and degree of urine protein excretion can be used to stratify CKD. These staging criteria are described in later chapters of this textbook.

Diagnostic Testing

Estimating GFR

● **Serum markers,** such as creatinine and blood urea nitrogen, are commonly used to track changes in GFR. They are inexpensive and convenient tools, but their limitations and shortcomings must be understood.

○ When used in isolation, serum markers can provide only general information about trends in renal function.

■ Levels of these markers rise when there is poor renal clearance and fall when clearance improves.

■ Levels need to be interpreted in the patient's clinical context, with particular attention to historical laboratory values, in order to provide meaningful information about the acuity or severity of renal impairment.

○ Certain patient characteristics and drug effects can alter the serum levels of markers without changing true renal function.

■ A slightly elevated serum creatinine level in an extremely muscular individual may reflect a higher degree of creatinine generation rather than an impairment in renal function.

■ Conversely, a normal serum creatinine may overestimate true renal function if a patient is extremely small or cachectic, since these individuals generate less creatinine than average.

■ Drugs such as cimetidine and trimethoprim inhibit tubular secretion of creatinine and can thus lead to elevations in serum creatinine without impairing GFR.

■ Comorbidities such as upper GI bleeding or steroid use can cause blood urea nitrogen levels to increase.

○ It is also important to recognize that the relationship between the change in creatinine and the change in renal function is *nonlinear*. For example, a change in creatinine from 1.0 to 1.4 mg/dL represents a greater decline in kidney function than a change from 3.0 to 3.4 mg/dL, even though there is a 0.4 mg/dL difference in both examples.

○ The most commonly used markers are summarized in Table 1-1 below. Of these, serum creatinine is utilized most frequently in day-to-day clinical practice.

● **Equation-based estimates of GFR** incorporate serum markers and patient-dependent variables such as race and gender into mathematical models that approximate GFR *in the steady state*. A variety of online calculators are available for each equation, as the math is not always easy to do mentally. These equations provide useful quantitative approximations of GFR, but, like serum markers, their limitations need to be appreciated.

○ **All estimates of GFR are only valid in the steady state.** In acute kidney injury, when creatinine levels are fluctuating or gradually reaching a plateau level, GFR cannot be approximated with these equations.

○ The **Cockcroft–Gault** equation is the oldest of the three equations and has several limitations attributable to the discrepancy between weight and muscle mass. However, this equation continues to be important since it was used in most drug dosing studies to approximate renal function.

○ The **MDRD** equation was initially derived in a nonhospitalized, nondiabetic population.[1] It loses accuracy when applied to obese patients and can underestimate GFR in patients with normal renal function.

TABLE 1-1 SERUM MARKERS OF RENAL FUNCTION

Serum Marker	What It Measures	Use and Limitations
Creatinine	Accumulation of a muscle-derived metabolite that is *predominantly* cleared by glomerular filtration.	A reduction in GFR results in a rise in serum creatinine. However: 1. Creatinine is highly dependent on muscle mass. Individuals at the extremes of muscle mass may have physiologic values that are lower or higher than the reference ranges. 2. Dietary intake and drugs that inhibit tubular secretion (notably cimetidine and trimethoprim) may falsely elevate creatinine levels.
Blood urea nitrogen (BUN)	Accumulation of urea, a product of protein metabolism.	Although BUN may rise in renal disease, an elevated BUN is not specific for renal impairment. Increased generation (upper GI bleed, steroid use) and renal reabsorption (volume contraction) are common confounders.
Cystatin C	Cystatin C is generated at a steady rate by nucleated cells. It is filtered at the glomerulus and metabolized (but not reabsorbed) in the tubules.	Equations that utilize cystatin C in combination with creatinine may be more accurate in estimating GFR than those that utilize creatinine alone.

- ○ The **CKD-EPI** equation performs better than either the Cockcroft–Gault or MDRD equations when estimating GFR in patients with a true GFR >60 mL/min/1.73 m².[2] As such, it is often preferred in the general population.
  - ○ See summary of equations to calculate renal function in Table 1-2.
- **Timed collections** are used to directly calculate *clearance*. Clearance describes the quantity of fluid that is completely cleared of a marker over a definite period of time. When a marker is removed exclusively by renal filtration, clearance = GFR.
  - ○ **Inulin** was considered the classic gold standard marker for such measurements. Inulin is cleared by glomerular filtration and is neither reabsorbed nor secreted by the renal tubules. Other substances with similar properties (iothalamate, ethylenediaminetetraacetic acid, and iohexal) are now used more commonly to obtain precise measurements of GFR. Although these methods are useful in obtaining a very accurate GFR measurement, they are neither cost-effective nor convenient for most purposes and are used only in specific situations that require more precision than estimates from creatinine clearance (CrCl).
  - ○ **The 24-hour CrCl**
    - ■ CrCl is *not* a perfect surrogate for GFR since creatinine is dependent on muscle mass and is partially cleared by tubular secretion. However, because creatinine is

TABLE 1-2 EQUATIONS TO ESTIMATE RENAL FUNCTION

Equation	What It Measures	Use and Limitations
Cockcroft–Gault	**Estimates CrCl** using age, weight, gender, and creatinine	Easy to calculate, but loses accuracy when weight does not correlate to muscle mass.
MDRD	**Estimates GFR** using age, race, gender, and creatinine	Less accurate in obese individuals and those with near-normal GFR.
CKD-EPI	**Estimates GFR** using age, race, gender, creatinine and/or cystatin	May perform better than other equations in patients with *higher GFR* (particularly when both creatinine and cystatin are used in the equation).

endogenously produced and relatively inexpensive to measure, it is a convenient and cost-efficient method of quantifying renal filtration.

■ **CrCl** can be measured by collecting a 24-hour urine sample and using the following formula: **CrCl = ([Cr]$_{Urine}$ × volume of urine in 24 hours/[Cr]$_{Plasma}$)/1440.** *Note: Volume of urine should be expressed in mL; 1440 is used as a conversion factor (1440 minutes in 24 hours).*

■ While timed collections and **CrCls** are helpful when a precise measurement of renal function is required, they are often confounded by the logistical difficulties of urine collection over a precise time period.

■ To rule out an over- or undercollection of urine, the total amount of creatinine excreted ([Cr]$_{Urine}$ × volume of urine collected) can be compared to the expected amount of creatinine produced in a day (20 to 25 mg/kg/day in men; 15 to 20 mg/kg/day in women).

Urinary Assessment
- Examining the chemical and microscopic composition of the urine is extremely useful in determining whether glomerular and tubular function is intact.[3]
- Evidence of renal disease may be present in the urinary assessment even before there are changes in the GFR.
- **Urinalysis:** When used properly, the urinalysis can offer innumerable insights. The urine properties that are assessed on most urine dipsticks are listed in Table 1-3.
- **Microscopic examination:** Cells, crystals, and casts are common findings on urine microscopy.
  ○ The presence of cells on urine microscopy can help clinicians identify the type of renal injury that is sustained.
    ■ Red blood cells (RBCs) suggest bleeding into the upper or lower genitourinary tract
      □ Microscopic hematuria has traditionally been defined as **more than two RBCs per high-power field** on microscopy.
      □ RBCs are typically 4 to 7 μm in diameter and have a characteristic red pigment with central opacity and smooth borders.
      □ In glomerular diseases, the RBCs often taken on a **dysmorphic** appearance (blebs or outpouchings along the cellular contour) which suggest physical deformation as it squeezes through defects in the glomerular filtration barrier.
    ■ White blood cells (WBCs) suggest inflammation or infection
      □ WBCs can be distinguished from RBCs by their larger size, lack of pigment, and cytoplasmic granulation.

TABLE 1-3	URINALYSIS	
Test	What It Measures	Differential Diagnosis
Specific gravity	Assesses the relative density of urine	**Values ≤1.010** indicate a dilute urine (e.g., water ingestion, diabetes insipidus). **Values ≥1.020** indicate a more concentrated urine (e.g., dehydration, volume contraction).
Urine pH	Assesses urine acidification. Ranges between 4.5 and 7.8	**Low urine pH** can be observed in large protein consumption, metabolic acidosis, and volume depletion. **High urine pH** may be seen in distal RTA.
Ketones	Detects acetoacetic acid (but not beta hydroxybutyrate)	Ketones are mainly seen in diabetic and alcoholic ketoacidosis, but can also be observed in starvation, vomiting, and strenuous exercise.
Glucose	Assess glucose reabsorption at the proximal tubule	**If plasma glucose >180–200 mg/dL,** positive results indicate overflow of glucose into the urine. **If plasma glucose <180 mg/dL,** positive results suggest proximal tubular defect.
Hemoglobin	Detects presence of heme pigment in the urine	A positive result suggests hematuria. **However, if microscopy shows no urinary RBCs,** assess for free hemoglobin/myoglobin (e.g., rhabdomyolysis).
Protein	Detects anionic proteins (albumin)	**Significant proteinuria suggests renal parenchymal disease affecting the glomerular filtration barrier.**
Leukocyte esterase	Detects WBC activity in the urine	Can be used in conjunction with nitrite test to identify urinary tract infections. A positive test may also suggest renal inflammation (e.g., interstitial nephritis).
Nitrites	Detects bacterial conversion of nitrates to nitrites	In conjunction with positive leukocyte esterase, can be used to identify UTI. **Note: Not all bacteria convert nitrates to nitrites.**

- WBCs in a clean urine sample are most commonly due to an infectious pathogen, allergic response, or inflammatory condition.
- Urine eosinophils are not easily identified unless special staining (Hansel stain) is used. Urine eosinophils are nonsensitive and nonspecific markers, and should not be used to distinguish various forms of renal injury.
- Epithelial cells
  - **Squamous epithelial cells:** Present in the urine because of shedding from the distal genital tract and essentially are contaminants.
  - **Transitional epithelial cells:** Seen intermittently with bladder catheterization or irrigation. Occasionally, they may be associated with malignancy, especially if irregular nuclei are noted.

TABLE 1-4 COMMON URINARY CRYSTALS

Crystal	Description
Calcium oxalate	While these commonly appear as octahedral "envelopes," they can also take a rectangular, dumbbell, and ovoid shape.
Triple phosphate	These are usually 3–6-sided prisms that resemble "coffin lids."
Calcium phosphate	These crystals usually have the appearance of a small rosette.
Uric acid	Uric acid can have a variety of appearances, including rhomboids, rosettes, and four-sided "whetstones."

- □ **Renal tubular epithelial cells:** May be seen in significant numbers with tubular injury. Tubular epithelial cells from the proximal tubule tend to be very granulated.
  - Organisms
    - □ **Bacteria** are frequently seen in urine specimens, given the fact that urine is typically collected under nonsterile conditions. Identification and susceptibilities of these organisms typically require high-powered magnification, staining, culture, and in vitro testing against antibiotics.
    - □ **Fungi:** Presence of **Candida** in urine is typically thought to be a contaminant from genital secretions or, in the presence of a long, indwelling bladder catheter, colonization. Candida UTIs can cause similar symptoms to that seen with a bacterial infection. Other infectious fungal agents, including Aspergillus, Cryptococcus, and Histoplasmosis, can be seen in the chronically ill or immunocompromised patients.
    - □ **Parasites:** Presence of *Trichomonas vaginalis* and *Enterobius vermicularis* in urine are typically thought of as contaminants stemming from genital secretions.
  - ○ Urinary crystals are often an incidental finding. However, they can be used to identify the composition of kidney stones. Descriptions of various urinary crystals are summarized in Table 1-4.
  - ○ Casts are formed when the contents of the renal filtrate are trapped by proteins secreted into the tubular lumen (typically the Tamm–Horsfall protein). Thus, a cast provides a snapshot of the tubular milieu at the time of its formation. Please see Table 1-5 for casts.

Imaging Studies
- The appearance of the kidney, particularly on ultrasound, can provide a number of insights into the presence, cause, chronicity, and irreversibility of renal disease.
- However, it is generally not used to provide detailed quantitative data about renal function.
- The following attributes are assessed on renal ultrasound:
  - ○ Anatomy
    - ■ Prior to a renal biopsy, an ultrasound is generally done to confirm the presence of two nonatrophic kidneys.
    - ■ Ultrasound can also easily identify the presence of hydroureter or hydronephrosis caused by obstructive lesions.
    - ■ Distortions of renal architecture by tumor or cystic infiltration (as seen in polycystic kidney disease) can also be easily appreciated on ultrasound.
  - ○ Size
    - ■ The average kidney is 10 to 13 cm in length.
    - ■ Kidney size is proportional to body height. A 13-cm kidney would be considered suspiciously large in an individual who is under 5 ft tall (despite being in the

TABLE 1-5 URINARY CASTS

Type of Cast	Appearance	Description and Interpretation
Hyaline casts	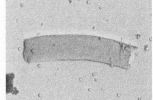	Acellular amalgam of Tamm–Horsfall protein, formed in concentrated, acidic urine.
Granular casts	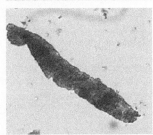	Encased tubular debris (resembles a tube of sand) consistent with *tubular* damage.
WBC casts	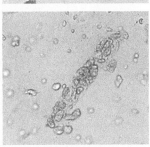	Encased WBCs suggest *interstitial* inflammation such as pyelonephritis.
RBC casts	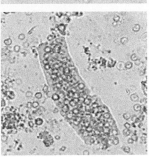	Encased RBCs suggest *glomerular* hematuria, an important finding in glomerulonephritis.

"normal" range). Likewise, a 10-cm kidney would be small for an individual greater than 6 ft tall.

- Small kidneys suggest atrophy attributable to a chronic disease process or aberration in development.
- Large kidneys (greater than 13 cm) can be seen with diabetic nephropathy, HIV-associated nephropathy, infiltrative disorders (amyloidosis, tumor infiltration), and inflammation (acute interstitial nephritis).
- Echogenicity
  - The renal parenchyma should be no more echogenic than the liver.
  - Increased echogenicity reflects an increase in tissue density, which is often associated with chronic parenchymal disease.
  - The combination of increased echogenicity and small kidney size is suggestive of chronic, irreversible damage.

Renal Biopsy

- Obtaining and examining renal tissue through a renal biopsy is the most definitive, yet most invasive, technique for diagnosing renal disease.
- **Indications**
  - Common indications for renal biopsy include acute renal failure of uncertain etiology, nephrotic syndrome, nephritic syndrome, rapidly progressive glomerulonephritis, acute or chronic renal allograft dysfunction.
  - Depending on other clinical features, renal biopsy can be considered in asymptomatic hematuria or proteinuria.
  - Studies have shown that ~40% of patients subjected to renal biopsy will have a change of diagnosis or management based on the results of the biopsy.[4]
- **Preprocedural evaluation**
  - **Renal imaging** should be performed to ensure that the patient has two kidneys of normal size and shape.
    - **Native kidney biopsy is relatively contraindicated for atrophic kidneys <9 cm in size,** as the risk of capsular hemorrhage increases in fibrotic kidneys (as does the risk of a low-yield biopsy result).
    - **Renal biopsy of a solitary native kidney should be undertaken only when absolutely necessary** to preserve renal function, as there is a risk of marked bleeding leading to nephrectomy.
  - **Blood pressure (BP)** should be optimally controlled, with diastolic BP <95 mm Hg, to minimize bleeding complications.
  - **Urine culture** should be sterile before a biopsy attempt.
  - **Blood coagulation parameters** should be normalized as much as possible before renal biopsy.
    - Systemic anticoagulants, including antiplatelet therapy, aspirin, and nonsteroidal anti-inflammatory drugs, should be discontinued ≥5 days before renal biopsy.
    - Prothrombin time (PT) should be <1.2 times control; activated partial thromboplastin time (aPTT) should be <1.2 times control.
    - In a patient with renal insufficiency and elevated blood urea nitrogen levels with a prolonged bleeding time, DDAVP, 0.4 mcg/kg IV for 2 to 3 hours, is usually given before biopsy.
    - Intravenous or subcutaneous unfractionated heparin should be stopped at least 6 hours prior to the procedure and should not be resumed until at least 18 to 24 hours after the procedure.
- **Complications**
  - **After a biopsy, patients should be observed for about 24 hours.**
    - The patient should remain supine for 6 hours and then remain at bed rest overnight.

- Vital signs and complete blood counts are closely monitored.
- To minimize the risk of bleeding, **BP** should ideally be well controlled (goal <140/90 mm Hg).

○ **Hematuria** and the formation of a perinephric hematoma occur to some degree in all patients after renal biopsy. A fall in hemoglobin of about 1 g/dL is not unusual after an uncomplicated renal biopsy.

○ **Blood loss requiring transfusion** occurs in about 2.2% of renal biopsies.[5]

- The most common site of significant blood loss is into the perinephric space, leading to a large perinephric hematoma.
- **Subcapsular bleeds** usually tamponade themselves. Rarely, a large subcapsular hematoma can compress the renal parenchyma and lead to pressure-induced ischemia and hypertension, a phenomenon referred to as a "Page Kidney."
- Significant bleeding into the urinary collecting system may also occur, which manifests as gross hematuria and may lead to ureteral obstruction.
- **Intervention to control bleeding,** such as embolization, is required in about 0.4% of cases.

○ **Hypotension** after renal biopsy can occur in 1% to 2% of patients and is usually fluid responsive.[6]

○ **Arteriovenous fistulas** can be detected radiologically in up to 18% of cases, but are rarely of clinical significance and usually resolve spontaneously.[7]

○ **Persistent pain** at the biopsy site may result from a subcapsular or perinephric hematoma or from renal colic as blood clots pass through the collecting system.

REFERENCES

1. Levey AS, Bosch JP, Lewis JB, et al. A more accurate method to estimate glomerular filtration rate from serum creatinine: a new prediction equation. Modification of diet in Renal Disease Study Group. *Ann Intern Med.* 1999;130(6):461–470.
2. Levey AS, Stevens LA, Schmid CH, et al. A new equation to estimate glomerular filtration rate. *Ann Intern Med.* 2009;150(9):604–612.
3. Perazella M, Coca S, Kanbay M, et al. Diagnostic value of urine microscopy for differential diagnosis of acute kidney injury in hospitalized patients. *Clin J Am Soc Nephrol.* 2008;3(6): 1615–1619.
4. Richards NT, Darby S, Howie AJ, et al. Knowledge of renal histology alters patient management in over 40% of cases. *Nephrol Dial Transplant.* 1994;9(9):1255–1259.
5. Lees J, McQuarrie E, Mordi N, et al. Risk factors for bleeding complications after nephrologist-performed native renal biopsy. *Clin Kidney J.* 2017;10(4):573–577.
6. Manno C, Strippoli GF, Arnesano L, et al. Predictors of bleeding complications in percutaneous ultrasound-guided renal biopsy. *Kidney Int.* 2004;66(4):1570–1577.
7. Harrison KL, Nghiem HV, Coldwell DM, et al. Renal dysfunction due to an arteriovenous fistula in a transplant recipient. *J Am Soc Nephrol.* 1994;5(6):1300–1306.

Approach to Proteinuria and Hematuria

Ryan Kunjal and Timothy Yau

2

Proteinuria

GENERAL PRINCIPLES

Definition

- The glomerulus functions as a barrier, preventing cells and large particles, such as proteins, from spilling into the urine.
- With an intact glomerulus, individuals excrete <150 mg of total protein and <30 mg of albumin in urine every 24 hours.
  - The urine protein found in normal individuals may derive from tubular secretion (Tamm–Horsfall proteins) or from minute amounts of filtered proteins that have escaped reabsorption and degradation by the renal tubular cells.
  - Higher rates of protein excretion (proteinuria) suggest glomerular disease.
- **Nephrotic range proteinuria is an excretion of >3500 mg of protein per 24 hours.** This can be associated with idiopathic glomerular conditions (e.g., minimal change disease, focal segmental glomerular sclerosis [FSGS]) or systemic diseases (e.g., diabetic nephropathy, lupus). When it coexists with hypoalbuminemia, hyperlipidemia, and edema, it forms the **nephrotic syndrome.**
- The degree of proteinuria is a component of the Kidney Disease Improving Global Outcomes (KDIGO) classification of chronic kidney disease (CKD).[1]
- Its importance is underscored by the following:
  - Proteinuria can be an early sign of kidney disease, often preceding a detectable change in glomerular filtration rate (GFR).
  - Significant excretion of the protein albumin is associated with subsequent risk of acute kidney injury (AKI), CKD progression, and cardiovascular mortality.
  - Interventions that reduce the amount of proteinuria may slow the progression of kidney disease and improve the prognosis of cardiovascular disease.

Classification

- Proteinuria mainly occurs due to glomerular dysfunction. Tubular dysfunction may also cause slight increase in proteinuria, but rarely to the nephrotic range (>3.5 g/day).
- **Glomerular proteinuria** results from disruption of the glomerular filtration barrier, leading to increased filtration of plasma proteins in amounts that exceed tubular reabsorption capacity. It is comprised mainly of albumin.
- **Tubular proteinuria** is due to inadequate reabsorption of filtered low–molecular-weight proteins (e.g., beta$_2$-microglobulin or lysozyme). It can coexist with glomerular proteinuria or be an isolated finding in the setting of defective proximal tubule function. Typically, tubular proteinuria is <1 g per 24 hours.
- **Overflow proteinuria** occurs when there is excessive systemic production of abnormal proteins of small molecular weight that exceeds the capacity of the tubule for reabsorption. Examples include urinary excretion of filtered free light chains in multiple myeloma and lysozymuria in acute monocytic leukemia.

Etiology

- **Transient (functional) proteinuria:**
  - Transient proteinuria is primarily seen in children and adolescents who are healthy and asymptomatic, and have normal renal function with bland urine sediment.
  - It is believed to result from alterations in renal hemodynamics in hyperadrenergic states like fever, exercise, congestive heart failure, seizures, use of vasopressors, pregnancy, and obstructive sleep apnea.
  - Transient proteinuria disappears on repeat testing and requires no further evaluation.
- **Orthostatic (postural) proteinuria:**
  - This syndrome is characterized by the excretion of abnormal quantities of protein in the upright position, with normal levels of protein excretion while in supine position.
  - This is demonstrated by a 24-hour split urine collection divided into a 16-hour daytime (upright) portion and an 8-hour overnight (supine) portion.
  - Exclusion may be possible with normal protein excretion in a first pass early morning urine protein to creatinine ratio (PCR) <0.15 mg/mg.
  - Most patients have rates of protein excretion <1 g per 24 hours.
  - It is present in up to 3% to 5% of adolescents and young men, aged mostly <30 years.
  - **It has not been associated with long-term adverse outcomes and also requires no further evaluation.[2]**
- **Persistent proteinuria:**
  - Persistent proteinuria is present regardless of position, activity level, or functional status. It is established by confirming proteinuria on subsequent testing days to weeks after the first positive test. This category comprises the majority of patients with proteinuria.
  - It may result from an isolated kidney disease or may be part of a multisystem process with renal involvement.
  - Patients with persistent proteinuria are typically classified as having nephrotic (>3.5 g/day) or nonnephrotic range proteinuria (<3.5 g/day), and by the presence or absence of features of the nephrotic syndrome.

DIAGNOSIS

A 24-hour urine collection for protein is the definitive means of demonstrating the presence of proteinuria but spot testing is usually more convenient. When spot testing is done, a random urine sample for urine protein and urine creatinine can be measured. The urine PCR roughly estimates the 24-hour excretion rate (with some exceptions below). For screening, the routine urine dipstick is usually the first sign that leads to further testing.

Semiquantitative Methods

- **Routine urine dipstick:**
  - The simplest and least expensive method, urine dipsticks may be limited by relatively poor diagnostic accuracy for proteinuria detection.
  - This dye-impregnated paper uses tetrabromophenol blue as a pH indicator. Urine albumin binds to the reagent and changes its pH, which then results in a spectrum of color changes depending on the degree of pH change. A typical scale for a positive test is shown in Table 2-1.
  - False-positive and false-negative results may occur because these semiquantitative estimates are concentration dependent. Therefore:
    - Highly concentrated urine may show an abnormal result even when the absolute daily protein excretion is normal.
    - Highly dilute urine may show normal or only modestly elevated results for protein concentration even when elevated amounts of protein are excreted. Even with 30 mg/dL of protein, the dipstick can be negative up to 50% of the time.

TABLE 2-1	SCALE FOR DETECTING PROTEINURIA ON ROUTINE URINE DIPSTICK

Negative

Trace: 15–30 mg/dL

1+: 30–100 mg/dL

2+: 100–300 mg/dL

3+: 300–1000 mg/dL

4+: >1000 mg/dL

- The dipstick **will not detect nonalbumin proteins,** such as immunoglobulins, and thus false-negative results may be seen in diseases such as multiple myeloma.
- **False-positive results** can occur in patients who receive contrast up to 24 hours before the test and when highly alkaline urine overwhelms the dye's buffer.
- **Albumin-sensitive tests:**
  - Test strips that are more sensitive to albumin are also available (Albustix).
  - Dye-impregnated strips and special immunoassays can detect albumin concentrations as low as 30 mg/day, which is far below the 300 mg/day threshold of the standard dipstick.
- **Implications of a positive dipstick:** Detection of proteinuria should **prompt an examination of urinary sediment and further quantification of the proteinuria.** Any evidence of hematuria, dysmorphic red blood cells (RBCs), RBC casts, or lipiduria should be noted and may be a sign of underlying pathology.

Quantitative Methods

- **Spot urine PCR:**
  - Urinary dilution will directly affect protein concentration. However, creatinine is excreted fairly constantly during the day and its concentration serves as an internal control for urine dilution. The PCR is therefore independent of urine concentration.
  - **A PCR ratio <150 mg/g is considered normal.**
  - Correlation with a 24-hour urine collection is based on the assumption that daily creatinine excretion is roughly 1 gram per 24 hours.
  - The accuracy of the ratio is diminished when creatinine excretion is either markedly increased (e.g., extremely muscular individuals where the ratio will underestimate proteinuria), or markedly reduced (e.g., acute kidney injury also leads to reduced Cr excretion, and may lead to false values).
- **Spot urine albumin to creatinine ratio (ACR):**
  - Like the PCR, it uses creatinine concentration as an internal control for urinary dilution.
  - **A value <30 mg/g is considered normal.**
  - Values from 30 to 300 mg/g were formerly termed microalbuminuria but are now referred to as moderately increased albuminuria (A2 in the KDIGO classification).
  - ACR >300 mg/g are detected by the routine dipstick and fall into the category of severely increased albuminuria (A3, formerly called macroalbuminuria).
  - ACR at least once annually, is the recommended screening tool for diabetic nephropathy in type 1 diabetics with duration of at least 5 years, in all type 2 diabetics, and in all patients with comorbid hypertension.
  - Falsely elevated values may be obtained with hyperglycemia, vigorous exercise, infection, and ketoacidosis.

TABLE 2-2	THE APPROXIMATE RELATIONSHIPS OF CATEGORIES OF ALBUMINURIA TO OTHER MEASURES OF ALBUMINURIA/PROTEINURIA		
	Category of Albuminuria		
Measure	Normal to Mildly Increased (A1)	Moderately Increased (A2)	Severely Increased (A3)
Dipstick	(−) to trace	Trace to (+)	(+) or greater
ACR	<30	30–100	>300
PCR	<150	150–500	>500
AER	<30	30–100	>300
PER	<150	150–500	>500

ACR, albumin to creatinine ratio (mg/g); PCR, protein to creatinine ratio (mg/g); AER, albumin excretion rate (mg/24 hrs); PER, protein excretion rate (mg/24 hrs).

- Table 2-2 shows the approximate relationships of categories of albuminuria to other measures as discussed below.
- **The 24-hour urine protein collection:**
  - Although this is the definitive method of urinary protein quantification, it is used less often because of frequent errors in collection, patient inconvenience, and the increased use of spot urine ratios.
  - A 24-hour urinary protein is preferable in patients in whom urine creatinine excretion is less reliable (e.g., nonsteady state renal function, high and low muscle mass).
  - To verify proper collection, **a 24-hour urine creatinine should always be measured in the same urine specimen.** Excretion of creatinine in male patients during a 24-hour period should be roughly 20 to 25 mg/kg and for female patients it should be ~15 to 20 mg/kg. If the amount of creatinine in the urine sample is quite different from the expected range, an error in the collection of the sample should be suspected.

CLINICAL APPROACH TO PROTEINURIA

- Once proteinuria has been detected on a dipstick, the next step is to confirm the abnormal result by repeat measurement after several weeks with a freshly voided specimen. If proteinuria is heavy on dipstick (2+ or greater), then no repeat confirmatory test is needed.
- The next step is to **quantify protein excretion by either the ACR or the PCR.** If there is concern about the validity of the spot quantification, a 24-hour urine collection for protein and creatinine excretion can be collected.
- The history and physical examination should include a search for symptoms and signs attributable to kidney disease and identify risk factors for kidney disease. Key issues to be addressed are:
  - The presence and duration of common causes of kidney disease such as diabetes and hypertension.
  - Features suggestive of a connective tissue disorder such as arthralgias, arthritis, skin rashes, and constitutional symptoms.
  - Clinical features of malignancy should be sought. For example, solid organ malignancies have been associated with membranous nephropathy, whereas lymphomas and leukemias have been associated with minimal change disease.

○ Features suggestive of infections such as hepatitis, endocarditis, syphilis, or human immunodeficiency virus should be explored. These disorders can lead to many different forms of glomerular disease.

○ A complete drug history detailing all prescription, illicit, herbal/alternative, and over-the-counter medications should be taken. For example, nonsteroidal anti-inflammatory drugs can cause a minimal change lesion.

○ A family history of kidney disease should be noted, such as hereditary nephritis or polycystic kidney disease.

○ Additional testing is determined by the clinical context. **In all cases, a urine sediment, GFR estimation, complete blood count, basic metabolic profile, and serum albumin are appropriate.** Urine protein electrophoresis and serum protein electrophoresis should be ordered if there is suspicion of an overflow proteinuria from myeloma, amyloidosis, or other paraprotein diseases. Dysmorphic RBCs in the sediment or nephrotic range proteinuria would potentially prompt a kidney biopsy if the clinical scenario does not point to an obvious etiology. An evaluation of the anatomy of the urinary tract is usually not needed unless there is significant hematuria or history of recurrent urinary tract infection.

○ Therapy for proteinuria will depend on the specific etiology determined.

Hematuria

GENERAL PRINCIPLES

Definition

• Hematuria is the presence of RBCs in the urine. A careful and logical approach is required as the causes range broadly from benign processes to genitourinary (GU) malignancies.

• Hematuria can be either gross or microscopic:
  ○ **Gross hematuria** is visible to the patient.
  ○ **Asymptomatic microscopic hematuria (AMH)** is the presence of three or more RBCs per high-powered field (HPF) on microscopic examination of a urine specimen (properly collected and noncontaminated). A urine dipstick that tests positive for blood is not diagnostic on its own.

Epidemiology

• Gross hematuria has an estimated community prevalence of 2.5%.

• AMH has a prevalence ranging from 2% to 31%, with higher rates found among older men and men with smoking histories.[3]

Etiology

• Causes of hematuria can be classified by site of origin—**glomerular or nonglomerular.**

• Glomerular hematuria occurs when RBCs traverse a defect in the glomerular filtration barrier.
  ○ Features that are suggestive of glomerular hematuria include:
    ▪ Concomitant proteinuria
    ▪ RBC casts
    ▪ Dysmorphic RBCs
  ○ Glomerular hematuria is a key characteristic of the **nephritic syndrome.**
    ▪ The nephritic syndrome presents with glomerular hematuria (gross or microscopic hematuria with dysmorphic RBCs and/or RBC casts), hypertension, and a reduction in GFR. Nonnephrotic proteinuria and edema are also typically present.

- Diseases presenting with the nephritic syndrome include anti-glomerular basement membrane (GBM) disease, infection-associated glomerulonephritis, lupus nephritis, IgA nephropathy, and vasculitis.
  - Nephritic syndrome requires early diagnosis and treatment as it can be aggressively progressive. **Rapidly progressive glomerulonephritis** is the most severe form of the nephritic syndrome and can cause renal failure in the span of a few days to weeks.
- **Nonglomerular hematuria can be further divided anatomically into upper and lower urinary tract causes.**
- The various etiologies are listed in Table 2-3.
- Of note 43% to 68% of AMH is due to unknown causes, while IgA nephropathy is the most common glomerular cause.[3]

Associated Conditions

- Malignancies are detected in up to 5% of patients with microscopic hematuria and in up to 30% to 40% of patients with gross hematuria.[3]
- However, the use of urinalysis as a screening tool for cancer detection in healthy, asymptomatic patients is not recommended.

DIAGNOSIS

Clinical Presentation

- In gross hematuria, urine may appear red, cola colored, or brown. It may be symptomatic with associated renal colic (e.g., nephrolithiasis) or painless, which has a stronger association with cancer. **All cases warrant further urologic investigation** to rule out an underlying GU malignancy even if it is self-limited.
- AMH is usually found incidentally on microscopic analysis of urine that tested positive for blood on dipstick. History, physical examination, and laboratory tests can rule out such benign causes as infection, menstruation, vigorous exercise, medical renal disease, viral illness, trauma, or recent urologic procedures. These insults should be removed or treated appropriately, and the urine retested after at least 48 hours. Persistent hematuria warrants a full workup.
- Figure 2-1 is an algorithm for the evaluation of AMH that has been adapted from the recommendations of the AUA.[4]

History

The following key points must be noted from the history:

- A history of gross hematuria is important as bleeding from malignancy may be intermittent.
- Associated symptoms such as **fever, dysuria, and flank pain suggest infection.** Attention must also be placed to collateral information which may rule out the other benign causes as listed above.
- Constitutional and systemic symptoms such as weight loss, rash, arthritis, or pulmonary symptoms suggest a variety of systemic illnesses, including malignancy and vasculitis.
- The presence of certain factors as shown in Table 2-4 can help identify those with AMH who are at increased risk of GU malignancy.
- Medications should be carefully reviewed as certain commonly prescribed drugs can cause hematuria (**nonsteroidal anti-inflammatory drugs, busulfan, aspirin, oral contraceptives, and warfarin**). Hematuria in patients who are taking anticoagulants requires further evaluation, regardless of type or level of anticoagulant therapy.
- **Travel history** may uncover a risk for schistosomiasis.
- **Family history** of hematuria can clue into Alport syndrome, thin basement membrane disease, sickle cell disease, and polycystic kidney disease.

TABLE 2-3 CAUSES OF MICROSCOPIC HEMATURIA

Origin	Causes
Glomerular	IgA nephropathy Thin basement membrane disease (benign familial hematuria) Hereditary nephritis (Alport syndrome) Loin pain hematuria syndrome (may also have gross hematuria) Glomerulonephritis
Nonglomerular	*Upper urinary tract* 　Infection/inflammation: 　　Interstitial nephritis 　　Pyelonephritis 　　Tuberculosis 　Masses/malignancies 　　Renal cell CA 　　Transitional cell CA 　Mineral deposition 　　Hypercalciuria, hyperuricosuria 　　Nephrolithiasis 　Nonglomerular renal diseases 　　Cystic diseases: Medullary sponge kidney, polycystic kidney disease 　　Papillary necrosis: Analgesic abuse, NSAIDs, sickle cell disease 　Ureteral stricture 　Vascular disorders 　　Arteriovenous malformation 　　Nutcracker syndrome 　　Renal infarction 　　Renal vein thrombosis *Lower urinary tract* 　Infection/inflammation 　　Cystitis, prostatitis, urethritis 　　*Schistosoma haematobium* in North Africans 　Masses/malignancies 　　Benign bladder and ureteral polyps and tumors 　　Bladder cancer 　　Prostate cancer/benign prostatic hypertrophy 　Trauma (catheterization/blunt urethral or bladder trauma)
Uncertain	Exercise hematuria Menstrual contamination Over anticoagulation (usually with warfarin) Sexual intercourse "Benign hematuria" (unexplained microscopic hematuria)

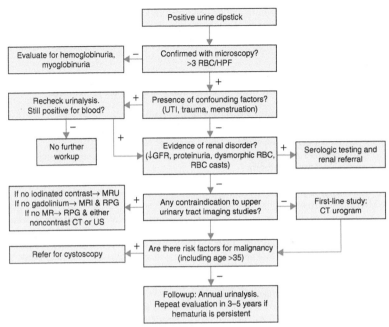

FIGURE 2-1. Algorithm for microscopic hematuria evaluation. RBC, red blood cell; CT, computed tomography; MRU, magnetic resonance urogram.

Physical Examination

- Hypertension can be a manifestation of glomerulonephritis.
- Edema may be a sign of proteinuria or nephrotic syndrome.
- Fever, costovertebral angle tenderness, and suprapubic tenderness are suggestive of an infectious etiology.
- A nonblanching purpuric rash may be another sign of vasculitis.
- Abdominal examination may reveal a mass, enlarged bladder, or polycystic kidneys.

TABLE 2-4	RISK FACTORS FOR SIGNIFICANT UROLOGIC PATHOLOGY IN PATIENTS WITH MICROSCOPIC HEMATURIA

Age >35 yrs
Male sex
Past or current smoking
History of gross hematuria
Occupational exposure to chemicals or dyes (benzenes or aromatic amines)
Chronic urinary tract infections
Irritative voiding symptoms
History of high-dose cyclophosphamide
Pelvic irradiation
Analgesic abuse

- A detailed GU examination should be performed to look for local sources of bleeding and to exclude rectal or vaginal bleeding.

Diagnostic Testing

Laboratories

- *Laboratory* evaluation usually begins with **urine dipstick testing followed by microscopic examination of the urine sediment and evaluation for proteinuria.**
- **Dipstick testing:**
  - High sensitivity (>90%) but lower specificity (65%) for hematuria.
  - False-negative results can be due to ingestion of large amounts of ascorbic acid or other reducing agents, low pH, or the presence of formaldehyde.
  - **False-positive results can be due to semen, high pH, presence of oxidizing agents, and myoglobinuria.**
  - When positive, the urine sample should be centrifuged and the sediment examined microscopically to count the number of RBCs per HPF.
- **Microscopic analysis:**
  - Allows for confirmation of RBCs as well as examination of RBC morphology and casts.
  - **Dysmorphic RBCs and RBC casts are indicative of a glomerular cause of hematuria.** Dysmorphic RBCs are variable in size and shape and have irregular borders compared with the normal, doughnut-shaped RBCs.
  - **Acanthocytes,** or doughnut-shaped RBCs with membrane blebs, have also been used as a marker for glomerular bleeding.
- **Urine culture** is obtained if pyuria or bacteriuria is present. Once appropriate treatment with antibiotics is given, urine dipstick test and microscopic examination should be repeated several weeks later. If the hematuria has resolved, no further evaluation is needed.
- **Quantification of proteinuria** with a spot PCR or ACR should follow the detection of coexistent proteinuria on dipstick testing. Presence of significant proteinuria suggests glomerular pathology rather than ureteral abnormalities.
- **Serum creatinine or blood urea nitrogen** should also be obtained. Any abnormality warrants further evaluation to determine the etiology of renal impairment (either independent of, or as it relates to the cause of hematuria).
- **Serologic testing** may be indicated based on the clinical scenario if glomerular causes are suspected. These may include antinuclear antibodies (ANA), antineutrophil cytoplasmic antibodies (ANCA), cryoglobulins, and Hepatitis B and C titers, among others.
- **Urine cytology** is less sensitive than cystoscopy in the detection of bladder cancer (48% vs. 87%) **and is no longer recommended in the routine evaluation of hematuria.**[2] Likewise, urine markers approved by the U.S. Food and Drug Administration for bladder cancer detection (NMP22 BladderChek, BTA stat, ImmunoCyt, or UroVysion FISH) are not recommended for patients with AMH. These may be useful, however, in patients with persistent microhematuria after a negative workup or with risk factors for cancer.

Imaging

- Radiologic imaging is indicated for evaluation of the upper urinary tract.
- **Multiphasic computed tomography urography (CTU):**
  - Consists of three phases:
    - (1) a noncontrast phase to diagnose hydronephrosis and urinary calculi
    - (2) a nephrogenic phase to evaluate the parenchyma for neoplasms and inflammation
    - (3) an excretory phase to detect filling defects caused by urothelial lesions
  - Multiphasic CTU is the CT imaging modality of choice in the evaluation of the upper urinary tract with high sensitivity (>91%) and specificity (94% to 97%).[2]

- **Magnetic resonance urography (MRU):**
  - An acceptable alternative if patients have contraindications to CTU (renal insufficiency, iodinated contrast allergy, pregnancy).
  - If gadolinium contrast is contraindicated, the combination of magnetic resonance imaging and retrograde pyelogram (RPG) allows for evaluation of the entire upper urinary tract. RPGs are invasive but can be used safely in renal impairment as it does not rely on renal excretion of contrast media.
  - If magnetic resonance imaging cannot be performed because of metal in the body, combining noncontrast CT or renal ultrasonography with RPG is recommended.
- **Intravenous urography:** Has been supplanted by CTU due to low sensitivity in detecting masses <3 cm in size. Even if lesions are detected, further imaging is needed to characterize the mass.

Diagnostic Procedures
- **Cystoscopy:**
  - Is the preferred modality for evaluation of the lower urinary tract.
  - Recommended in patients with AMH over the age of 35 or any patients with risk factors of urinary tract malignancy (Table 2-4) regardless of age.
  - Disadvantages of cystoscopy include its invasive nature, risk for iatrogenic infection, and patient discomfort.
- **Ureterorenoscopy:**
  - Once the above radiologic tests are performed and are negative, fiberoptic imaging of the upper urinary tract and the kidney may be performed.
  - It is very invasive and not a recommended first-line procedure.

MONITORING/FOLLOW-UP

- A minority of patients who initially have a negative workup for microscopic hematuria eventually develop significant disease.
- Annual urinalysis is recommended in patients with persistent AMH. If clinical suspicion remains low, this may be discontinued after two consecutive negative results.
- Patients with persistent or recurrent hematuria after a negative initial evaluation warrant repeat evaluation within 3 to 5 years.

REFERENCES

1. KDIGO 2012 Clinical Practice Guideline for the evaluation and management of chronic kidney disease. *Kidney Int Suppl.* 2013;3(1):1–150.
2. Springberg P, Garrett L, Thompson A, et al. Fixed and reproducible orthostatic proteinuria: results of a 20-year follow-up study. *Ann Intern Med.* 1982;97(4):516–519.
3. Sharp VJ, Barnes KT, Erickson BA, et al. Assessment of asymptomatic microscopic hematuria in adults. *Am Fam Physician.* 2013;88:747–754.
4. Davis R, Jones JS, Barocas DA, et al. Diagnosis, evaluation and follow-up of asymptomatic microhematuria (AMH) in adults: AUA guideline. *J Urol.* 2012;188(6 Suppl):2473–2481.

Disorders of Water Balance

Usman Younus and Steven Cheng

3

GENERAL PRINCIPLES

- Disorders of sodium (hypo- or hypernatremia) reflect abnormalities in water homeostasis.
- Antidiuretic hormone (ADH) is the key regulator of renal free water excretion.
  - ADH controls water permeability at the collecting duct of the nephron, allowing water to be conserved or excreted as needed.
  - ADH is secreted in response to an increase in plasma osmolality, decreased effective circulatory volume, and other factors such as pain, nausea, and certain medications.
  - Disruption in ADH release or signaling, along with alterations in water intake, all contribute to the development of hypo- or hypernatremia.
- Both hypo- and hypernatremia are associated with increased morbidity and mortality.
- Rapid correction of hypo- and hypernatremia can also contribute to adverse outcomes.

Hyponatremia

GENERAL PRINCIPLES

Definition

- Hyponatremia is defined as a serum or plasma sodium concentration <135 mmol/L.
- Acute hyponatremia is defined as a fall in sodium over a period of <48 hours.

Classification

- The causes of hyponatremia can be categorized based on plasma osmolality.
- Hyponatremia with normal plasma osmolality is termed **pseudohyponatremia** (isotonic hyponatremia). This is most commonly attributable to a laboratory error caused by severe elevations of plasma lipids or proteins. A marked increase in plasma lipids or plasma proteins essentially "dilutes" the sodium concentration, as measured by flame photometry. Alternate methods, using ion-specific electrodes, specifically measure the concentration in the aqueous portion of plasma and are thus unaffected by lipid or protein aberrations.
- **Hypertonic hyponatremia** occurs when the plasma osmolality is increased, drawing water from the intracellular to the extracellular space. The increase in the aqueous fraction of plasma thereby lowers the serum sodium concentration.
- **Hypotonic hyponatremia** occurs when the plasma osmolality is decreased and is the most common form encountered in clinical practice. This is primarily due to increased water intake and/or impaired water excretion.

Epidemiology

- Hyponatremia is the most common electrolyte abnormality among hospitalized patients.

- The prevalence of hyponatremia is lower in the general ambulatory population but is still associated with poor outcomes.
- Hyponatremia is an independent predictor of mortality, even at mildly reduced levels.

Etiology

- Isotonic hyponatremia:
  - As described previously, pseudohyponatremia is due to elevated lipids or proteins.
  - The absorption of sodium-free isotonic surgical irrigants (glycine, sorbitol, mannitol) can also result in isotonic hyponatremia.
- Hypertonic hyponatremia:
  - Hypertonic hyponatremia results in a shift of water from intracellular to extracellular spaces, thus reducing the serum sodium concentration.
  - Hypertonic hyponatremia is most commonly caused by hyperglycemia. Serum sodium levels decrease by ~2.4 mmol/L for every 100 mg/dL increase in the plasma glucose.
  - Other causes of hypertonic hyponatremia include mannitol and intravenous immunoglobulin (IVIG).
- Hypotonic hyponatremia:
  - Hypotonic hyponatremia can be further characterized by whether renal free water clearance is intact (excretion of dilute urine) or impaired (suboptimal urinary dilution). See Figure 3-1.
  - An appropriately dilute urine has a low urine osmolality (<100 mOsm/L). This occurs when the intake of water simply exceeds the capacity for renal water excretion. Causes include primary polydipsia, severe malnutrition, and beer potomania.
  - Impaired urinary dilution is reflected by a urine osmolality >100 mOsm/L. This finding suggests that ADH is present, due to either an appropriate physiologic stimulus (such as a reduction in circulating volume) or an inappropriate state of oversecretion

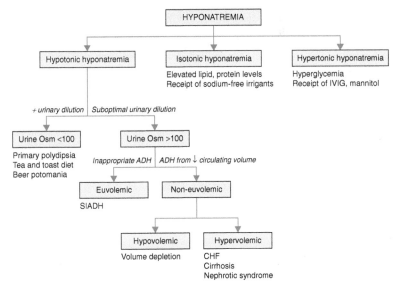

FIGURE 3-1. Causes of Hyponatremia.

TABLE 3-1	COMMON CAUSES OF SIADH
CNS disorders	Hemorrhage, psychosis, infection, alcohol withdrawal
Malignancy (ectopic ADH)	Small-cell lung carcinoma (most commonly implicated), CNS disease, leukemia, Hodgkin disease, duodenal cancer, pancreatic cancer
Pulmonary	Infection, acute respiratory failure, mechanical ventilation
Miscellaneous	Pain, nausea (powerful stimulator of ADH), HIV (multifactorial), general postoperation state
Pharmacologic agents (either mimic or enhance ADH)	Cyclophosphamide, vincristine, vinblastine, NSAIDs, tricyclics and related agents, selective serotonin reuptake inhibitors, chlorpropamide, nicotine, bromocriptine, oxytocin, DDAVP

ADH, antidiuretic hormone; CNS, central nervous system; HIV, human immunodeficiency virus; NSAID, nonsteroidal anti-inflammatory drug.

(such as the syndrome of inappropriate antidiuretic hormone [SIADH]). Common causes of SIADH are listed in Table 3-1.

Pathophysiology

- As plasma sodium falls, cells in the brain readjust intracellular osmolality by lowering the osmotic content. If changes occur rapidly or in the face of severe hyponatremia, this adaptation fails, leading to cerebral edema, altered mental status, and seizures.
- Hyponatremia can be fatal should brainstem herniation result.
- Patients with underlying disorders such as cirrhosis or pre-existing neurologic disease may be at particular risk of severe complications in acute hyponatremia.
- Central pontine myelinolysis (osmotic demyelination) is thought to be due to rapid correction of chronic hyponatremia. Alcoholic patients and those with severe malnutrition appear to be at increased risk of this potentially devastating condition. Cognitive, behavioral, and movement disorders due to the occurrence of osmotic demyelination may not be apparent for days after the correction of hyponatremia, and visible changes on magnetic resonance imaging scan may take weeks to appear.

RISK FACTORS

- Psychiatric illnesses which lead to primary polydipsia
- Comorbid conditions: congestive heart failure, cirrhosis, nephrotic syndrome, renal failure, alcoholism, and malignancy
- Medications:
  ○ Diuretics can induce volume contraction, and thiazide diuretics impair free water excretion
  ○ Selective serotonin reuptake inhibitors (SSRIs) are associated with SIADH
  ○ Desmopressin, which is sometimes used for incontinence and von Willebrand disease, can increase water reabsorption

DIAGNOSIS

Clinical Presentation

- Hyponatremia is usually asymptomatic until serum sodium <125 mmol/L, although fatalities have been reported with an extremely rapid decrease from a normal [Na$^+$] to the 120- to 128-mmol/L range.[1]
- Symptoms include central nervous system (CNS) effects, such as confusion, weakness, headache, obtundation, or seizures, with acute hyponatremia.
- Chronic hyponatremia (developing over >48 hours) is generally fairly well tolerated. Symptoms include cognitive defects as well as nausea, vomiting, weakness, and headache.

History

A thorough history should include the estimated duration of inciting factors and an assessment of signs or symptoms suggesting that immediate intervention may be necessary (mental status change, lethargy, coma, seizure). Management of a patient with hyponatremia depends on whether the process is considered to be *acute* or *chronic* and the severity of symptoms.

Physical Examination

- The physical examination should be geared toward assessing the volume status of the patient.
- Elevated blood pressure, an S3 heart sound, or increased jugular venous pressure indicates volume excess often in the setting of early congestive heart failure. Edema in the lower extremities or presacral region or evidence of pulmonary edema indicates increased extracellular fluid volume in heart failure and kidney disease.
- Conversely, orthostatic hypotension, decreased skin turgor, dry mucosal membranes, and decreased jugular venous pressure suggest intravascular volume depletion.

Diagnostic Testing

Laboratories

- Blood tests:
  - A basic metabolic panel and plasma osmolarity are essential for the evaluation of hyponatremia.
  - Additional laboratory tests include the following:
    - Uric acid, which is generally increased in volume depletion, can be helpful if the patient's volume status is difficult to ascertain.
    - Thyroid-stimulating hormone and cortisol levels should be checked in euvolemic hypotonic hyponatremia.
    - An osmolar gap is extremely helpful in the evaluation of hypertonic hyponatremia.
      - Calculated plasma osmolarity = 2 × [Na] + (BUN/2.8) + (glucose/18)
      - Osmolar gap = Measured − calculated plasma osmolarity
- Urine tests:
  - Urine osmolarity is important in determining whether the kidneys are appropriately diluting the urine (urine osmolality <100 mOsm/L) or whether water is being reabsorbed by ADH (urine osmolality >100 mOsm/L).
  - Urine sodium is low in volume depletion and can be used when intravascular volume status is difficult to determine.

Imaging

- Head computed tomography (CT) should be ordered if the patient has neurologic symptoms.
- In cases of SIADH where a malignancy is suspected, a chest x-ray can be ordered to evaluate for lung cancer.

TREATMENT

Asymptomatic Hyponatremia

- Hypervolemic hyponatremia is generally asymptomatic and reflects the severity of the underlying disease, such as heart failure or cirrhosis.
  - Optimal management of the underlying disease is required.
  - The presence of hyponatremia in heart failure and cirrhosis often portends to poor outcomes.
- Hypovolemic hyponatremia can be managed with fluid resuscitation. Expansion of the extracellular compartment with normal saline will attenuate the production of ADH and lower urine osmolality.
- Euvolemic hyponatremia can be seen in patients with SIADH. When asymptomatic, these patients can often be managed with fluid restriction.
  - The ratio of (**urine sodium + urine potassium**)/**plasma sodium** can be used to guide the degree of fluid restriction.[2]
    - 1: No free water
    - 0.5 to 1.0: 500 mL
    - 0.5: 1000 mL
  - When necessary, pharmacologic agents can be used when hyponatremia persists despite attempted fluid restriction.
    - Salt tablets, urea tablets, or a diet rich in salt and protein all increase the renal solute load and result in an obligate increase in urine volume, since urine osmolality is relatively fixed in SIADH. However, fluid restriction remains important for this to be successful.
    - Loop diuretics decrease the medullary concentration gradient required for the reabsorption of water, and thus can reduce water reabsorption even in the presence of ADH. They should be cautiously given the potential side effect of intravascular contraction.
    - Vasopressin antagonists can be used in SIADH and other states of ADH excess. While they effectively promote a water diuresis, they must be titrated extremely carefully to avoid overcorrection of serum sodium.

Acute and/or Symptomatic Hyponatremia

- Hyponatremia—acute or chronic—presenting with significant symptoms, may necessitate emergent therapy with hypertonic saline.
- The initial rate of correction generally should be 1 to 2 mmol/L/hr, unless persistent symptoms such as continued seizure activity justify a faster reversal rate.
- Once symptoms have been controlled, the rate of correction is adjusted to no more than a total of 8 mmol/L in the first 24 hours. More rapid correction increases the risk of osmotic demyelination, especially in chronic hyponatremia.
- There are various ways to dose hypertonic saline in order to achieve this targeted rate of correction:
  - Hypertonic saline can be given in small, discrete boluses (generally 100 cc each) until the goal is achieved (up to 3 doses).
  - Alternatively, the Adrogue–Madias equation can be used to determine the predicted change in serum sodium after 1 L of hypertonic saline.
    - $\Delta[Na^+] = (513 - [Na]s)/(TBW + 1)$
    - [Na]s is the current serum sodium, and TBW is the estimated total body water
    - Dividing the desired rate of correction (mEq/L/hr) by the calculated $\Delta[Na^+]$ (mEq/L/L of fluid) gives you the appropriate rate of administration (liter of fluid per hour)

- The human body is not a closed system and one must take into account the introduction of solute (including potassium replacement, which can increase serum sodium levels) as well as ongoing urinary losses of electrolytes and insensible water losses.
- No equation can sufficiently take into account these dynamic changes, so frequent reassessment of the serum sodium (even every 1 to 2 hours initially) is mandatory to avoid overcorrection.[3]
- If the rate of correction is exceeded, the serum sodium should be brought back down to ensure a correction of no more than 8 mmol/L over the 24-hour period. This can be accomplished by administering free water (D5W) and/or ADH analogs.

Hypernatremia

GENERAL PRINCIPLES

Definition

Any increase in the serum sodium to >145 mmol/L automatically increases hypertonicity, leading to intracellular dehydration.

Classification

- Unlike hyponatremia, all cases of hypernatremia are true hyperosmolar states.
- Although the serum sodium is elevated, intravascular volume may be low or high, depending on the etiology.

Epidemiology

- The overall incidence of hypernatremia is significantly lower than hyponatremia.
- Patients admitted with hypernatremia were more likely to be elderly, whereas those with hospital-acquired hypernatremia had similar ages to the general hospital population.
- The presence of hypernatremia is also associated with an increased risk of poor outcomes.

Etiology

Figure 3-2 summarizes an approach to the common causes of hypernatremia.

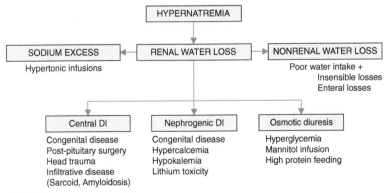

FIGURE 3-2. Hypernatremia.

Pathophysiology

- As the sodium concentration increases, water leaves the intracellular space causing a loss of cellular volume.
- The changes seen in hypernatremia are associated with substantial morbidity and mortality. However, just as with hyponatremia, chronic development of hypernatremia is better tolerated than an equivalent acute change.
- Cerebrospinal fluid movement into the interstitial areas of brain tissue, as well as an increased generation of intracellular effective osmoles, protects the brain cells from the chronic effects of hypernatremia.

DIAGNOSIS

Clinical Presentation

Symptoms are primarily a reflection of CNS involvement and include lethargy, irritability, weakness, confusion, and progression to coma. These findings are generally not apparent until the sodium concentration has increased to >160 mmol/L.

History

- As with hyponatremia, determining the duration of neurologic symptoms is critical, as it will determine how quickly the serum sodium should be corrected.
- The patient's fluid intake should be carefully reviewed. Decreased thirst and poor access to water account for a large proportion of hypernatremia cases among the elderly and institutionalized.
- Any changes in urine output should also be reviewed. Polyuria and polydipsia may indicate free water losses from diabetes insipidus.

Physical Examination

- The patient's volume status should be a key focus of the physical examination. Volume depletion may be suggested by orthostatic hypotension, dry mucous membranes, and reduced skin turgor. Volume overload may be suggested by elevated blood pressures, jugular venous distention, and edema.
- A full neurologic examination is often necessary to rule out other causes of the CNS symptoms.

Diagnostic Testing

- Blood tests:
  - A basic metabolic panel is required to identify changes in the serum sodium in the context of other serum electrolytes.
  - The serum sodium can also be used to calculate the free water deficit: Free water deficit = TBW × ([Na]s/140 − 1), where [Na]s is the serum sodium and TBW is the total body water, estimated as 0.5 × body weight in kg.
- Urine tests:
  - Urine osmolarity is a crucial test that differentiates renal from nonrenal sources of free water loss.
  - Urine sodium and urine potassium can assist in the assessment of intravascular volume (urine sodium is low with volume contraction). In the context of hypernatremia, these tests are also used to help calculate the electrolyte-free water clearance. $C_{H_2O} = V(1 - [U_{Na} + U_K]/P_{Na})$, where U_{Na} and U_K are urinary sodium and potassium, respectively, and P_{Na} is plasma sodium.

TREATMENT

- In order to normalize the sodium concentration, the free water deficit must be determined (as shown above) and corrected with the administration of water.
- As previously noted, humans are not static systems, and ongoing water losses frequently complicate free water replacement. In addition to the water required to correct the static free water deficit, additional water should be given to keep pace with the daily insensible losses and renal free water clearance.
- As with hyponatremia, chronic hypernatremia should be corrected slowly and deliberately. Frequent laboratory checks should be used to guide the rate of water replacement, with a target corrective rate of approximately 0.5 mmol/L/hr. Faster correction rates can prevent adequate time for intracellular adjustment of tonicity, leading to cellular swelling.
- In patients with hemodynamic instability, volume resuscitation with normal saline takes precedence. Lesser degrees of clinical volume depletion can be treated with 0.45% saline solution.
- Once the volume status has been restored satisfactorily, D5W alone should be used to correct hypernatremia. The dextrose component is metabolized as long as insulin deficiency is not present, leaving free water.

REFERENCES

1. Waikar SS, Mount DB, Curhan GC. Mortality after hospitalization with mild, moderate, and severe hyponatremia. *Am J Med.* 2009;122(9):857–865.
2. Furst H, Hallows KR, Post J, et al. The urine/plasma electrolyte ratio: a predictive guide to water restriction. *Am J Med Sci.* 2000;319(4):240–244.
3. Mohmand HK, Issa D, Ahmad Z, et al. Hypertonic saline for hyponatremia: risk of inadvertent overcorrection. *Clin J Am Soc Nephrol.* 2007;2(6):1110–1117.

Disorders of Potassium Balance

4

Pooja Koolwal and Andreas Herrlich

GENERAL PRINCIPLES

- Total body potassium (K^+) is about 50 mEq/kg, 98% of which is intracellular. Intracellular [K^+] are about 140 mEq/L, approximately 35 times the normal extracellular (or plasma) value of about 4 mEq/L.
- Normal daily K^+ intake can vary widely and requires tight regulation of plasma concentration. Changes in plasma [K^+] may occur due to K^+ shifting into or out of cells, independent of body K^+ stores, see Table 4-1.
- K^+ elimination primarily occurs through the kidneys, though some stool elimination occurs (about 10 mEq/day) as well. Minimal K^+ is lost through sweat.
- **Renal potassium regulation:**
  - Potassium is freely filtered at the glomerulus and 67% is reabsorbed at the proximal convoluted tubule, while 20% is reabsorbed in the thick ascending loop of Henle. Tight regulation occurs in the distal tubule and collecting duct.
  - Aldosterone plays a central role in [K^+] regulation by stimulating its excretion in the cortical collecting duct of the nephron.
  - Hyperkalemia also directly stimulates renal K^+ secretion, which is dependent on adequate tubular flow in the distal nephron.
  - Decreased effective circulating volume (ECV) will increase aldosterone production and increase potassium secretion in exchange for sodium retention. But decreased ECV also decreases distal flow rate, which leads to reduced K^+ excretion. This

TABLE 4-1 FACTORS AFFECTING TRANSCELLULAR K^+ SHIFT

Physiologic	Pathologic
Na^+/K^+ ATPase • Maintains high intracellular K^+ gradient **Catecholamines** • α-adrenergic—impairs K^+ entry into cells • β_2-adrenergic—promotes K^+ entry into cells **Insulin** • Promotes K^+ entry into cells • Insulin deficiency impairs K^+ entry into cells **Exercise** • Causes K^+ release from cells for local vasodilation and increased blood flow	**Extracellular pH** • Acidosis—pH decreases and H^+ will move into cells in exchange for *K^+ shifting out of cells* • Alkalosis—pH increases and H^+ will move out of cells in exchange for *K^+ shifting into cells* **Hyperosmolarity** • Increased intracellular [K^+] drives K^+ out of cells down chemical gradient **Cell turnover** • Increase cell breakdown—K^+ released from cells • Increased cell production—K^+ is rapidly taken up by cells

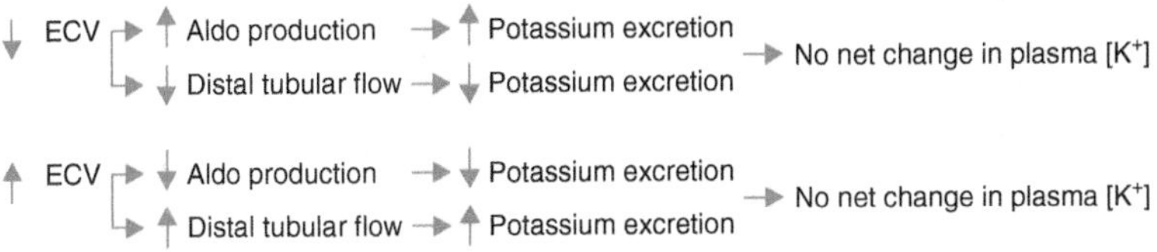

FIGURE 4-1. Extracellular volume effect on potassium concentration.

generally allows plasma [K$^+$] to remain at stable concentrations within certain limitations (please see Fig. 4-1). However, when potassium secretion is impaired by, for example, an angiotensin receptor blocker (ARB) or angiotensin-converting enzyme (ACE) inhibitor, or if dehydration is severe because the patient is taking a diuretic, these limitations can become relevant and plasma [K$^+$] can rise above normal levels.

Hypokalemia

GENERAL PRINCIPLES

Definition
Hypokalemia is defined as [K$^+$] <3.5 mEq/L.

Pathophysiology
Hypokalemia may result from decreased intake, intracellular shift, or increased renal or gastrointestinal (GI) losses.
- **Decreased intake:** In the setting of decreased intake, the normally functioning kidney can decrease K$^+$ excretion to <25 mEq/day. Moderate dietary K$^+$ restriction alone does not cause hypokalemia.
- **Intracellular shift:** Please refer back to Table 4-1.
  - **Alkalosis**—promotes K$^+$ shift into cells and H$^+$ movement out of cells.
  - **Stimulation of the Na$^+$/K$^+$-ATPase pump**—activity can be increased by catecholamines, particularly β_2-adrenergic stimulation and insulin. It can also mediate hypokalemia often seen with refeeding syndrome.
  - **Treatment of anemia or neutropenia**—increased hematopoiesis after vitamin B$_{12}$/folic acid for megaloblastic anemia or granulocyte-macrophage colony-stimulating factor (GM-CSF) for neutropenia can cause increased K$^+$ uptake.
  - **Hypokalemic periodic paralysis**—results from rapid K$^+$ shifting into skeletal muscle cells (often after exercise, large carbohydrate meal, or insulin dose). It results from a defect in dihydropyridine-sensitive calcium channels of skeletal muscles, which can either be inherited in an autosomal dominant pattern or acquired, as in thyrotoxicosis.
  - **Hypothermia.** Hypothermia is believed to cause an influx of potassium into the intracellular space. Of note, in severe hypothermia, hyperkalemia can be seen due to tissue ischemia and is highly correlated to terminal hypothermia.
- **Increased GI losses** (normal fecal K$^+$ losses are around 10 mEq/day):
  - With normal dietary K$^+$ intake, if fecal losses exceed ~55 mEq/day, the kidney's ability to conserve K$^+$ can be exceeded and K$^+$ depletion will occur.
  - **Large volume stool output** of any cause may thus cause hypokalemia.
  - Gastric secretions contain very little K$^+$. **In the case of significant vomiting or large-volume nasogastric suction, hypokalemia is NOT due to K$^+$ loss in the**

gastric fluid. Proton loss and volume contraction cause metabolic alkalosis. Although some intracellular shift of K^+ from alkalemia occurs, the key factor in the development of hypokalemia in these cases is bicarbonaturia and hypovolemia-induced aldosterone release, which enhances K^+ excretion in the distal nephron.

- **Increased renal losses:**
  - **Diuretics:** Loop and thiazide diuretics increase distal nephron sodium delivery and water excretion. The ensuing hypovolemia induces aldosterone secretion. Both of these effects lead to hypokalemia. Bartter and Gitelman syndromes are loss-of-function mutations in furosemide- and thiazide-sensitive channels, respectively.
  - **Syndromes of mineralocorticoid excess:**
    - **Primary hyperaldosteronism (Conn syndrome)** due to adrenal adenoma or hyperplasia
    - **Secondary hyperaldosteronism** due to renal artery stenosis, fibromuscular dysplasia, renin-secreting tumor (rare)
    - **Apparent mineralocorticoid excess**
      - **11β-Hydroxylase deficiency**—cortisol is a potent mineralocorticoid, but is inactivated in the kidney by 11β-hydroxysteroid dehydrogenase. Licorice (found in chewing gum and tobacco) can inactivate this enzyme, thereby increasing cortisol activity.
      - **Cushing syndrome**—hypokalemia results from the excess production of steroids that are normally metabolized by 11β-hydroxysteroid dehydrogenase enzyme.
    - **Liddle syndrome,** a gain-of-function mutation of distal epithelial Na^+ channels (ENaC), increases sodium reabsorption in the collecting duct and enhances the excretion of potassium
    - **Glucocorticoid remediable hyperaldosteronism** is the result of a mutation that causes aldosterone production to be stimulated by ACTH. This results in increased aldosterone production, remediable by suppressing ACTH synthesis using glucocorticoids
  - **Increased distal nephron flow:** This can result from saline diuresis, diuretics, salt-wasting nephropathy, and glucosuria (diabetes mellitus or Fanconi syndrome).
  - **Nonreabsorbable anion:** The presence of a nonreabsorbable anion in the distal nephron creates negative charge in the lumen, promoting K^+ secretion. This phenomenon can be seen with bicarbonaturia (metabolic alkalosis) and urinary hippurate (from glue sniffing).
  - **Tubular toxins:** Amphotericin, gentamicin, hypercalcemia, and cisplatin all cause tubular damage, impairing K^+ reabsorption.
  - **Hypomagnesemia:** Hypomagnesemia can cause urinary K^+ wasting and refractory hypokalemia. Adequate renal potassium retention cannot take place before a magnesium deficit is corrected. Hypomagnesemia is often seen with alcoholism, diuretics, diarrhea, malnutrition, aminoglycosides, and cisplatin use.

DIAGNOSIS

Clinical Presentation

- Mild hypokalemia (3.0 to 3.5 mEq/L) is generally asymptomatic, although it does pose an increased risk of arrhythmias and increased mortality in patients who also have cardiovascular disease or who are on digitalis.
- **Weakness and muscle pain or cramps,** usually occur initially involving the lower extremities and can develop as the $[K^+]$ drops below 3 mEq/L.
- Decrease in K^+ to below 2.5 mEq/L can lead to **paralysis,** including respiratory muscle paralysis. Some patients can present with an ileus due to effects of hypokalemia on smooth muscle. Rhabdomyolysis can occur with severe hypokalemia. However,

rhabdomyolysis in itself elevates plasma [K⁺] and prevents further decrements, possibly masking the underlying etiology. Checking serum creatine phosphokinase (CPK) levels may aid in the diagnosis of suspected hypokalemia-induced rhabdomyolysis.

- Hypokalemia can impair renal water reabsorption and cause nephrogenic diabetes insipidus.
- Prolonged hypokalemia can cause irreversible interstitial nephritis, renal cysts, hypertension, and glucose intolerance.

History

The history should try to elicit common causes such as vomiting, diarrhea, laxative abuse, and diuretic use. A family history of hypokalemia may suggest inherited disorders such as Bartter, Gitelman, or Liddle syndrome. A history of weakness after adrenergic stimuli, insulin, or high-carbohydrate meals suggests hypokalemic periodic paralysis. Concurrent hyperthyroidism may represent thyrotoxic periodic paralysis.

Physical Examination

Physical examination findings should focus on signs of volume depletion (volume contraction may lead to metabolic alkalosis and hypokalemia) or hypertension (suggesting mineralocorticoid excess).

Diagnostic Testing

Laboratories

- **Urine potassium excretion:** In the hypokalemic state, expected renal K⁺ excretion should fall to <25 mEq/day. Random urine [K⁺] can be misleading when the urine is very dilute and falsely low values would suggest extrarenal causes of K⁺ loss. A 24-hour urine K⁺ is ideal but may be difficult to obtain.
- If there is concern for increased urinary potassium losses, **a plasma renin and aldosterone level should be obtained** (please see Table 4-2). **Assessment of urinary potassium and renin/aldosterone activity does not always differentiate between all specific causes of hypokalemia.**[1] Clinical history remains vital in pinpointing the cause.
- **Acid–base status:** Hypokalemia with metabolic alkalosis is usually due to diuretics, vomiting, or mineralocorticoid excess. Hypokalemia with metabolic acidosis is less common; type I and II renal tubular acidosis (RTA), salt-wasting nephropathy, and diabetic ketoacidosis (DKA) (especially after insulin administration has caused intracellular shift of K⁺) should be considered.
- **Magnesium:** As mentioned, hypomagnesemia can cause urinary K⁺ wasting and refractory hypokalemia, if it remains uncorrected.

TABLE 4-2	INTERPRETATION OF SERUM RENIN AND ALDOSTERONE LEVELS IN HYPOKALEMIA	
	High Renin	Low Renin
High aldosterone	Usually indicates diuretic use, salt-wasting nephropathies, GI volume loss, or renovascular disease. Rarely, renin-secreting tumors can also cause this.	Indicates primary hyperaldosteronism due to either adrenal adenoma or hyperplasia. Adrenal CT scan or MRI may guide further management.
Low aldosterone		Indicates nonaldosterone mineralocorticoid effect—for example, 11β-hydroxylase deficiency or Liddle syndrome.

Electrocardiography

Electrocardiography (EKG) changes due to hypokalemia: Prominent U waves, diminished or inverted T waves, and ST-segment depression may be seen. With extremely low [K^+] levels, there may be lengthened PR and QRS intervals, which can lead to ventricular fibrillation. EKG changes do not correlate well with the degree of hypokalemia.

TREATMENT

- At a plasma [K^+] of 3 mEq/L (not caused by an acute transcellular shift but by chronic losses), total body potassium deficit ranges from 200 to 400 mEq. This is the amount that needs to be replaced in addition to ongoing daily losses.
- **As the plasma level decreases to <3 mEq/L, deficits can be >600 mEq,** but the degree of deficit is difficult to predict due to ongoing transcellular shifts and K excretion. This is classically seen in hyperglycemic states, such as DKA, in which the combination of hyperglycemia, glucosuria, ketonuria, and insulin treatment affect transcellular [K^+] shift and K^+ secretion, and plasma K^+ levels can change dramatically during the course of treatment.
- **Potassium replacement should be given orally whenever possible** due to the potential for cardiac arrhythmias, vein sclerosis, and the increased cost in using intravenous (IV) administration.
  - ○ Oral doses of 40 mEq of potassium are well tolerated up to every 4 hours.
  - ○ Potassium chloride is usually administered, as the chloride component helps correct the often-coinciding alkalosis and bicarbonaturia.
  - ○ Potassium citrate can be given if hypokalemia associated with acidemia is present.
  - ○ IV potassium can be administered in concentrations of 40 mEq/L via a peripheral line or 60 mEq/L via a central line.
    - The rate of infusion should not exceed >10 mEq/hr unless absolutely necessary.
    - IV potassium should be administered in a saline solution rather than with dextrose; insulin release in response to the dextrose can further decrease [K^+].
- **Correction of metabolic alkalosis will help prevent renal K^+ wasting that accompanies bicarbonaturia.** In cases of vomiting, H_2-blockers or proton pump inhibitors can reduce the acidity of gastric secretions and prevent acid loss. In hypovolemic patients with a contraction alkalosis, isotonic IV fluids should be used for volume repletion.
- In the **treatment of hypokalemia due to hyperaldosteronism or diuretic use** (e.g., for congestive heart failure [CHF], hypertension), potassium-sparing diuretics are useful.
  - ○ **Spironolactone** reduces aldosterone synthesis and is commonly used in patients with CHF and cirrhosis with ascites.
  - ○ **Amiloride and triamterene** block the ENaC channel in the distal nephron. Amiloride is favored as triamterene carries a significant risk of nephrolithiasis and possible renal insufficiency. In states of aldosterone excess, doses of 20 to 40 mg/day PO of amiloride may be needed; otherwise, doses of 5 to 10 mg/day may suffice. Amiloride is also the treatment of choice for Liddle and Gitelman syndrome.

Hyperkalemia

GENERAL PRINCIPLES

Definition

Hyperkalemia is defined as [K^+] >5 mEq/L.

Pathophysiology

- **Acute hyperkalemia typically reflects transcellular potassium shifts.**
  - **Pseudohyperkalemia:** It is due to release of potassium from cellular elements (white blood cells, platelets, hemolyzed red blood cells [RBCs]) after sample collection. Spurious [K$^+$] elevations can also result from repeated fist clenching or prolonged tourniquet application during phlebotomy.
  - **Very large oral or IV K$^+$ load:** Normally, oral K$^+$ loads of up to 135 to 160 mEq are well tolerated, producing only small increases above the normal K$^+$ plasma level of about 3.5 mEq/L. Potassium release from RBCs after massive transfusions can also result in hyperkalemia, which can be prevented by washing the RBCs. Citrate anticoagulant used in RBC storage can cause concurrent hypocalcemia, increasing the potential for arrhythmia.
  - **Decreased cellular uptake:** usually due to insulin deficiency or nonselective beta-blockade. Digitalis toxicity also impairs Na$^+$/K$^+$ ATPase activity.
  - **Extracellular K$^+$ release:** can be caused by trauma, tissue necrosis, rhabdomyolysis, tumor lysis syndrome, severe exercise, or depolarizing neuromuscular blockers (e.g., succinylcholine).
  - **Metabolic acidosis (due to inorganic acids):** Metabolic acidosis due to organic acids (e.g., ketoacids and lactic acid) usually do NOT cause hyperkalemia. The extracellular K$^+$ shift seen in, for example, DKA and nonketotic hyperosmolar state, is thought to be due to hyperosmolality from hyperglycemia and insulin deficiency and not metabolic acidosis.
  - **Hyperkalemic periodic paralysis:** In some cases this is due to a mutation in the skeletal muscle Na$^+$ channel.
- **Chronic hyperkalemia** *implies decreased renal K$^+$ excretion,* usually due to decreased aldosterone effect or decreased flow in the distal nephron. In chronic kidney disease, decreased nephron mass is to some degree compensated for by increased K$^+$ secretion per nephron.
  - **Decreased aldosterone effect**
    - **Decreased aldosterone synthesis**
      - **Medications** that disrupt the renin–angiotensin–aldosterone (RAAS) axis will decrease synthesis of aldosterone. These include ACE inhibitors, ARBs, and renin inhibitors. Nonsteroidal anti-inflammatory drugs and heparin are also known to reduce aldosterone synthesis.
      - A variety of **medical conditions** decrease aldosterone production, including adrenal insufficiency (acquired immune deficiency syndrome, and Addison disease), diabetes mellitus, and type II pseudohypoaldosteronism (PHA) (also known as Gordon syndrome/chloride shunt).
    - **Aldosterone resistance**
      - **Medications** such as aldosterone antagonists (amiloride, triamterene, spironolactone, eplerenone, and trimethoprim) and cyclosporine decrease the response to aldosterone.
      - **Type I PHA** is caused by loss-of-function mutation of either the mineralocorticoid receptor (renal PHA type I) or the amiloride-sensitive epithelial Na$^+$ channel (multiple target organ defect PHA type I).
      - **Type IV RTA** is a term used to describe the nonanion gap metabolic acidosis and hyperkalemia that occur in the setting of decreased aldosterone effect. Usually it is caused by fibrosis affecting the distal nephron, for example, in diabetic kidney disease.
  - **Decreased distal flow:** A marked reduction in distal flow can be seen with severe volume contraction or intense vasoconstriction, as seen in CHF, cirrhosis, renal artery stenosis, and hypovolemia. Ordinarily, volume contraction stimulates the secretion of aldosterone and enhances K$^+$ secretion. However, this homeostatic mechanism can be

overwhelmed with severe reductions in distal flow and/or concurrent predisposition toward hyperkalemia (from medications such as ACE inhibitors, ARBs, or aldosterone antagonists, for example).

DIAGNOSIS

Clinical Presentation

The two principal clinical manifestations of hyperkalemia are **muscle weakness** and **cardiac conduction disturbances.** Hyperkalemia raises the resting membrane potential of muscle cells. Although muscle contraction is normally associated with membrane depolarization, persistent elevation of membrane potential inactivates Na^+ channels, resulting in muscle weakness.

- In hyperkalemia, first confirm true hyperkalemia by **checking whole-blood [K⁺]** and **assess the EKG for conduction abnormalities that warrant immediate treatment** (see below). Once the patient is stabilized, investigate the underlying cause.
- **Review of medications and medical history** often make the diagnosis. Diabetes mellitus may suggest hyporeninemic hypoaldosteronism (HRHA), and chronic kidney disease implies limited ability to excrete K^+. **A dietary history of high-K^+ foods** (bananas, tomatoes, potatoes, oranges, melons, avocados, meats, kiwis, milk, spinach, apricots, lima beans, papayas, cucumber) or K^+-containing salt substitutes should be sought. History of trauma may indicate rhabdomyolysis (elevated CPK). Recent chemotherapy should raise the possibility of tumor lysis syndrome (hyperphosphatemia, hyperuricemia). If the cause of hyperkalemia is still not obvious, then an evaluation of urinary potassium excretion should follow.

Diagnostic Testing

Laboratories
- **Pseudohyperkalemia** should be ruled out by checking whole-blood [K⁺].
- The **transtubular K^+ gradient** (TTKG) is no longer recommended for use in hyperkalemia since its underlying assumption that osmolar reabsorption does not occur distal to the collecting duct has been found to be untrue.[2]
- **Acid–base status:** Nonanion gap acidosis along with low urine pH is often seen along with decreased aldosterone effect (type IV RTA). The hyperkalemic variant of type I RTA also presents with nongap acidosis, but the urine pH will be high.
- Please refer to Table 4-3 for interpretation of renin and aldosterone levels in hyperkalemia.

Electrocardiography
At [K⁺] levels >6 mEq/L, EKG will classically show increased amplitude and narrowing of the T wave and shortening of the QT interval. As [K⁺] rises to >7 to 8 mEq/L, the PR

TABLE 4-3	RENIN AND ALDOSTERONE LEVELS IN HYPERKALEMIA	
Disorder	Renin	Aldosterone
Primary hypoaldosteronism	↑	↓
Aldosterone receptor blockade, pseudohypoaldosteronism type I	↑	↑
Hyporeninemic hypoaldosteronism	↓	↓

↓, decreased; ↑, increased.

interval increases, and loss of the P wave can occur along with widening of the QRS. This sine-wave pattern can rapidly lead to ventricular fibrillation or asystole if untreated. The level at which EKG changes occur in any particular patient is highly variable. Chronic hyperkalemia is more likely to present with normal EKG. Additional electrolyte abnormalities, such as hypocalcemia or hyponatremia, amplify the effects of hyperkalemia on cardiac conduction.

TREATMENT

- The treatment of hyperkalemia must be initiated in the context of the [K^+], and the presence or absence of neuromuscular symptoms and EKG changes. A significant [K^+] elevation in the absence of symptoms or EKG changes should raise concern for pseudo-hyperkalemia (prompting whole-blood K^+ testing) or chronic hyperkalemia (in which cellular adaptation has taken place).
- Correction of concurrent acidemia, hypocalcemia, and hyponatremia decreases the hyperkalemic effects on the cell membrane.
- **Methods to stabilize the cell membrane or shift potassium into the cell are only temporizing measures. Potassium removal is needed to resolve the total body excess.**
  - ○ **IV calcium is the first treatment in severe hyperkalemia,** because it stabilizes the myocardial membrane. It is only recommended if EKG changes are present.
    - ■ Calcium chloride contains 13.6 mEq (272 mg) of elemental calcium per gram, while calcium gluconate contains 4.7 mEq (93 mg) per gram. Thus, 1 g of calcium chloride may be sufficient, but 2 g of calcium gluconate may be required.
    - ■ Because there is risk of tissue necrosis with extravasation (especially with calcium chloride), administration through a central vein is preferred. Each gram of calcium should be given slowly, over 5 to 10 minutes.
  - ○ **Insulin** rapidly lowers serum [K^+] (within minutes) by causing intracellular shift, and the effect can last up to a few hours.
    - ■ It is usually given as a dose of 10 units of regular insulin IV along with 25 to 50 g of dextrose (1 to 2 ampules of 50% dextrose).
    - ■ A peak reduction in serum [K^+] of 1 to 1.5 mEq/L can be expected.
    - ■ If the patient already has hyperglycemia, insulin can be given alone. Patients who are normoglycemic may become hypoglycemic when 10 units of regular insulin is administered with only 25 g of dextrose.
    - ■ In nondiabetic patients, glucose administration can result in endogenous insulin secretion, which will lower serum [K^+]. In insulin-dependent diabetics, glucose alone can produce hyperkalemia due to increased serum osmolality.
  - ○ **β_2-Adrenergic agents** will also promote intracellular shift of potassium.
    - ■ **Albuterol** is classically given in a dose of 5 to 20 mg by nebulizer or 0.5 mg IV. With IV administration, the onset of action is similar to insulin, but the effect is slightly delayed when given by nebulizer. The magnitude and duration of effect is similar to that of insulin administration.
    - ■ Owing to the risk of precipitating coronary events secondary to beta-agonist–induced tachycardia, alternate agents are preferred in patients with known or suspected significant coronary heart disease.
  - ○ **Renal elimination** is preferred when possible and is often the only measure necessary for mild to moderate hyperkalemia. **Increasing distal delivery of sodium** and poorly reabsorbed anions (e.g., bicarbonate) will increase K^+ excretion; this can be accomplished by sodium chloride, sodium bicarbonate, or diuretic (especially loop diuretic) administration.

- Patients with volume depletion may respond readily to fluid administration alone. Euvolemic patients may be given simultaneous saline and loop diuretics, while the volume-overloaded patient may respond to diuretics alone.
- Patients with PHA type II respond dramatically to thiazide diuretics.
- Although IV sodium bicarbonate will raise extracellular pH and causes a very modest K^+ shift into cells, the primary mechanism by which bicarbonate lowers serum $[K^+]$ is through stimulating aldosterone production and renal K^+ excretion.[3] It is administered as 50 mEq (one ampule) IV over several minutes. Administration is often limited by complications of sodium loading in patients with CHF or chronic kidney disease, particularly when larger repeated doses are given. It should be used with caution in patients with hypocalcemia.

○ **Cation-exchange resins** eliminate potassium by exchanging it with another cation in the GI tract.

- **Sodium polystyrene sulfonate** (SPS or Kayexalate) exchanges potassium for sodium in the GI tract. It can be given orally or rectally. Although the rectal preparation has a faster onset of action than the oral preparation, the oral route is preferable, given recent reports of intestinal necrosis, particularly in patients with recent abdominal surgery, bowel injury, or intestinal dysfunction. However, intestinal necrosis can in principle occur in anybody and is thought to be due to sorbitol-induced osmotic necrosis. The normal dose is 15 g PO q6h or 30 to 50 g PR, as needed. Each gram removes up to 1 mEq of potassium. In exchange, 1 to 2 mEq of sodium is absorbed. There is no role for SPS in patients with impending dialysis treatments as it will cause them to have loose bowel movements during their treatment.
- **Patiromer (Veltassa)** binds potassium in exchange for calcium in the gut. It was studied in chronic kidney disease patients with hyperkalemia who were receiving RAAS inhibitors and was effective in decreasing potassium levels and recurrence of hyperkalemia.[4] Dosing should start at 8.4 g PO daily and maximum dose is 25.2 g/day. Due to concerns for decreased absorption of other medications, it should not be taken within 3 hours of any other medication.

○ **Dialysis:** If hyperkalemia is severe, especially when renal and GI routes of elimination are not feasible, dialysis can be lifesaving.

- Peritoneal dialysis (PD) can lower $[K^+]$ as well, but not nearly as rapidly as hemodialysis (HD).
  - □ If PD is chosen, several rapid exchanges (~60- to 70-minute dwell time per exchange) may be performed conveniently using a cycler.
  - □ In a patient with plasma $[K^+]$ of 6.0 mEq, four rapid exchanges can be expected to remove a total of ~25 to 30 mEq of K^+ (similar to two doses of SPS), which may be enough to get the patient out of danger.
- In more severe hyperkalemia or conditions in which continued K^+ influx into plasma is expected, HD may be necessary.
  - □ If HD is used, a dialysate $[K^+]$ of 2 mEq/L is often sufficient.
  - □ In severe hyperkalemia, dialysate $[K^+]$ of 1 mEq/L may be used for the first 30 to 60 minutes, with close monitoring of whole-blood $[K^+]$.
  - □ If one anticipates HD will be started in a timely manner, IV calcium may be the only treatment necessary; treatment with insulin and beta-agonist might be indicated initially but will reduce efficacy of HD somewhat by driving K^+ into cells, where it cannot be removed by the dialyzer. Similarly, use of SPS should be avoided prior to anticipated HD.
  - □ It is important to remember that immediate post-HD plasma $[K^+]$ represents a nadir, and intracellular K^+ will subsequently shift to the extracellular space (called "rebound"). Thus, potassium repletion for a serum $[K^+]$ that appears to have overcorrected after dialysis is seldom appropriate. A recheck a few hours later will reveal the true $[K^+]$ at steady state.

- Chronic hyperkalemia is often associated with diabetic-associated HRHA, renal failure, or CHF. The serum potassium in this setting is usually stable and ≤6 mEq/L. Many of these patients are appropriately maintained on medications to treat the underlying condition(s), such as ACE inhibitors or spironolactone. Not infrequently these medications are discontinued due to mild elevations in [K^+]. In almost all cases, a moderate reduction in potassium intake, the use of diuretics as indicated, and a tolerance for stable mild to moderate hyperkalemia (usually below ≤6 mEq/L) allows successful continuation.

REFERENCES

1. Cely CM, Contreras G. Approach to the patient with hypertension, unexplained hypokalemia, and metabolic alkalosis. *Am J Kidney Dis.* 2001;37(3):E24.
2. Kamel KS, Halperin ML. Intrarenal urea recycling leads to a higher rate of renal excretion of potassium. *Curr Opin Nephrol Hypertens.* 2011;20(5):547–554.
3. Palmer BF. Regulation of potassium homeostasis. *Clin J Am Soc Nephrol.* 2015;10(6):1050–1060.
4. Weir MR, Bakris GL, Bushinsky DA, et al. Patiromer in patients with kidney disease and hyperkalemia receiving RAAS inhibitors. *N Engl J Med.* 2015;372(3):211–221.

Disorders of Calcium and Phosphorus Balance

5

Miraie Wardi and Daniel Coyne

GENERAL PRINCIPLES

- The average daily intake of calcium is widely variable, ranging from 400 to 1500 mg/day, much of which is supplemented with oral calcium.
  - From that, 20% to 40% is absorbed in the small intestine; the remaining calcium is excreted in the stool along with a small amount of calcium from colonic secretions.
  - Maintenance of calcium balance involves buffering in the skeletal system and tightly controlled excretion in the kidneys.
    - In the kidney, 80% to 85% of the calcium load is reabsorbed along the proximal nephron. In the ascending loop of Henle, calcium is reabsorbed passively through the tight junction protein, paracellin-1.
    - Although a smaller percentage is reabsorbed in the distal tubule, distal calcium reabsorption is actively regulated by the actions of parathyroid hormone (PTH).
- Over 99% of total calcium in the adult body is stored in the bone complexed as hydroxyapatite crystals. The remaining total body calcium remains in the extracellular fluid (ECF).
- The normal total calcium range in the ECF is 8.6 to 10.3 mg/dL. In the ECF:
  - 50% of calcium is in the ionized state.
  - 40% is bound to albumin; this form is not filterable in the kidney.
  - 10% is bound to anions like citrate, sulfate, and phosphate as a filterable complex.
- The ionized fraction is physiologically active and plays an important role in neuromuscular activity, secretion, and signal transduction; therefore it is tightly regulated in a narrow range (4.5 to 5.1 mg/dL) by the following mechanisms:
  - **PTH**
    - PTH is released in response to hypocalcemia. The parathyroid gland senses the drop in the ECF ionized calcium concentration via a calcium-sensing receptor, which stimulates the release of PTH.
    - PTH maintains calcium homeostasis via three mechanisms.
      - **Increases 1-α hydroxylase activity** in the proximal tubule, which stimulates the production of **calcitriol.** Calcitriol increases **intestinal** calcium and phosphorus absorption.
      - Enhances proximal tubular **reabsorption of calcium** and decreases proximal tubular reabsorption of phosphorus.
      - Simulates **bone turnover** and a release of calcium and phosphorus into the ECF.
  - **Vitamin D** is a fat-soluble vitamin present in diet and produced in the skin in the presence of ultraviolet light. 25-Hydroxylase in the liver forms calcidiol.
  - **Calcitriol** is formed in the proximal tubule from 1-α hydroxylation of calcidiol. It can also be formed in activated macrophages.
    - Calcitriol has multiple actions that are crucial in calcium homeostasis:
      - It **stimulates** calcium absorption **in the intestines.**
      - It inhibits PTH synthesis and secretion **at the parathyroid gland.**
      - **It promotes** osteoclastic bone resorption leading to a release of calcium and phosphorus from the bone.

- In the bone, calcitriol also increases the production of fibroblast growth factor 23 (FGF23), a key regulator of serum phosphorus levels.
- Calcitriol is inactivated by 24-hydroxylase. Activity of this enzyme is increased by calcitriol and decreased by PTH.
- **FGF23** plays a central role in the control of serum phosphorus, but it also contributes significantly to calcium homeostasis as a key regulator of calcitriol and inhibitor of PTH secretion.

Hypercalcemia

GENERAL PRINCIPLES

- Clinically significant hypercalcemia can be due to increased bone resorption, increased intestinal absorption, and decreased renal clearance. Primary hyperparathyroidism and malignancy account for the majority (>90%) of cases (please see Table 5-1).
- Increased bone resorption
  - **Primary hyperparathyroidism** (sporadic, familial, MEN1, MEN2, lithium therapy) is the **most common cause of hypercalcemia in ambulatory patients.**
    - An adenoma of a single gland is found in 85% of cases and 15% of cases are due to hyperplasia of all four glands.
    - Parathyroid carcinoma is responsible for <1% of the cases.
    - Most patients are asymptomatic with modest hypercalcemia (<11 mg/dL) found incidentally.
    - These patients remain at risk for long-term consequences of hyperparathyroidism such as nephrolithiasis and osteopenia.

TABLE 5-1 CAUSES OF HYPERCALCEMIA

Increased Bone Resorption
Primary hyperparathyroidism
MEN1 and MEN2A
Malignancy
Postrenal transplant
Immobilization
Familial hypocalciuric hypercalcemia
Thyrotoxicosis
Paget disease
Vitamin A intoxication
Lithium
Adrenal insufficiency

Increased Intestinal Absorption
Milk-alkali syndrome
Granulomatous disease
Vitamin D intoxication

Decreased Renal Excretion
Thiazide diuretics
Acute renal failure
Volume depletion
Vasoactive intestinal polypeptide tumors (VIPoma)
Pheochromocytoma

	TABLE 5-2	MALIGNANCY-RELATED HYPERCALCEMIA	

Cause	Mechanism	Implicated Malignancies
Osteolytic hypercalcemia	Cytokines produced by the tumor act locally to stimulate bone resorption.	Breast cancer, non–small-cell lung cancer, myeloma, lymphoma
Humoral hypercalcemia	Tumor products act systemically to stimulate bone resorption (PTHrP).	Squamous cell carcinomas and renal, bladder, ovarian cancers
Tumoral calcitriol production	Tumor promotes activation of calcitriol.	Lymphomas

○ **Malignancy** is responsible for the majority of cases of hypercalcemia among *hospitalized* patients. Malignancy induces hypercalcemia in three ways (please see Table 5-2).

○ **Tertiary hyperparathyroidism:** Long-term dialysis patients may develop parathyroid hyperplasia and an autonomous secretion of PTH.

○ **Immobilization:** Prolonged bed rest leads to an increase in bone resorption and may lead to hypercalcemia.
  ■ This is typically seen in critically ill patients, patients with spinal cord injuries, and those in full body casts.
  ■ Mobilization corrects hypercalcemia.

○ **Familial hypocalciuric hypercalcemia** (FHH) is an autosomal dominant disorder in which mutations in the calcium-sensing receptor lead to decreased receptor activity.
  ■ Patients have a mild hypercalcemia, hypophosphatemia, and normal or mildly elevated PTH levels.
  ■ FHH can be differentiated from primary hyperparathyroidism by a low urinary calcium level.
  ■ Parathyroidectomy is not indicated.

○ Thyrotoxicosis may stimulate osteoclastic bone resorption, causing a mild hypercalcemia. Concurrent hyperparathyroidism can also occur.

○ **Vitamin A intoxication** (doses >50,000 IU/day) can be associated with hypercalcemia secondary to increased osteoclast bone resorption.

● **Increased intestinal absorption**
  ○ **Milk-alkali syndrome** due to ingestion of large quantities of calcium carbonate–based antacids. It is characterized by hypercalcemia, alkalemia, nephrocalcinosis, and renal failure.
  ○ **Granulomatous disease:** Granulomatous diseases such as sarcoidosis, tuberculosis, and leprosy cause hypercalcemia due to exogenous production of 1-α hydroxylase which converts calcidiol to calcitriol. Treatment of the underlying disease corrects the hypercalcemia.
  ○ **Vitamin D intoxication:** May be observed in dialysis patients overtreated with vitamin D analogs. Hypercalcemia is usually mild and improves with dose adjustment or discontinuation of the drug.

● **Decreased renal excretion**
  ○ Acute renal failure
  ○ Volume depletion
  ○ Thiazide diuretics can be associated with a mild hypercalcemia likely due to increased proximal reabsorption from volume contraction.

DIAGNOSIS

Clinical Presentation

- Mild hypercalcemia is often asymptomatic and incidentally discovered on routine blood tests. Long-term manifestations include osteoporosis, nephrolithiasis, and chronic kidney disease (CKD).
- Severe hypercalcemia is often associated with neurologic and gastrointestinal (GI) symptoms.
  - **GI symptoms** include anorexia, nausea, vomiting, and constipation.
  - **Neurologic symptoms** include weakness, fatigue, confusion, stupor, and coma.
  - **Renal manifestations** include polyuria and nephrolithiasis. Polyuria combined with nausea and vomiting can cause volume depletion, resulting in impaired calcium excretion and worsening of hypercalcemia.

Diagnostic Testing

- The first step in the evaluation of presumed symptomatic hypercalcemia is measurement of **calcium** level. This should be interpreted in the context of the plasma albumin concentration (corrected calcium) or an **ionized calcium** should be measured.
- Confirmed hypercalcemia can then be divided into PTH and non–PTH-related mechanisms with the measurement of **intact PTH.**
- Intact PTH levels are either elevated or inappropriately normal such as seen in primary hyperparathyroidism, FHH, tertiary hyperparathyroidism, and lithium-induced hypercalcemia.
- **Urinary calcium** should be ordered to distinguish FHH from primary hyperparathyroidism. Low urinary calcium concentrations (<200 mg calcium per 24 hours or fractional excretion of calcium <1%) are suggestive of FHH.
- Non–PTH-related hypercalcemia can be due to PTH-related peptide or **vitamin D metabolite**–related mechanisms.
  - $1,25(OH)_2D_3$ (calcitriol) levels are elevated in granulomatous disorders and calcitriol overdose.
  - $25(OH)D$ levels are elevated with noncalcitriol vitamin D intoxication (rare).
- **Phosphorus** may be low in settings of elevated PTH (primary hyperparathyroidism) or PTHrP (e.g., humoral hypercalcemia of malignancy). Phosphorus may be high in vitamin D toxicity or increased bone resorption without hyperparathyroidism (Paget disease).

TREATMENT

- **Volume repletion**
  - **Correction of hypovolemia is the initial goal** and often requires at least 3 to 4 L of 0.9% saline in the first 24 hours.
  - Continuing maintenance IV fluids after restoring ECF volume promotes further calcium excretion.
  - Electrolyte concentrations should be monitored every 8 to 12 hours during induction and maintenance of diuresis.
- While repleting intravascular volume is the mainstay of hypercalcemia management, drug therapy is indicated in certain situations.
- **Dialysis:** Both **hemodialysis** and **peritoneal dialysis** using dialysate with low calcium are very effective means of treating hypercalcemia. Very low calcium dialysis baths should be used with caution as rapid development of hypocalcemia can occur.

- Parathyroidectomy in cases of hyperparathyroidism is indicated if the following criteria are met:
  - Corrected plasma calcium >1 mg/dL above upper limit of normal
  - Hypercalciuria >400 mg/day
  - Renal insufficiency
  - Reduced bone mass (T-score <−2.5 by DEXA)
  - Age <50 years
  - Nephrolithiasis
  - Lack of feasibility of long-term follow-up

Hypocalcemia

GENERAL PRINCIPLES

- Hypocalcemia can result from either decreased calcium absorption from the GI tract or decreased calcium resorption from bone.
- **Decreased calcium absorption**
  - **Vitamin D deficiency:** Vitamin D (calcidiol) deficiency is common, mainly due to limited exposure to sunlight. Vitamin D deficiency can also be due to malabsorption syndromes and anticonvulsant use because of increased calcidiol metabolism.
  - Deficiency of vitamin D can lead to rickets and osteomalacia.
  - **CKD:** The loss of functional renal mass and reduced activity of 1-α hydroxylase from phosphorus retention contribute to the decreased renal conversion of calcidiol (25[OH]D) to calcitriol (1,25[OH]2D3). With decreasing levels of calcitriol, patients with CKD are prone to developing hypocalcemia. However, the balance is partly maintained by increasing levels of PTH as glomerular filtration rate (GFR) declines.
  - **Vitamin D–dependent rickets:** This condition can be classified into two types:
    - **Type 1:** due to impaired hydroxylation of calcidiol to calcitriol
    - **Type 2:** due to end-organ resistance to calcitriol
- **Decreased PTH level or effect:**
  - **Hypoparathyroidism** can be associated with acquired and inherited diseases that result from either impaired synthesis or release of PTH. Etiologies of hypoparathyroidism include the following:
    - Polyglandular autoimmune syndrome type I associated with chronic mucocutaneous candidiasis and primary adrenal insufficiency
  - Autoimmune diseases: pernicious anemia, diabetes mellitus, vitiligo, and autoimmune thyroid disease
    - Iatrogenic after thyroidectomy
    - Secondary to radiation, infiltrative disorders, or deposition of metals such as iron, copper, or aluminum
  - **Hypomagnesemia** results in decreased PTH secretion and hypocalcemia.
  - **Familial hypocalcemia** results from activating mutations in the calcium-sensing receptor. Subsequent downregulation of PTH transcription leads to hypocalcemia from inappropriately low PTH levels due to receptor malfunction.
  - **Pseudohypoparathyroidism** (Albright hereditary osteodystrophy) is a hereditary disorder in which the target cell response to PTH is decreased. Renal calcium excretion is increased and the PTH level is increased. Phenotypic characteristics include short stature, obesity, shortened metacarpals and metatarsals, and heterotopic calcification.
  - **Calcimimetics** have been used for the control of elevated PTH levels in patients with secondary hyperparathyroidism and may induce hypocalcemia.

- **Extravascular deposition/intravascular chelation:**
  - **Hungry bone syndrome:** A profound reduction in calcium concentration can occur after surgical removal of parathyroid.
    - This "hungry bone syndrome" is due to a rapid bone mineralization in the absence of PTH.
    - Symptoms can occur soon after surgery, and patients' calcium levels should be carefully monitored (q4h to q6h).
    - Hypocalcemia also occurs after thyroid surgery (5% of cases).
  - **Hyperphosphatemia:** High concentrations of phosphorus form complexes with extracellular calcium, resulting in hypocalcemia.
    - This phenomenon can occur during rapid release of intracellular phosphorus, as seen in rhabdomyolysis and tumor lysis syndrome (TLS).
    - Iatrogenic causes of this can occur during the administration of intravenous (IV) phosphorus or phosphorus-containing enemas.
  - **Acute pancreatitis:** The release of pancreatic lipase digests retroperitoneal and omental fat. The fatty acids, once released, bind to the calcium. The hypocalcemia is aggravated by the hypoalbuminuria and hypomagnesemia associated with acute pancreatitis.
  - **Citrate-containing blood products:** Massive transfusions of citrate-containing blood products can cause intravascular chelation of calcium, leading to hypocalcemia. The use of citrate in continuous renal replacement therapy or plasma exchange can also cause this.
  - **Gadolinium-based contrast agents:** Gadodiamide and gadoversetamide may interfere with assays for serum calcium, and unexpected hypocalcemia detected immediately after the administration of these agents should be rechecked before action is taken.[1]
- **Septic shock:** Endotoxic shock has been associated with hypocalcemia through unclear mechanisms. Hypocalcemia may be partially responsible for the hypotension, as myocardial function correlates with ionized calcium levels.

DIAGNOSIS

Clinical Presentation

- **Symptoms** depend not only on the degree of hypocalcemia but also on the rate of decline of the plasma calcium concentration.
  - Precipitation of symptoms is also influenced by plasma pH and the presence or absence of concomitant hypomagnesemia, hypokalemia, or hyponatremia.
  - Neuromuscular excitability symptoms are most common.
    - The patient may experience circumoral and distal extremity paresthesias or carpopedal spasm.
    - Other manifestations include mental status changes, irritability, and seizures.
- On physical examination, hypotension, bradycardia, laryngeal spasm, and bronchospasm may be present.
  - Neurologic examination is significant for latent tetany, elicited as classical **Chvostek** (facial twitch elicited by tapping on the facial nerve just below the zygomatic arch with the mouth slightly open) and **Trousseau** sign (development of wrist flexion, metacarpophalangeal joint flexion, hyperextended fingers, and thumb flexion after a blood pressure cuff has been inflated to 20 mm Hg above systolic pressure for a duration of 3 minutes).
  - Cardiovascular effects include hypotension, prolonged QT interval, and impaired excitation contraction coupling, leading to congestive heart failure.
  - Long-standing hypocalcemia can also be associated with subcapsular cataracts.

Diagnostic Testing

- **Total calcium concentration should be corrected to the serum albumin.** Decreased total plasma calcium concentration is found in hypoalbuminemia without changes in the ionized calcium level. In general, for every 1.0 g/dL decrement in plasma albumin, there is a 0.8 mg/dL decline in the reported total plasma calcium level.
- **Magnesium** deficiency should be ruled out.
- **Phosphorus** will be low in conditions associated with low vitamin D activity, except for kidney failure, where there is decreased renal clearance of phosphorus. The plasma phosphorus will be increased in rhabdomyolysis or TLS.
- **PTH** that is low or inappropriately normal in the setting of hypocalcemia is indicative of hypoparathyroidism. A high PTH is often found with vitamin D deficiency states, CKD, and pseudohypoparathyroidism.
- **25(OH)D and 1,25(OH)$_2$D$_3$** levels are useful in assessing for vitamin D deficiency and vitamin D–dependent rickets, respectively.

TREATMENT

- For patients with symptomatic hypocalcemia or a corrected calcium concentration of <7.5 mg/dL, **IV calcium gluconate should be administered** (100 to 300 mg, or 1 to 3 mL of 10% calcium gluconate solution, over 10 to 15 minutes). The first ampule can be administered over several minutes followed by a constant infusion at a rate of 0.5 to 1.0 mg/kg/hr.
  - ○ Adjustments in the rate should be based on serial plasma calcium determinations.
  - ○ Treatment of hypocalcemia is ineffective without adequate treatment of hypomagnesemia.
  - ○ In the setting of metabolic acidosis, hypocalcemia should be corrected before the acidosis.
- Mild hypocalcemia can be treated with **oral calcium supplements.** 1 to 3 g/day of elemental calcium can be given between meals to maximize enteric absorption.
- Vitamin D supplementation can also be given and is generally required for patients with hypoparathyroidism.
  - ○ Cholecalciferol and ergocalciferol are used to replace low levels of 25-hydroxy vitamin D. They are inexpensive, but less effective than calcitriol.
  - ○ **Calcitriol** is a potent **active vitamin D** preparation and has a fast onset and short duration of action. A dose of 0.5 to 1.0 mcg/day is usually required in patients with hypoparathyroidism.
  - ○ Patients who are receiving calcium and vitamin D replacement therapy should be monitored for hypercalciuria, nephrolithiasis, and nephrocalcinosis since the filtered calcium load may exceed the capacity for renal excretion in patients with hypoparathyroidism.

Disorders of Phosphorus Metabolism

GENERAL PRINCIPLES

- The average diet contains 1000 to 1400 mg of phosphorus, mainly from high-protein foods and dairy products; between 60% and 70% of this is absorbed in the gut. The remainder is lost in the stool, with an additional 200 mg/day that is secreted into the colon.
- The vast majority of the body's phosphorus content is stored in the skeletal framework. Of the 700 g of phosphorus found in the average individual, 85% of it is in the skeleton and 15% in soft tissues. ECF contains 1% of total body phosphorus.

- There is a dynamic capture and release of phosphorus that allows regulation of the serum phosphorus levels.
- Most inorganic phosphorus is freely filtered in the glomerulus. The proximal tubule is the primary site of active reabsorption of phosphorus, with 70% to 80% of the filtered phosphorus reabsorbed in the proximal tubule. The remaining 20% to 30% reabsorbed in the distal tubule.
- Plasma phosphorus levels are regulated by a number of mechanisms that control the skeletal stores of phosphorus as well as renal handling of phosphorus. Of central importance are:
  - PTH: The major role of PTH is to preserve constant serum calcium concentration.
    - At the level of proximal tubule, PTH acts on receptors at apical and basolateral sodium-phosphate cotransporters to promote phosphorus wasting.
    - PTH also acts directly on bone to increase phosphate entry into the ECF and indirectly on the intestine by stimulating the synthesis of calcitriol.
  - **Vitamin D** increases plasma phosphate because of enhanced intestinal phosphorus absorption by increasing sodium-phosphate cotransport across the apical brush border membrane.
  - **FGF23:** This molecule belongs to a group of substances called phosphatonins. Their main effect is to promote renal excretion of phosphate and lower plasma phosphorus levels.
    - In contrast to PTH, FGF23 also leads to decreased production of calcitriol and, therefore, has a net effect of reducing plasma phosphorus concentration.
    - The reduction of GFR in kidney disease, which leads to subsequent phosphorus retention, is a potent stimulus for FGF23 release.
  - **Insulin** stimulates an intracellular shift in plasma phosphate, thus lowering the plasma phosphorus concentrations.

Hyperphosphatemia

GENERAL PRINCIPLES

Definition

Hyperphosphatemia is defined by a plasma phosphorus concentration that exceeds the normal range of 2.3 to 4.3 mg/dL.

Pathophysiology

- The **three main mechanisms** that lead to hyperphosphatemia are impaired renal excretion, transcellular shift into the ECF, and increased phosphate intake (please see Table 5-3).
- **Impaired renal excretion**
  - **Renal failure:** With declining GFR, the fractional excretion of phosphate begins to increase and reabsorption is suppressed. Once GFR reaches around ≤25 mL/min, it can no longer keep up with the dietary intake and the plasma phosphorus level begins to rise. Hence, hyperphosphatemia is a frequent finding in advanced CKD.
  - **Decreased PTH effect:** Because PTH decreases proximal tubular reabsorption of phosphate, deficiency of this hormone (hypoparathyroidism) or a resistance to its actions (pseudohypoparathyroidism) leads to increased tubular transport of phosphate, resulting in hyperphosphatemia.
  - **Direct stimulation of proximal tubule reabsorption:** Conditions such as acromegaly, tumoral calcinosis, and the administration of bisphosphonates are known to

TABLE 5-3   CAUSES OF HYPERPHOSPHATEMIA

Impaired Renal Excretion
Renal failure (acute and chronic)
Hypoparathyroidism
  Developmental
  Autoimmune
  After surgery/radiation
  Activating mutation in calcium-sensing receptor
Parathyroid suppression with **hypercalcemia**
  Vitamin D or A intoxication
  Granulomatous disease
  Bone metastasis
  Immobilization
Pseudohypoparathyroidism
Acromegaly
Tumoral calcinosis
Bisphosphonates
Heparin
Magnesium abnormalities (hyper and hypo)

Transcellular Shift
Rhabdomyolysis
Tumor lysis syndrome
Massive hemolysis
Acidosis
Hypoinsulinemia
Hyperthermia
Hemolytic anemia
Fulminant hepatic failure

Increased Phosphate Intake or Absorption
High phosphate diet (in the setting of CKD)
Flee® enemas
Vitamin D intoxication
Rapid administration of IV phosphorus supplementation

CKD, chronic kidney disease; IV, intravenous.

directly stimulate renal phosphorus reabsorption. In the case of acromegaly, this is thought to be mediated by elevated levels of insulin-like growth factor 1.

- **Transcellular shift: Acidosis** and **hypoinsulinemia** both reduce phosphate entry into cells.
- **Increased phosphate load**
  ○ Dietary indiscretion by the patient with CKD
  ○ Iatrogenic (e.g., use of phosphorus-containing enemas in CKD patients)
  ○ Vitamin D intoxication can result in increased intestinal absorption of phosphorus.
  ○ Increased release of phosphorus from cellular stores
     ▪ **Rhabdomyolysis** can cause severe hyperphosphatemia acutely, which precipitates hypocalcemia secondary to malignant calcium phosphate deposition in soft tissues.
     ▪ **TLS** usually follows chemotherapy for hematologic malignancies or rapidly growing solid tumors.
     ▪ **Massive hemolysis**

DIAGNOSIS

Clinical Presentation

- Symptoms of acute hyperphosphatemia are generally **attributable to accompanying hypocalcemia** and include **tetany, seizures,** and **dysrhythmias.**
- Hypocalcemia is thought to result from tissue deposition of calcium once calcium × phosphate product reaches >55.
- Tissue deposition of calcium can occur in blood vessels, skin, kidneys, and other organs.
- Calciphylaxis is the term used for tissue ischemia that may result from the calcification and subsequent thrombosis of small blood vessels.
- Chronic hyperphosphatemia contributes to renal osteodystrophy.

Diagnostic Testing

- **Plasma creatinine** provides a general assessment of renal clearance.
- **Intact PTH** is elevated in CKD, but is low in the setting of hypoparathyroidism.
- **Creatine kinase** is markedly elevated in rhabdomyolysis.
- **Uric acid levels** are often markedly elevated in TLS.
- **Markers of hemolysis** (lactate dehydrogenase, haptoglobin, bilirubin, and so forth) are helpful in the appropriate setting.
- **Calcium** levels are usually low in acute hyperphosphatemia but should only be treated if symptoms occur, as treatment can precipitate calcium phosphate deposition.

TREATMENT

- **Acute hyperphosphatemia** in patients who do not have renal insufficiency can be managed with saline diuresis and correction of the underlying cause.
- **Chronic hyperphosphatemia** is almost always a result of CKD, and the treatment is aimed at reducing the intestinal absorption of phosphate.
  - **Reduce enteric absorption of phosphorus:**
    - **Dietary restriction of phosphate.** The first step is to institute dietary restriction of phosphate to 600 to 900 mg/day.
    - **Niacinamide.** Niacinamide is the amide form of vitamin B and has been shown to reduce phosphorus levels in the dialysis population by decreasing the phosphorus uptake in the gut.[2]
  - **Calcium-based phosphate binders**
    - Binders are agents that form insoluble complexes with dietary phosphorus to prevent absorption of phosphorus in the gut.
    - Calcium-based binders are often used as first-line agents in patients with CKD who are not on dialysis, as they are widely accessible and inexpensive. However, adding a calcium load to a population at risk for vascular calcification should be done with great caution and frequent monitoring. In patients who already have hypercalcemia or evidence of vascular calcification, an alternative should be utilized.
      - **Calcium carbonate** (TUMS®) starting at 500 mg (200 mg elemental calcium) TID with meals to a maximum of 3750 mg/day (1500 mg elemental calcium).
      - **Calcium acetate** (PHOSLO®) starting at 667 mg (167 mg elemental calcium) TID with meals to a maximum of 6000 mg/day (1500 mg elemental calcium).
    - **Non–calcium-based binders** are effective agents that avoid the risk of calcium loading in CKD patients. However, they are generally more expensive and associated with GI discomfort.

- □ **Sevelamer carbonate** (RENVELA®) starting at 800 mg TID with meals; maximum dose 7200 mg/day.
        - □ **Lanthanum carbonate** (FOSRENOL®) starting at 250 mg TID with meals; maximum dose 3000 mg/day.
    - ○ **Hemodialysis**
        - ■ In the dialysis population, elevated phosphorus levels may reflect dietary indiscretions, binder noncompliance, or frequently missed dialysis treatments. Resumption of all of the above is often sufficient to improve plasma phosphorus concentrations.
        - ■ Among dialysis modalities, daily nocturnal home hemodialysis is even more effective than intermittent hemodialysis in phosphorus removal.
        - ■ In the acute setting, dialysis may be warranted in patients with symptomatic hypocalcemia from severe hyperphosphatemia in conjunction with renal failure.

Hypophosphatemia

GENERAL PRINCIPLES

Definition

Hypophosphatemia is defined as plasma phosphorus levels below the normal range of 2.3 to 4.3 mg/dL.

Pathophysiology

- Three main mechanisms for hypophosphatemia are redistribution of extracellular phosphate into the intracellular space, decrease in intestinal absorption of phosphate, or increase in renal excretion of phosphate.
- **Redistribution of extracellular phosphate** (especially important in hospital setting):
    - ○ **Respiratory alkalosis** leads to a rise in intracellular pH, which in turn stimulates glycolysis, and phosphate is incorporated into adenosine triphosphate (ATP).
    - ○ **Refeeding syndrome** can occur in chronically malnourished individuals due to rapid intracellular shifts of phosphorus.
    - ○ **Treatment of diabetic ketoacidosis** (DKA) with IV insulin leads to rapid flux of phosphorus into the cells.
    - ○ **Hungry bone syndrome** after partial parathyroidectomy causes movement of phosphate into the cells, leading to hypophosphatemia.
- **Decreased intestinal absorption** (uncommon)
    - ○ **Malnutrition:** Poor intake alone is very rarely sufficient to cause hypophosphatemia, but if the quantity of phosphorus ingested remains less than the amount lost in colonic secretions for a prolonged period of time, hypophosphatemia may ensue. Typically, this occurs in conjunction with one of the following exacerbating conditions.
    - ○ **Malabsorption syndromes:** In addition to poor intake and absorption of phosphorus and vitamin D, the accompanying diarrhea also contributes to significant GI losses.
    - ○ **Oral phosphate binders:** Indiscriminate use of phosphate binders in end-stage renal disease patients who may not be eating very well may lead to low phosphorus levels.
    - ○ **Vitamin D deficiency:** Severe deficiency of this vitamin can lead to hypophosphatemia. The secondary hyperparathyroidism resulting from vitamin D deficiency contributes further to hypophosphatemia through increasing renal phosphate excretion.
    - ○ **Alcoholism:** Alcoholics often have poor intake of both phosphate and vitamin D, resulting in total body phosphorus depletion. Use of dextrose-containing IV fluids leads to insulin secretion, which further lowers plasma phosphate by intracellular redistribution, as discussed above.

- **Increased renal excretion**
  - **Hyperparathyroidism:** Persistently elevated levels of PTH lead to renal phosphorus wasting.
    - Hypophosphatemia is usually mild in primary hyperparathyroidism because PTH also stimulates calcitriol synthesis, resulting in increased intestinal absorption of phosphate.
    - However, in severe vitamin D deficiency, the resultant increase in PTH is not accompanied by the compensatory rise in calcitriol levels and hypophosphatemia can be severe.
  - **After renal transplant:** Renal phosphate wasting is common after successful renal transplant due to persistently elevated PTH.
  - **Osmotic diuresis:** In DKA or recovering acute tubular necrosis (ATN), excessive phosphate losses occur in urine, along with other solutes.
  - **Fanconi syndrome:** A defect in proximal tubular reabsorption will cause phosphorus wasting. Although congenital forms of Fanconi syndrome are very rare in adults, the syndrome can be a manifestation of proximal tubule toxicity from light chains in multiple myeloma.
  - **Familial X-linked hypophosphatemic rickets** (XLH) is caused by mutations in the PHEX gene. The condition is characterized by growth retardation, renal phosphate wasting, hypophosphatemia, and rickets. Plasma concentrations of calcitriol are low.
  - **Autosomal dominant hypophosphatemic rickets** has a similar phenotype to XLH but is inherited in an autosomal dominant fashion. Mutations in the FGF23 are responsible for the disease.
  - **Oncogenic osteomalacia:** Paraneoplastic production of FGF23 by mesenchymal tumors is responsible for phosphaturia in cases of oncogenic osteomalacia.

DIAGNOSIS

Clinical Presentation

- Symptoms and signs of hypophosphatemia are due to inability to make ATP and occur if total body phosphate depletion is present and the plasma phosphorus level is <1 mg/dL.
- **Neuromuscular symptoms:** weakness, rhabdomyolysis, impaired diaphragmatic function, paresthesias, dysarthria, confusion, seizures, and coma.
- **Hematologic symptoms:** hemolysis and platelet dysfunction.
- Chronic hypophosphatemia leads to rickets in children and osteomalacia in adults.

Diagnostic Testing

- **Fractional excretion of phosphorus and 24-hour urine phosphorus:**
  - Fractional excretion of phosphorus >5% or a urine phosphate excretion of >100 mg per 24 hours in the setting of hypophosphatemia indicates excessive renal loss.
  - Excretion rates are lower in states of impaired intestinal absorption or hypophosphatemia from transcellular shifts.
  - One exception is vitamin D deficiency, which causes phosphaturia from secondary hyperparathyroidism.
- **Plasma calcium** is typically low in secondary hyperparathyroidism from vitamin D deficiency, but high or normal in primary hyperparathyroidism.
- **25(OH) vitamin D level:** Low levels suggest vitamin D deficiency.
- **PTH** is elevated in primary or secondary hyperparathyroidism.
- **Hypomagnesemia** and **hypokalemia** accompany hypophosphatemia in the setting of refeeding syndrome.

TREATMENT

- **Moderate hypophosphatemia** (1 to 2.5 mg/dL):
  - ○ This is usually asymptomatic and can be managed primarily by treating the underlying cause. **Oral agents** can be used to help restore serum phosphorus to normal levels.
    - ▪ **Neutra-Phos** (250 mg phosphorus and 7 mEq each sodium and potassium per capsule)
    - ▪ **Neutra-Phos K** (250 mg phosphorus and 14 mEq potassium per capsule)
    - ▪ **K-Phos Neutral** (250 mg phosphorus, 13 mEq of sodium, and 1 mEq of potassium per tablet)
- **Severe hypophosphatemia (<1 mg/dL):**
  - ○ Most often requires IV phosphate.
  - ○ **Potassium phosphate** (1.5 mEq potassium per mmol phosphate)
  - ○ **Sodium phosphate** (1.3 mEq sodium per mmol phosphate)
  - ○ IV infusion should be stopped when the plasma phosphorus level is >1.5 mg/dL or when PO therapy is possible.
  - ○ Because of the need to replenish intracellular stores, 24 to 36 hours of phosphate infusion may be required.
  - ○ Hyperphosphatemia must be avoided, as it can cause hypocalcemia and ectopic calcification.
  - ○ IV phosphate should be given cautiously in renal failure.

REFERENCES

1. Gandhi MJ, Narra VR, Brown JJ, et al. Clinical and economic impact of falsely decreased calcium values caused by gadoversetamide interference. *Am J Roentgenol.* 2008;190(3):W213–W217.
2. Cheng S, Young D, Huang Y, et al. A randomized, double-blind, placebo-controlled trial of niacinamide for reduction of phosphorus in hemodialysis patients. *Clin J Am Soc Nephrol.* 2008;3(4):1131–1138.

Acid–Base Disorders

Owais Bhatti and Steven Cheng

6

GENERAL PRINCIPLES

The body maintains acid–base homeostasis through three primary mechanisms:
- Chemical buffering by extracellular and intracellular buffers.
- Controlling pCO_2 through modulation of alveolar ventilation.
- Altering net acid excretion or the reabsorption of HCO_3^-.

Definitions
- An **acid** is a substance that donates H^+ ions and a base is a substance that accepts H^+ ions.
  - **Physiologic balance of the acid–base status** can be described by the following equation:

$$CO_2 + H_2O \leftrightarrow H_2CO_3 \leftrightarrow H^+ + HCO_3^-$$

  - Acids and bases may be "strong" or "weak" depending on the degree of ionization in the human body.
  - The **Henderson–Hasselbalch equation** shows the pH as a mathematical relationship between HCO_3^- and pCO_2.

$$pH = 6.1 + \log[HCO_3^-]/(0.03 \times pCO_2)$$

- **Acidemia** is an increase in the $[H^+]$ and a decrease in the pH.
- **Alkalemia** is a decrease in the $[H^+]$ and a rise in the pH.

Classification
- Acid and base disturbances are generally classified by the genesis of the disorder.
  - Changes in the pCO_2 are referred to as "Respiratory" processes.
    - A decrease in pH due to an increase in pCO_2 is termed "Respiratory Acidosis."
    - An increase in pH due to a decrease in pCO_2 is termed "Respiratory Alkalosis."
  - Changes in the $[HCO_3^-]$ are referred to as "Metabolic" processes.
    - A decrease in pH due to a decrease in $[HCO_3^-]$ is termed "Metabolic Acidosis."
    - An increase in pH due to an increase in $[HCO_3^-]$ is termed "Metabolic Alkalosis."

Pathophysiology
- Acid–base homeostasis is under constant challenge. For example, the typical Western diet generates 1 mEq of acid/kg/day. The human body is well adapted to maintain pH within a narrow range (please see Fig. 6-1).
- **Buffering:**
  - HCO_3^- is the most important physiologic buffer in the extracellular fluid (ECF) space.
  - HCO_3^- can combine with free H^+ to form H_2CO_3, which can subsequently convert to CO_2 and H_2O (see ventilatory response, below)
  - Intracellular buffers include proteins, phosphates, and hemoglobin.
  - Bone can also absorb a significant acid load and, on dissolution, release buffer compounds such as calcium carbonate and calcium bicarbonate.

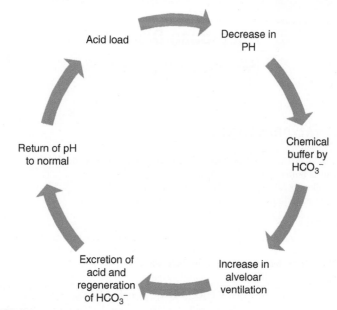

FIGURE 6-1. Physiologic response to acid load.

- **Ventilatory response:**
  - The ability to sense changes in pH and control pCO_2 via alveolar ventilation allows the body to further respond to the acid–base imbalance.
  - In response to an acid load, a reduction in pCO_2 attenuates the change in pH by shifting the equation toward the generation of CO_2 and H_2O.
    - The normal pCO_2 is 40 mm Hg.
    - The level falls with increased ventilation, and rises with decreased ventilation.
- **Excretion:**
  - Ultimately, net acid excretion and reabsorption/regeneration of HCO_3^- is required to return the system to balance.
  - This is accomplished through the renal elimination of titratable acids (dihydrogen phosphate) and nontitratable acids (ammonium).
  - Bicarbonate reabsorption must also be maximized to excrete the daily acid load.
    - The majority of bicarbonate reabsorption occurs at the proximal tubule.
    - Bicarbonate reabsorption is regulated by plasma HCO_3^- levels and effective circulating volume.
- Acid–base disorders arise when the capacity for resisting change in pH is exceeded or when mechanisms used to maintain physiologic pH are impaired (see Fig. 6-2).
- **Acidosis can occur from any of the following:**
  - **Metabolic insults:**
    - **A large acid load**
    - Exogenous sources, such as ethylene glycol or other alcohols
    - Endogenous sources during conditions such as lactic acidosis or ketoacidosis
  - **A loss of bicarbonate buffer**
    - Gastrointestinal (GI) loss (diarrhea).
    - Renal loss (proximal renal tubular acidosis [RTA]).

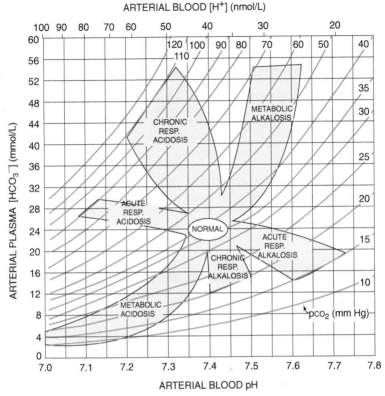

FIGURE 6-2. Acid–base map. HCO_3^-, bicarbonate; pCO_2, partial pressure of CO_2; resp., respiratory. (Adapted from DuBose TD, Cogan MG, Rector FC Jr. Acid–base disorders. In: Brenner BM, ed. *Brenner and Rector's The Kidney.* 5th ed. Philadelphia, PA: WB Saunders; 1996:949.)

- ○ **An inability to excrete the acid load (distal RTA).**
- ○ **Respiratory failure** causes acidosis through the elevation of pCO_2.
- • **Alkalosis can occur from any of the following:**
  - ○ **Metabolic insults:**
    - ▪ Loss of H^+-rich fluids
    - ▪ Alkali ingestion
    - ▪ Renal bicarbonate reabsorption
    - ▪ Volume contraction, hypochloremia, and hypokalemia all impair renal excretion of excess alkali and contribute to the perpetuation of the alkaline state
  - ○ **A decrease in pCO_2 due to hyperventilation (respiratory alkalosis).**
- • **Compensation:**
  - ○ Compensatory responses minimize the change in pH by minimizing the alteration in the $[HCO_3^-]$ to $[pCO_2]$ ratio.
  - ○ Expected values for compensatory responses are found in Table 6-1.

TABLE 6-1	EXPECTED COMPENSATORY RESPONSES FOR PRIMARY ACID–BASE DISTURBANCES	
Disorder	Primary Change	Compensatory Response
Metabolic acidosis	Decreased HCO_3^-	1.2 mm Hg decrease in pCO_2 for every 1 mEq/L fall in HCO_3^-
Metabolic alkalosis	Increased HCO_3^-	0.7 mm Hg increase in pCO_2 for every 1 mEq/L rise in HCO_3^-
Acute respiratory acidosis	Increased pCO_2	1 mEq/L increase in HCO_3^- for every 10 mm Hg rise in pCO_2
Chronic respiratory acidosis	Increased pCO_2	3.5 mEq/L increase in HCO_3^- for every 10 mm Hg rise in pCO_2
Acute respiratory alkalosis	Decreased pCO_2	2 mEq/L decrease in HCO_3^- for every 10 mm Hg fall in pCO_2
Chronic respiratory alkalosis	Decreased pCO_2	4 mEq/L decrease in HCO_3^- for every 10 mm Hg fall in pCO_2

Metabolic Acidosis

GENERAL PRINCIPLES

- Metabolic acidosis is a clinical disorder characterized by low pH and low HCO_3^-.
- The appropriate respiratory compensation is hyperventilation resulting in low pCO_2.

DIAGNOSIS

Metabolic acidosis is further categorized into those that have an increased anion gap (AG, also known as an **AG acidosis**) and those that have a normal AG (also known as a **non-AG acidosis**).

Diagnostic Testing
- Differentiating the various forms of metabolic acidosis is critical for management.
- **Step 1: AG versus non-AG**
  - In patients with an AG acidosis, the acid dissociates into H^+ and an "unmeasured" anion.
  - Detection of this "unmeasured anion" is possible through the AG, a simple difference between the measured cations and anions that predominate in the ECF space.
    - $AG = [Na^+] - ([Cl^-] + [HCO_3^-])$
    - Normal AG is 10 ± 3 mEq/L
      - This normal AG typically reflects the presence of unmeasured negative charges from plasma albumin.
      - Because of this, a fall in serum albumin of 1 g/dL (from normal of 4 g/dL) decreases the AG by 2.5 mEq/L.
  - An increase in the AG reflects an accumulation of other unmeasured anions, such as lactate and acetate, from the various causes of an AG acidosis.
  - The amount by which the AG increases (ΔAG) typically approximates the amount by which the serum HCO_3^- decreases (ΔHCO_3).

- The relationship between $\Delta AG/\Delta HCO_3$ is often referred to as the **delta ratio.**
- A significant disparity between the ΔAG and the ΔHCO_3 suggests a superimposed metabolic disorder.
  ○ When $\Delta AG \ll \Delta HCO_3$, the disproportional reduction in serum HCO_3 should raise suspicion of a superimposed nongap metabolic acidosis.
  ○ When $\Delta AG \gg \Delta HCO_3$, the decrease in serum HCO_3 has been attenuated by another process, and one should look for sources of a superimposed metabolic alkalosis or a pre-existing chronic respiratory acidosis with a compensatory increase in serum bicarbonate.
- **Step 2 (Non-AG): renal versus GI etiology**
  ○ In a non-AG acidosis, the differential includes renal causes (RTA) and enteric bicarbonate losses (diarrhea). A carefully obtained history is often sufficient to differentiate these causes. When necessary, the urine AG can be used to assess appropriate renal acidification.
  ○ The urine AG is calculated with the following formula:

$$\text{Urine AG} = [Na^+] + [K^+] - [Cl^-]$$

  ○ In physiologic states with normal acid–base handling, the urine AG is slightly positive.
  ○ In acidemia, the normal renal response is to increase ammonia production to allow enhanced excretion of the acid load. The higher urine ammonium concentration is balanced by higher Cl levels, and the urine AG becomes negative because the chloride concentration exceeds Na + K.
  ○ If urinary acidification is inadequate due to RTA, the urine ammonium levels are low and the urine AG remains positive.

Differential Diagnosis

Please see Table 6-2 for common causes of non-AG metabolic acidosis.

Anion Gap Metabolic Acidosis

AG metabolic acidosis encompasses disorders of organic acidosis resulting from increased acid production.
- **Lactic acidosis:**
  ○ Under normal conditions, humans produce relatively small amounts of lactate.
  ○ An **increase in production** can occur due to various reasons.
  ○ Treatment of lactic acidosis must be directed at the underlying cause. Therapy with HCO_3^- has not been found to be effective clinically and may even have deleterious effects.
- **Diabetic ketoacidosis (DKA):**
  ○ In insulin deficiency, fatty acids are oxidized to ketoacids (β-hydroxybutyric and acetoacetic acids), resulting in acid–base disturbance.

TABLE 6-2 COMMON CAUSES OF NON-ANION GAP METABOLIC ACIDOSIS

Non-Anion Gap Metabolic Acidosis

GI Causes:
- Diarrhea
- Intestinal fistula
- Ureterosigmoidostomy

Renal Causes:
- Renal tubular acidosis
- Carbonic anhydrase inhibitors

○ Diagnosis of DKA is made by the combination of **AG metabolic acidosis, hyperglycemia, and the presence of serum or urine ketones.**
  ■ Diagnostic tests which use a nitroprusside reagent react with acetoacetate only.
  ■ In early DKA, the ratio of β-hydroxybutyric acid to acetoacetic acid is 5:2.
  ■ During treatment of DKA, the formation of acetoacetate is favored, so the nitroprusside test may falsely demonstrate a rise in ketones as this ratio varies.
○ Mainstays of therapy for DKA are insulin, volume repletion, and the management of electrolyte abnormalities.

- **Alcohol or starvation ketoacidosis:**
  ○ This should be considered in all patients with a history of alcohol abuse who present with an unexplained high-AG metabolic acidosis.
  ○ Combination of alcohol ingestion and poor dietary intake is the cause of the ketoacidosis.
  ○ Ratio of β-hydroxybutyric acid to acetoacetic acid is up to 20:1. Therefore, the nitroprusside test may grossly underestimate the degree of ketoacidemia in these patients.
  ○ Therapy consists of vigorous volume, glucose, and electrolyte repletion.

- **Toxic alcohol ingestions:**
  ○ Examples include **methanol** and **ethylene glycol ingestion.**
  ○ Initial acid–base status may be normal soon after ingestion. However, an **increased osmolar gap** may be an early clue to the diagnosis.
  ○ Osmolar gap = measured serum osmolality − calculated osmolality
    ■ Calculated serum osmolality = $2[Na^+] + [glucose]/18 + [urea]/2.8$
    ■ A difference of >15 to 20 mOsm/kg suggests toxic alcohol ingestion.
    ■ An osmolar gap can also be due to other conditions that are not associated with a high-AG acidosis, including ethanol and isopropyl alcohol.
  ○ Patients with methanol poisoning present with abdominal pain, vomiting, headache, and visual disturbances (optic neuritis).
  ○ Ethylene glycol intoxication is similar to that of methanol, but does not produce optic neuritis. Calcium oxalate crystals in the urine are suggestive.
  ○ Most morbidity of methanol and ethylene glycol results from damage mediated by metabolites, formate and glycolate.
    ■ Fomepizole blocks alcohol dehydrogenase, thereby retarding metabolism of methanol and ethylene glycol.
    ■ Hemodialysis may also be required to clear toxic metabolites and correct severe metabolic abnormalities.

- **Salicylate overdose:**
  ○ Symptoms include nausea, vomiting, tinnitus, altered mental status, coma, and death.
  ○ Symptoms correlate poorly with plasma levels, but almost always are present with very high levels (>50 mg/dL).
  ○ Treatment:
    ■ Alkalinizing the urine with HCO_3^- infusion may reduce symptoms and promote renal excretion.
    ■ Hemodialysis should be considered for patients with extremely high levels, severe symptoms, significant renal failure, or refractory acidosis.

- **Additional causes are listed in** Table 6-3.

Nongap (Hyperchloremic) Metabolic Acidosis

- GI loss:
  ○ Diarrhea and enteric fistulas account for the majority of nongap metabolic acidosis.
- RTA:
  ○ They are a heterogeneous group of disorders defined by the presence of metabolic acidosis due to diminished renal acid excretion.

TABLE 6-3	COMMON CAUSES OF ANION GAP METABOLIC ACIDOSIS

Anion Gap Metabolic Acidosis

Endogenous acid generation and accumulation
- Lactic acidosis
- Ketoacidosis
- Poor clearance of organic anions in renal failure (phosphates, sulfates)

Exogenous acid exposure and toxic accumulation
- Alcohols—Ethylene glycol, Methanol
- Salicylate
- 5-Oxoproline (from acetaminophen)
- Propylene glycol

○ On the basis of pathophysiologic mechanisms, RTA can be classified as type I, type II, and type IV, which are shown in Table 6-4.

TREATMENT

- Treatment of metabolic acidosis is usually **best accomplished by treating the underlying disease.**
- In non-AG metabolic acidosis, a persistent bicarbonate deficit can be replaced with oral or intravenous bicarbonate.
- The amount of HCO_3^- required to correct the acidemia can be estimated by the HCO_3^- deficit:

$$HCO_3^-\ deficit = HCO_3^-\ space\ (L) \times (desired\ HCO_3^- - actual\ HCO_3^-)$$

TABLE 6-4	RENAL TUBULAR ACIDOSIS		
	Type I (Classic Distal)	Type II (Proximal)	Type IV (Distal Hyperkalemic)
Basic defect	Decreased distal acidification	Diminished proximal HCO_3^- reabsorption	↓ Aldosterone, ↓ ammoniagenesis
Urine pH	>5.3	Variable: >5.3 if above reabsorptive threshold; <5.3 if below	Usually <5.3
Plasma HCO_3^-	<10 mEq/L	14–20 mEq/L	>15 mEq/L
Plasma K⁺	Usually reduced or normal	Usually reduced or normal	Elevated
Associated conditions	Sjögren syndrome, nephrocalcinosis, drugs (amphotericin)	Multiple myeloma, Fanconi syndrome	Diabetes mellitus

where HCO_3^- space (theoretic volume of HCO_3^- distribution) = 0.5 – 0.8 × body weight in kg.

○ The HCO_3^- space is not constant, but increases with increasing severity of the acidosis.

○ In normal state, this space is 50% of body weight, but increases to as high as 80% in severe acidosis (bicarbonate <10 mEq/L). This results from greater use of nonbicarbonate buffers as acidosis worsens.

○ In acute settings, intravenous (IV) sodium HCO_3^- (50 mEq in 50-mL ampules) can be given as a bolus or continuous infusion (two to three ampules mixed in D5W).

○ In chronic metabolic acidosis, oral alkali can be given as sodium bicarbonate tablets or as sodium or potassium citrate solution.

• In AG metabolic acidosis (e.g., lactic acidosis or DKA), alkali therapy may be deleterious and should be reserved for **patients with severe acidosis (pH <7.1) in order to maintain cardiovascular stability.**

Metabolic Alkalosis

GENERAL PRINCIPLES

Metabolic alkalosis is a clinical disorder characterized by elevated pH due to an increase in HCO_3^-. Compensatory hypoventilation results in a rise of pCO_2.

DIAGNOSIS

• The kidney is able to excrete large amounts of bicarbonate. Because of this, exposure to a bicarbonate load is generally insufficient to cause a persistent metabolic alkalosis.

• However, maintenance of the alkalemia will occur if renal filtration is compromised (low GFR) or if an underlying condition leads to increased tubular reabsorption of bicarbonate (volume contraction, hyperaldosteronism, hypokalemia, and chloride depletion).

• Disorders of metabolic alkalosis can be conveniently divided into *chloride-responsive*, *chloride-resistant*, and *unclassified* categories (Table 6-5).

TABLE 6-5	TYPES OF METABOLIC ALKALOSIS	
Chloride Responsive	Chloride Resistant	Unclassified
Vomiting	Hyperaldosteronism	Alkali administration
Gastric drainage	Cushing syndrome	Milk-alkali syndrome
Villous adenoma	Bartter/Gitelman syndrome	Massive transfusion of blood products
Chloride diarrhea		
Diuretics	Black licorice	Hypercalcemia
Posthypercapnia cystic fibrosis cation-exchange resins (e.g., antacids)	Profound potassium depletion	Refeeding syndrome

Diagnostic Testing

- Chloride-responsive metabolic alkalosis occurs in volume-depleted states with low urine chloride levels (<25 mEq).
- Chloride-resistant metabolic alkalosis occurs in euvolemic states and is associated with elevated urine chloride levels (>40 mEq/L).

Differential Diagnosis

- **Chloride-responsive metabolic alkalosis:**
  - **Vomiting or gastric drainage:**
    - This is one of the most common causes of metabolic alkalosis.
    - Gastric secretions contain as much as 100 mmol/L of acid. Gastric parietal cells generate one HCO_3^- molecule for each H^+ secreted.
    - Maintenance of metabolic alkalosis occurs due to the subsequent volume contraction.
  - **Diuretics:**
    - Loop and thiazide diuretics stimulate H^+ secretion in the cortical collecting duct.
    - In addition, these diuretics maintain metabolic alkalosis by volume depletion.
  - **Posthypercapnic state:** The HCO_3^- retained by the kidney during chronic hypercapnia can cause a rise in serum pH when hypercapnia is quickly corrected.
- **Chloride-resistant metabolic alkalosis:**
  - **Primary hyperaldosteronism:**
    - Aldosterone stimulates distal H^+ and potassium secretion, coupled with sodium reabsorption, in the cortical collecting duct. This leads to hypokalemic metabolic alkalosis, often with concomitant hypertension and mild volume expansion.
  - **Corticosteroid excess:**
    - Many corticosteroids have considerable mineralocorticoid effect, leading to hypokalemic metabolic alkalosis.
    - Sources of excess corticosteroid include:
      - Exogenous administration.
      - Overproduction of endogenous corticosteroid (i.e., Cushing syndrome).
      - Apparent mineralocorticoid excess, resulting from impaired enzymatic conversion of cortisol to cortisone due to inherited or acquired (i.e., glycyrrhizic acid from black licorice) defects.
  - Bartter syndrome is a rare condition presenting in children with increased renin levels and hyperaldosteronism without hypertension or sodium retention.
    - The disease occurs due to mutations which impair activity of the $Na^+/K^+/2Cl^-$ channel in the thick ascending limb of the loop of Henle, leading to Na^+, K^+, and Cl^- wasting.
    - Bartter syndrome may be difficult to distinguish from surreptitious diuretic use and may require screening urine for presence of diuretics.
- **Unclassified metabolic alkalosis:**
  - Administration of HCO_3^- or organic anions that metabolize into HCO_3^- (citrate or acetate) can lead to metabolic alkalosis, especially in patients with renal insufficiency.
  - **Milk-alkali syndrome** is seen in patients who consume a large amount of antacids containing calcium and alkali (e.g., calcium carbonate).
    - Hypercalcemia decreases parathyroid-hormone–mediated HCO_3^- loss and also causes alkalosis through volume contraction.
    - Patients may present with metabolic alkalosis, hypercalcemia, and often a reduction in renal function.
  - **Massive transfusion of blood products** (>10-U packed RBCs) can produce moderate metabolic alkalosis secondary to elevated citrate that metabolizes into HCO_3^-.
  - Similarly, metabolic alkalosis may be seen in patients undergoing **plasmapheresis**, as replacement plasma has citrate.

TREATMENT

- For nonurgent cases, therapy is based on whether the case is chloride responsive or chloride resistant.
- **Chloride-responsive metabolic alkalosis:**
  - It typically **responds to the administration of oral or IV sodium chloride** in 0.9% or 0.45% solution with potassium supplements.
    - This lowers the plasma HCO_3^- level by reversing the contraction alkalosis, decreasing sodium retention, and promoting HCO_3^- excretion.
    - In edematous states (e.g., patient with heart failure), the administration of saline may not be an option.
      - Acetazolamide (250 to 375 mg PO daily or bid) is a carbonic anhydrase inhibitor that decreases proximal sodium reabsorption while increasing renal excretion of HCO_3^-.
  - Concurrent hypokalemia must be corrected for metabolic alkalosis to resolve.
  - The use of H_2-blockers or proton-pump inhibitors can minimize proton loss in gastric secretions.
- **Chloride-resistant metabolic alkalosis:**
  - It does not respond to the administration of volume.
  - For mineralocorticoid excess states, successful treatment requires restoration of normal mineralocorticoid activity, including surgical removal of an adrenal adenoma or by the use of potassium-sparing diuretics in addition to potassium supplements.
  - Bartter syndrome may respond to nonsteroidal anti-inflammatory drugs, potassium-sparing diuretics, and potassium supplements.
- In acute and severe metabolic alkalosis, hydrochloric acid can be administered extremely cautiously to attenuate the dramatic rise in pH, but the potential complications warrant serious consideration before attempted use. Alternatively, hemodialysis can be used to rapidly lower the pH in severe metabolic alkalosis (pH >7.6).

Respiratory Acidosis

GENERAL PRINCIPLES

- Acute respiratory acidosis results from acute alveolar hypoventilation when only the buffering defense is available.
- Chronic respiratory acidosis is caused by chronic decreased effective alveolar ventilation. Over time, the renal compensatory mechanisms operate at maximal capacity.

DIAGNOSIS

- Respiratory acidosis is a disorder caused by processes that increase pCO_2, resulting in a decrease in pH and a compensatory increase in HCO_3^-.
- The increase in pCO_2 is due to decreased alveolar ventilation. The physiologic buffer systems generate the immediate response to the low pH during the acute phase.
- Over the next several days, renal compensation is initiated through an increase in net acid excretion termed the *chronic phase.*
- The third response to respiratory acidosis is the restoration of effective ventilation.
- **The causes of acute respiratory acidosis** include neuromuscular abnormalities, airway obstruction, thoracic–pulmonary disorders, vascular disease, respiratory muscle fatigue, and mechanical ventilation.

- **The causes of chronic respiratory acidosis** include thoracic–pulmonary disorders (e.g., chronic obstructive pulmonary disease) and neuromuscular abnormalities.
- When a patient in a steady state of chronic hypercapnia suffers a new insult, the pCO_2 acutely rises. This is termed acute respiratory acidosis superimposed on chronic respiratory acidosis.
- When patients with steady state of chronic hypercapnia suffer an acute renal insult, they lose their renal compensation which results in worsening of their acidosis.

TREATMENT

- Treatment is restoration of effective ventilation.
- In chronic respiratory acidosis, treatment is difficult, but maximizing pulmonary function may lead to significant improvement.

Respiratory Alkalosis

GENERAL PRINCIPLES

- **Acute respiratory alkalosis** results from acute alveolar hyperventilation when only the buffering defense is available.
  - Patients may present with paresthesias, muscle cramps, tinnitus, and even seizures.
- **Chronic respiratory alkalosis** is caused by chronic increased effective alveolar ventilation. During this period, the renal compensatory mechanisms are fully exerted.

DIAGNOSIS

- Respiratory alkalosis is the most common acid–base disorder in seriously ill patients.
- Respiratory alkalosis is a disorder caused by processes that decrease pCO_2, resulting in an increase in pH and a compensatory decrease in HCO_3^-. The decrease in pCO_2 is due to increased alveolar ventilation.
- The buffering response constitutes the acute phase, and the renal response defines the chronic stage of respiratory alkalosis.
- The third response to respiratory alkalosis is the restoration of appropriate ventilation.
- Causes of respiratory alkalosis include central stimulation of respiration (e.g., fever, anxiety, head trauma), peripheral stimulation of respiration (e.g., pulmonary embolism and pneumonia), liver insufficiency, sepsis, and mechanical ventilation.

TREATMENT

- The key to therapy is treating the underlying cause. **Correcting significant hypoxemia may be more important than the acid–base disturbance.**

Approach to the Patient with Acute Kidney Injury

Fadi Tohme

7

GENERAL PRINCIPLES

- Acute kidney injury (AKI) is among the most commonly encountered clinical syndromes in the hospital setting, with an incidence rate approaching 20%.
- Sepsis, major surgery, hypovolemia, and heart failure are the four major causes of AKI in hospitalized patients.
- In the acute setting, small changes in serum creatinine (SCr; 0.3 mg/dL) or in urine output are independently associated with increased mortality and substantial financial cost to the health care system.
- Awareness of AKI is limited by the sensitivity of SCr, the standard biomarker of kidney damage, and therefore requires clinical context to either anticipate or mitigate the disease course.
- Early recognition of AKI by the physician is essential to the care of the hospitalized patient.

Definition

An abrupt reduction in kidney function as measured by one of the following criteria, based on the 2012 Kidney Disease: Improving Global Outcomes (KDIGO) guidelines[1]:
- **Rise in SCr by ≥0.3 mg/dL within 48 hours**
- **1.5-fold increase in SCr compared to baseline within the prior 7 days**
- **Documented oliguria of <0.5 mL/kg/hr for more than 6 hours.**

Classification

- Criteria for AKI are standardized to facilitate communication between practitioners and to clarify the results of outcome-based analyses.
- A staging system compiled by the KDIGO group that categorizes the severity of AKI is shown in Table 7-1.
- AKI is commonly subclassified into **prerenal, postrenal, and intrinsic renal injuries.**
- Inclusion of novel biomarkers in the definition of AKI allows use of an alternate terminology: functional, subclinical, and structural AKI.
- Intrinsic renal injury can be from **glomerular, vascular, interstitial, or tubular** causes.
- The different intrinsic etiologies of AKI, as well as cardiorenal and hepatorenal syndromes, and specific management strategies, will be discussed in the following chapter. Glomerulonephritis and vasculitis are discussed elsewhere.

Epidemiology

- Generally, AKI is a disease of the hospitalized patient, with 13% to 21% of all hospitalized patients meeting the diagnostic criteria for AKI depending on the definition used. As can be expected, the number is much higher (approaches 50%) in patients with multiorgan failure and in the intensive care unit (ICU). In contrast, only ~1% of all patients presenting to the emergency room have the diagnosis of AKI.

TABLE 7-1 CLASSIFICATION/STAGING SYSTEM FOR AKI

Stage	Serum Creatinine Criteria	Urine Output Criteria
1	Rise in SCr ≥0.3 mg/dL (within 48 hrs) or ≥150–200% from baseline (within the prior 7 days)	<0.5 mL/kg/hr for >6 hrs
2	Rise in SCr >200–300% from baseline	<0.5 mL/kg/hr for >12 hrs
3	Rise in SCr >300% from baseline, or SCr >4 mg/dL with an acute increase of at least 0.5 mg/dL, or initiation of renal replacement therapy	<0.3 mL/kg/hr for >24 hrs or anuria >12 hrs

AKI, acute kidney injury; SCr, serum creatinine.

- AKI is associated with high mortality, which has not changed significantly in the last 60 years. The average mortality in an ICU patient with AKI is quoted anywhere from 45% to 60%. Studies have demonstrated that AKI is an independent factor contributing to the mortality and not just an innocent bystander, as previously believed.[2]
- Some of the possible **reasons for the persistent poor survival in AKI** include:
  - **Delay in diagnosis of AKI:** By the time a patient's SCr increases 0.3 mg/dL, renal function would have declined by at least 25%. Creatinine remains a late marker of AKI and is being challenged by more sensitive and biologically significant biomarkers.
  - **Absence of effective therapies to reverse AKI:** Management of AKI remains largely supportive and focuses on prevention of further injury. There are no pharmacologic therapies yet known to hasten recovery of renal function after AKI.
  - **Inability of dialysis to provide actual renal replacement:** The endocrine, cytokine, and immunologic functions of the kidney are not being replaced with dialysis.

DIAGNOSIS

- The initial diagnostic evaluation of a patient suspected to have AKI is triggered by either an **increase in** SCr or **decrease in urine output over several hours.**
- A stepwise approach should always focus on delineating whether AKI is the result of prerenal or postrenal processes, with the understanding that intrinsic renal injury will likely take a more thorough battery of testing and may not be forthcoming by evaluation of the patient's volume status and urinary outlet alone.
- By definition, **prerenal and postrenal lesions** impose functional restraints on renal performance and anticipate dramatic improvement in solute clearance after removal of such lesions, if achieved in a timely fashion.
- In contrast, **intrinsic AKI** is *not* expected to reverse swiftly and the clinical course and prognosis depend on the underlying cause.
- In the ICU, the most common cause is acute tubular necrosis (ATN), usually due to both ischemic and toxic insults (multifactorial ATN).

Clinical Presentation

The following questions should be answered by the end of the history and physical examination in a patient with AKI.

- Is the patient volume depleted?
- Does the patient have a urinary tract obstruction?

- Has this patient been exposed to a major nephrotoxin (medications, IV contrast, over-the-counter agents, herbal products, and so forth)?
- Could this patient have intrinsic renal disease?
- Does the patient have a pre-existing condition (e.g., decompensated congestive heart failure, liver cirrhosis, diabetes, peripheral vascular disease) increasing vulnerability to renal injury?
- Is there a need for further serologic testing and/or renal biopsy?

History
- **Urine patterns and frequency**
  - Estimate daily urine volumes and recent trends (1 "Dixie" cup = 75 mL, 1 coffee cup = 225 mL, 1 soda can = 350 mL, 24-hour urine container = 2.5 L).
  - Elicit any history of hematuria, dysuria, or pyuria.
  - Urgency, frequency, dribbling, and incontinence, especially in elderly men, may point toward prostatic disease.
  - Onset of urinary symptoms may also provide a temporal clue to the duration of illness.
  - For hospitalized patients, a careful review of the intake, output, and daily weights is essential.
- **Volume status**
  - History of dizziness, orthostatic instability, dependent lifestyle, prolonged nursing home residence, and unmonitored chronic diuretic use, may point toward intravascular depletion, whereas weight gain, edema, or periorbital swelling (especially in the mornings) may signify fluid retention.
  - Consider the possible mechanisms of fluid loss—hemorrhage, diarrhea, polyuria, and situations leading to excessive insensitive losses (e.g., fever or diminished intake due to dysphagia, surgical wounds closing by secondary intention)—as they all predispose to volume depletion.
  - Review the patient's records or hospital chart in detail for episodes of blood pressure swings.
  - For postoperative patients with AKI, it is essential to review the intra- and post-operative records. These provide important information such as perioperative hemodynamic changes, cardiopulmonary bypass time (cardiac surgery), and aortic cross-clamp time (vascular surgery).
- **Medications**
  - A thorough review of the patient's medications is essential in pinpointing the correct diagnosis.
  - This **includes over-the-counter medicines** (nonsteroidal anti-inflammatory drugs [NSAIDs], high-dose acetaminophen), herbal products, and other health and food supplements.
  - Scout for **nephrotoxins** in the hospital chart (e.g., NSAIDs, renin–angiotensin–aldosterone system inhibitors, aminoglycosides, cisplatin, methotrexate, proton-pump inhibitors).
  - In hospitalized patients, exclude covert nephrotoxic exposure, such as iodine-based IV contrast media with radiologic studies and angiograms.
  - Some drugs may precipitate or exacerbate urinary retention and should be considered as possible causes of postrenal AKI (e.g., tricyclic antidepressants, carbidopa, disopyramide, and certain antihypertensive agents).
  - Several herbal products, such as herbal appetite suppressants (*Hoodia gordonii*) and herbal diuretics (*Radix Tripterygium*), have been implicated in AKI because of volume depletion.
  - Herbal products containing aristolochic acid may cause interstitial nephritis and tubular necrosis.

- **Infections**
  - The source and severity of infection, as well as the treatment strategies for the infection, in a patient with AKI must be carefully reviewed.
  - **Sepsis** initiates an innate immune response and can lead to renal vasoconstriction and ATN. Sepsis can also cause tubular damage independently of renal blood flow and perfusion. It is associated with endothelial and microvascular dysfunction, leading to an excessive inflammatory response and subsequent stress and damage to the tubular epithelial cells.[3]
  - Some infectious organisms **directly** lead to renal involvement: For example, *Legionella* infection can cause an interstitial nephritis.
  - **Indirect causes** include bacterial endocarditis or hepatitis C with cryoglobulinemia, both of which can cause an immune complex deposition glomerulonephritis.
  - Finally, the many different **antibiotics** in use today can cause nephrotoxicity, either directly or by causing acute allergic interstitial nephritis.
- **Other potential etiologies**
  - Patients should be carefully questioned for other symptoms of systemic diseases.
  - Severe myalgias, dark urine (with or without decreased urine output), and appropriate clinical scenarios (exercise, crush injury, recent surgery, drug or alcohol use, medications, immobilization, and so forth) may point toward **rhabdomyolysis.**
  - Arthralgias, arthritis, skin rash, oral ulcers, hair loss, and significant cytopenias in the past may suggest the possibility of a **connective tissue disorder** (e.g., systemic lupus erythematosus).
  - Sinusitis, cough, and hemoptysis may suggest diseases such as **Wegener granulomatosis** or **Goodpasture syndrome.**
  - A history of recent sore throats or significant skin infections may suggest acute **poststreptococcal glomerulonephritis.**
  - Bone pain and anemia may suggest underlying **multiple myeloma.**
  - Also important is a history of chronic liver disease. Common causes of AKI in cirrhosis include prerenal AKI (sepsis from spontaneous bacterial peritonitis, diarrhea associated with lactulose use, decreased oral intake, diuretics, hepatorenal syndrome) and intrinsic renal disease (ATN, membranoproliferative glomerulonephritis with or without cryoglobulinemia in patients with hepatitis C).
- **Risk factors**
  - Appraisal of a patient's **comorbidities** may identify a handicapped autoregulatory system.
  - For example, in decompensated heart failure, a patient's increased sympathetic tone may cause an increased susceptibility to nephrotoxic radiocontrast.
  - Similarly, the presence of hypertension, diabetes, or significant peripheral vascular disease should also raise the possibility of dysfunctional microvasculature due to increased atherosclerotic burden, intimal hyperplasia, and decreased arterial capacitance.

Physical Examination
- **Volume status**
  - Determination of the patient's **volume status** by a thorough examination is an absolute prerequisite in the examination of the renal patient.
  - Check the patient's pulse and blood pressure. If blood pressure is normal or high, evaluate for orthostatic hypotension in the sitting and standing positions, paying careful attention to the pulse as well.
  - Check for dry mucous membranes and decreased skin turgor
  - Assess for jugular venous distention and edema in the dependent areas.
  - Perform a passive leg raise test: >10% change in cardiac output or arterial pulse pressure is expected when both legs are passively raised to 45 degrees for about a minute in a hypovolemic patient.

- **Cardiac examination**
  - This should focus on the location and character of apical impulse, presence of S_3 (volume overload) or S_4 (pressure overload), and functional regurgitant murmurs suggesting valve ring dilatation because of volume overload.
  - The presence of dyspnea and tachypnea suggests fluid overload. Acidosis may induce Kussmaul respiration, but this deep-sighing character is not to be confused with the dyspnea of pulmonary edema.
  - Inspiratory crackles at the lung bases occur in pulmonary edema.
- **Abdominal examination**
  - Hepatomegaly, splenomegaly, and ascites can occur due to passive congestion in fluid overload states.
  - The liver may be pulsatile if volume overload has resulted in severe functional tricuspid regurgitation.
  - A distended and firm abdomen should raise the suspicion for abdominal compartment syndrome. Bladder pressures can help establish this diagnosis. These should be checked using a pressure transducing system that is connected to an indwelling urinary catheter, after injection of 25 cc of normal saline while the patient is in a supine position.
  - Exclude obstruction by assessing bladder distention, performing a prostate examination, and placing a Foley catheter if indicated.
- **Other systemic signs**
  - Rash (e.g., vasculitis, atheroemboli, interstitial nephritis, lupus), arthritis (e.g., vasculitis, connective tissue disorders), and pulmonary hemorrhage (vasculitis, lupus) can also provide diagnostic clues.
  - Large lower extremity muscle groups tender to palpation may alert the physician to a developing compartment syndrome and rhabdomyolysis.
  - A complete and thorough examination is required in addition to the above to elicit possible causes of the AKI, to assess the degree of compensation, and to detect features suggestive of uremic syndrome.

Diagnostic Testing

Laboratories

- **Examination of urine**
  - Urinalysis and microscopic examination of the urine sediment **by a trained physician** is probably the most important test in the evaluation of AKI.
  - The urinalysis should be bland, not reveal protein, blood, cells, or casts in prerenal azotemia and in uncomplicated postrenal failure, unless there is underlying chronic kidney disease.
  - The urinalysis and sediment may help to not only separate renal causes from pre- and postrenal etiologies but also to differentiate between a tubular, glomerular, or interstitial process (Table 7-2).
  - Presence of granular casts and tubular epithelial cells in the urine sediment correlates with prognosis for renal recovery.
  - If the urine dipstick tests strongly positive for blood but no red blood cells are seen, **myoglobinuria or hemoglobinuria** should be suspected, suggesting rhabdomyolysis or severe intravascular hemolysis leading to AKI.
  - It must be kept in mind that in certain diseases that affect the preglomerular blood vessels, such as thrombotic microangiopathies (e.g., thrombotic thrombocytopenic purpura or hemolytic uremic syndrome), the urine sediment may be bland despite a bona fide renal etiology.
  - The overall clinical presentation must therefore always be kept in mind. Indeed, the urine can be bland despite the diagnosis of ischemic ATN. This is typical in the

TABLE 7-2 URINALYSIS IN AKI

	UA Protein	UA Blood	FENa(%)	Sediment
Prerenal	No	No	<1	Bland; hyaline casts
Acute tubular necrosis	+	+	>1	Muddy brown granular casts; epithelial cells and epithelial cell casts
Glomerulonephritis	++	++	<1	Dysmorphic RBCs; RBC casts
Acute interstitial nephritis	+	+	>1	Eosinophils; WBCs and WBC casts; rarely, RBC casts
Postrenal	+/−	+/−	>1	Monomorphic RBCs and WBCs or crystals may be seen

AKI, acute kidney injury; FENa, fractional excretion of sodium; RBC, red blood cell; UA, urinalysis; WBC, white blood cell.

elderly patients with underlying dilated cardiomyopathy. Details of various types of casts and interpretations can be found in Chapters 1 and 2.

- **Urinary indices**
  - In **oliguric AKI,** the differentiation of prerenal failure from ATN is critical in guiding the decision to restrict or resuscitate the fluid.
  - Various parameters in the urine have been evaluated to make such a differentiation. The basic principle of these parameters is uniform: **In the face of diminished perfusion, the intact renal parenchyma tries to conserve as much sodium as possible** to restore extracellular fluid volume and, hence, renal perfusion. Thus, the **urine is very concentrated and allows excretion of very little sodium.**
  - However, once the renal parenchyma is damaged, the tubules lose their ability to concentrate the urine and to conserve sodium. It must be kept in mind that these indices are usually not useful in nonoliguric states.
  - The urinary indices are not helpful in the critically ill population who tend to have multifactorial AKI.
  - Some of these indices are presented in Table 7-3.

$$FENa = [(urine\ Na/plasma\ Na)/(urine\ creatinine/plasma\ creatinine)] \times 100$$

  - Although fractional excretion of sodium (FENa) is useful in distinguishing prerenal AKI from ATN, its sensitivity diminishes in the setting of diuretic use.

$$FEUrea = [(urine\ urea\ nitrogen/blood\ urea\ nitrogen\ )/ \\ (urine\ creatinine/plasma\ creatinine)] \times 100$$

  - FEUrea calculation takes advantage of urea transporters that are not altered by loop diuretic action, with a sensitivity near 85%, specificity of 92%, and positive predictive value of 98%. FEUrea >50 is consistent with ATN; <35 is consistent with prerenal injury.

TABLE 7-3 URINE DIAGNOSTIC INDICES IN THE DIFFERENTIATION OF PRERENAL AZOTEMIA FROM RENAL AZOTEMIA

	Typical Findings	
Diagnostic Index	Prerenal Azotemia	Acute Tubular Necrosis
Fractional excretion of sodium (%)	<1	>1
U_{Na}	<20	>20
Urine osmolality	>500	Variable
Plasma BUN to SCr ratio	>20	<10–15

Note that these indices are not reliable indicators to distinguish between prerenal AKI and ATN in critically ill patients.

BUN, blood urea nitrogen; SCr, serum creatinine; U_{Na}, urine sodium.

- **Blood counts and coagulation screen**
  - In addition to complete blood count, a peripheral smear must be examined where indicated.
  - The presence of schistocytes in cases of AKI suggests thrombotic thrombocytopenic purpura, hemolytic uremic syndrome, and disseminated intravascular coagulation as possible etiologies.
- **Chemistry panel**
  - Review of laboratory values, including blood urea nitrogen, creatinine, electrolytes, and acid–base balance, is essential to establish the previous baseline and trend leading to the current abnormality.
  - If severe metabolic acidosis is present, **anion and osmolar gaps should** be evaluated to not miss a severe metabolic derangement or toxic ingestion causing the AKI.
  - Elevated plasma **blood urea nitrogen out of proportion to SCr (>20:1)** should prompt an investigation of gastrointestinal bleeding, recent use of high-dose corticosteroids, leading to protein breakdown, or parenteral or enteral high-protein feeding.
  - In rhabdomyolysis, profound hyperkalemia and hyperphosphatemia (due to release from damaged myocytes), hypocalcemia (due to calcium–phosphorus binding), and a disproportionate elevation of the creatinine in relation to blood urea nitrogen may develop. **Creatinine kinase (CK) elevation** happens within 12 hours after the injury, and the rise is in proportion to the severity and extent of the muscle injury. Kidney injury has been reported with CK levels >5000 IU/L, but is typically seen with values >25,000 IU/L.

Imaging

- Assessment of obstruction should be given high priority in the patient presenting to emergency room with AKI.
- **Renal ultrasound (US)** is readily available and extremely accurate in excluding urinary tract obstruction as a cause of AKI.
  - Ultrasonography is useful in **delineating renal sizes and echo texture** and should be obtained early in the workup of AKI in patients presenting to the emergency room or hospital with hyperkalemia after a Foley catheter has been placed.
  - In the intensive care setting, where obstruction is an unlikely cause of AKI, the yield from renal US is very low and it should not be ordered routinely.
- Point-of-care ultrasonography (POCUS) can provide useful information about volume status and has become increasingly used in the ICU setting.[4] Table 7-4 lists commonly used measurements that help assess volume status and fluid responsiveness.

| TABLE 7-4 | USEFUL ULTRASOUND MEASUREMENTS OF HYPOVOLEMIA AND FLUID RESPONSIVENESS |

Measurement	% Change With Inspiration	Measurement Technique
IVC diameter decrease	>50%	Spontaneously breathing patients
IVC diameter increase	>12%	Mechanically ventilated patients
IJV diameter increase	>18%	Mechanically ventilated patients
VTI (measured at the LVOT) increase	>12%	Mechanically ventilated patients

IJV, internal jugular vein; IVC, inferior vena cava; LVOT, left ventricular outflow tract; VTI, velocity time integral.

- Computerized tomography and magnetic resonance imaging are alternative modalities to rule out obstruction due to microcalculi or a fibrotic process, in cases where dilatation of calyces may not be seen on US.

Diagnostic Procedures

- **Serologic profile and special tests**
  In situations suggestive of intrinsic renal disease, various serologic tests (Table 7-5) are indicated to delineate the etiology. These tests are discussed in detail in other chapters covering vasculitis, lupus nephritis, and intrinsic causes of AKI.
- **Tissue diagnosis**
  ○ **Renal biopsy is usually not required** to establish the diagnosis of ATN.
  ○ However, if the cause of AKI is not apparent, or if there is a suspicion of **rapidly progressive glomerulonephritis,** then renal histology is required to make a diagnosis and aid in management.
  ○ Renal biopsy must be done in a timely fashion, as certain disease processes irreversibly destroy renal parenchyma if they are not treated expeditiously.
  ○ In cases of suspected acute interstitial nephritis with a clear inciting agent, discontinuation of the agent and observation of the renal function can be chosen over a kidney biopsy, especially in patients with higher bleeding risk.
  ○ In cases of suspected glomerulonephritis (based on historical features, urine abnormalities, and blood and serologic tests), a renal biopsy is necessary before immunosuppressive therapy is instituted. For instance, even when diagnosis of lupus nephritis is obvious, most nephrologists obtain a tissue diagnosis to correctly define and classify the disease, and to outline progression and future therapy options.
- **Newer biomarkers**
  ○ There is great interest in the development of newer serum and urine markers for early diagnosis of AKI, as SCr is neither a true biomarker nor an early marker of disease.
  ○ SCr slowly identifies renal injury and does so indirectly, because it is derived from muscle filaments and not kidney structure.
  ○ An ideal biomarker would instead reflect actual cellular injury derived from the kidney (like troponin for myocardial infarction), and detect such injury within hours of the event.
  ○ If therapy can be started in the early stages of AKI (initiation phase), then this can potentially prevent the continued deterioration of renal function.
  ○ Serum and urine neutrophil gelatinase–associated lipocalin (NGAL) and kidney injury molecule-1 (KIM-1) are released from the injured proximal tubular cells and

TABLE 7-5	EXAMPLES OF SEROLOGIC OR SPECIAL TESTS ASSOCIATED WITH CAUSES OF AKI

Test	Associated Condition
1. ANA, double-stranded DNA	1. Lupus nephritis
2. C-ANCA (often + proteinase 3 ab)	2. Granulomatosis with polyangiitis (GPA)
3. P-ANCA (often + myeloperoxidase ab)	3. Microscopic polyangiitis, Churg–Strauss syndrome
4. Rheumatoid factor	4. Vasculitis, cryoglobulinemia, MPGN, rheumatoid arthritis
5. Cryoglobulins	5. Cryoglobulinemia-associated MPGN, vasculitis
6. Anti-GBM antibodies	6. Goodpasture syndrome
7. Antistreptolysin-O titer	7. PSCGN
8. Complement levels (low)	8. PSCGN, cryoglobulinemic MPGN I, LN, shunt nephritis, GN with SBE, atheroemboli
9. Hepatitis B and C antibodies	9. Membranous GN or MPGN
10. HIV antibody	10. Collapsing FSGS
11. Urine and serum protein electrophoresis and immune fixation and serum-free light chains	11. Myeloma kidney (cast nephropathy), monoclonal deposition disease, amyloidosis

ANA, antinuclear antibody; AKI, acute kidney injury; C-ANCA, cytoplasmic antineutrophil cytoplasmic antibody; FSGS, focal segmental glomerulosclerosis; GBM, glomerular basement membrane; GN, glomerulonephritis; HIV, human immunodeficiency virus; LN, lupus nephritis; MPGN, membranoproliferative glomerulonephritis; P-ANCA, perinuclear antineutrophil cytoplasmic antibody; PSCGN, poststreptococcal glomerulonephritis; SBE, subacute bacterial endocarditis.

can be classified as "damage biomarkers." NGAL increases as early as 1 hour after coronary artery bypass grafting in patients who later develop AKI.

○ Urinary insulin-like growth factor–binding protein 7 (IGFBP7) and tissue inhibitor of metalloproteinases-2 (TIMP-2) are classified as "stress biomarkers" and are thought to detect kidney stress prior to the incurrence of damage. (TIMP-2)•(IGFBP7) (trade name NephroCheck®) is a urine test with relatively short turnaround time that was cleared by the U.S. Food and Drug Administration in 2014 and is currently available for clinical use.

○ Other molecules of interest include cystatin C, interleukin-18, liver-type fatty acid–binding protein (L-FABP) and glutathione S-transferase (α and π-GST).[5]

○ Further studies are underway to determine if any of these biomarkers or a combination of several markers will improve the diagnostic algorithm of AKI.

NONDIALYTIC MANAGEMENT OF AKI

- Management of AKI **depends on the underlying etiology** and will be discussed under each category.
- However, some uniform guidelines that are noted below cover all diagnoses.
- **Avoid additional nephrotoxic agents.**
- **Avoid hypotension and hemodynamic instability.**

- **Hyperkalemia** and **metabolic acidosis** are frequently encountered in AKI and should be managed appropriately as described elsewhere. In the setting of AKI, these two conditions are the foremost reasons to initiate renal replacement therapy (RRT).
- **Nutritional support**
  - Nutrition is one of the important facets of supportive care.
  - AKI is a stressful, catabolic state, and adequate nutrition is essential with enteral or parenteral support and should be initiated in a timely manner.
  - Unlike CKD, where protein restriction is recommended, protein requirements in AKI vary from 1.0 g/kg (prior to dialysis initiation or during hemodialysis) to 2.5 g/kg (in continuous RRT).
- **Dose adjustment of medications**
  - **Adjusting doses of concurrent medications** to the renal function is **essential in preventing further renal injury** as well as **avoiding systemic toxicity.**
  - Even seemingly, innocuous medications such as magnesium-containing antacids and phosphorus-containing enemas (Fleet®) can be damaging in the setting of renal dysfunction.
  - Various guidelines are available to make recommended dose adjustments for the level of renal function. The pharmacist is also a valuable resource in making medication adjustments in renal failure.
  - If the patient requires initiation of hemodialysis or continuous RRT, then dose adjustments are again necessary in some cases to ensure adequate drug levels.
- **The diuretic challenge** is often used in patients with oliguric AKI from tubular injury, in an attempt to convert them to a nonoliguric state.
  - **Diuretics do not improve survival or hasten renal function recovery in AKI.**
  - The use of diuretics to convert from an oliguric to nonoliguric state should not sway the physician away from early nephrology consultation or institution of RRT in a timely fashion.
- If diuretics are used, then **doses utilized must be high enough to reach the loop of Henle** in order to be effective in the setting of reduced glomerular filtration rate (GFR). For example, with a GFR of <30 mL/min, a 160 to 200 mg IV bolus of furosemide might be needed.
- If there is a diuretic response, then it can be continued as intermittent doses or as a continuous infusion. Studies have not shown a difference in outcome with either method.
- Volume status should be ascertained carefully prior to and during diuretic administration, to avoid intravascular volume depletion.
- In one study, urinary output in response to intravenous furosemide determined prognosis for renal recovery and survival. The furosemide stress test (FST) protocol required administration of IV furosemide 1 mg/kg to patients with stage 1 and 2 AKI, with monitoring of urine output. Urine output of less than 200 mL in 2 hours was associated with poor prognosis.[6]

RENAL REPLACEMENT THERAPY IN AKI

- RRT is required in patients with AKI when the residual native function is insufficient to maintain volume, electrolyte, and acid–base balance, or prevent uremic complications.
- The **conventional factors that trigger initiation of RRT** include the following:
  - Metabolic acidosis
  - Hyperkalemia
  - Volume overload
  - Ingestion of toxins
  - Uremia

TABLE 7-6	COMMON INDICATIONS FOR INITIATION OF RENAL REPLACEMENT THERAPY IN ACUTE KIDNEY INJURY

- Volume overload refractory to diuretics
- Hyperkalemia refractory to medical therapy
- Metabolic acidosis refractory to medical therapy
- "Uremic" syndrome
  - Anorexia, nausea, vomiting
  - Serositis
  - Seizures, confusion
  - Neuropathy
  - Bleeding
- Overdoses/intoxications (e.g., ethylene glycol, methanol, lithium, theophylline, barbiturates)
- Refractory hypercalcemia
- Refractory hyperuricemia (e.g., tumor lysis syndrome)

- The exact definition of "uremia" is vague. Uremic manifestations do not correlate with blood urea nitrogen levels and may vary from mental status changes to uremic pericarditis.
- The important indications for initiation of hemodialysis in AKI are provided in Table 7-6.
- The timing of initiation of RRT in AKI remains controversial. Two recent trials, AKIKI and ELAIN, gave conflicting results regarding timing of RRT in AKI.[7,8] An ongoing multinational study, Standard vs. Accelerated Initiation of RRT in AKI (STARRT-AKI), will help to guide the optimal timing of initiation of RRT (https://clinicaltrials.gov/ct2/show/NCT02568722).
- RRT should be dosed appropriately based on evidence-based data.
- There are different modalities available to patients.
- RRT should be carefully supervised by the treating nephrologist, and every attempt should be done to minimize complications and adverse events.

Patients should be carefully monitored for signs of renal recovery such as increasing urine output in addition to downtrending of SCr.

Prerenal Acute Kidney Injury

GENERAL PRINCIPLES

- Prerenal azotemia is the most common cause of AKI. Rapid restoration of effective circulatory volume usually leads to prompt and complete resolution of AKI (Fig. 7-1).
- A complete examination of the urine, including the sediment, in addition to a thorough history and physical examination is essential in ascertaining the accurate diagnosis.

Definition

- Prerenal kidney injury is characterized by a state in which renal parenchymal function is preserved and is responding appropriately to diminished perfusion. Because the integrity of the renal parenchymal tissue is preserved, timely restoration of perfusion and glomerular ultrafiltration pressure should correct GFR.
- There is a continuum from compensated renal hypoperfusion, without a change in GFR, to prerenal injury with reduced GFR to ischemic ATN.

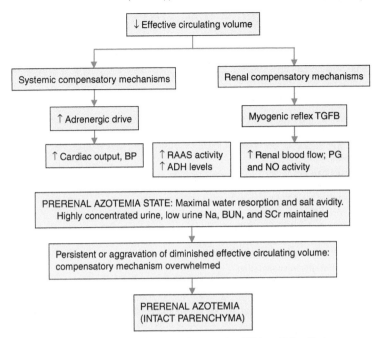

FIGURE 7-1. Pathophysiology of prerenal azotemia. ADH, antidiuretic hormone; BP, blood pressure; BUN, blood urea nitrogen; NO, nitric oxide; PG, prostaglandin; RAAS, renin–angiotensin–aldosterone system; SCr, serum creatinine; TGFB, tubuloglomerular feedback.

Etiology

The important causes of prerenal AKI are summarized in Table 7-7.

Management

- The fundamental problem in most cases of prerenal azotemia is diminished effective circulatory volume. Prompt and effective restoration improves renal blood flow (RBF), leading to increased GFR and improvement or normalization of renal function.
- In most cases of prerenal injury (except for those associated with volume overload), administration of intravenous fluids is the mainstay of therapy.
- The initial fluid of choice is administration of a crystalloid solution to restore the euvolemic state. Normal saline or isotonic fluids are the most effective choices.
- Prolonged prerenal state will lead to tubular injury.

Postrenal Acute Kidney Injury

GENERAL PRINCIPLES

Definition

- Obstructive uropathy describes an impediment to urine flow due to structural or functional change anywhere from the renal pelvis to the tip of the urethra. This resistance to

TABLE 7-7	MAJOR CAUSES OF PRERENAL ACUTE KIDNEY INJURY

Decrease in effective circulating volume

Hemorrhage: traumatic, surgical, gastrointestinal, postpartum

Gastrointestinal losses: vomiting, nasogastric suction, diarrhea, short gut syndrome

Renal losses: drug-induced or osmotic diuresis, diabetes insipidus, adrenal insufficiency

Skin and mucous membrane losses: burns, hyperthermia, other causes of increased insensible losses

"Third-space" losses: pancreatitis, intestinal obstruction, severe crush injury, hypoalbuminemia

Decreased cardiac output

Congestive heart failure

Pericardial tamponade/large pericardial effusion

Aortic or mitral valve disease

Afferent arteriolar vasoconstriction

Drugs: NSAIDs, calcineurin inhibitors

Electrolyte disturbances: hypercalcemia

Efferent arteriolar vasodilatation

ACEI

ARB

Common clinical scenarios that acutely impair autoregulation and decrease GFR

ACEIs or ARBs in the setting of bilateral renal artery stenosis

Underlying CKD on ACEI or ARB and sudden volume depletion (e.g., vomiting or diarrhea)

Use of ACEIs or ARBs in conjunction with NSAIDs or COX-2 inhibitors (e.g., elderly patient on ACEI started on NSAIDs for gout)

Use of NSAIDs in the setting of volume depletion

ACEI, angiotensin-converting enzyme inhibitor; ARB angiotensin II receptor blocker; CKD, chronic kidney disease; COX-2, cyclooxygenase 2; GFR, glomerular filtration rate; NSAID, nonsteroidal anti-inflammatory drug.

flow increases pressure proximal to the point of obstruction. Renal parenchymal damage may or may not be associated.

- Obstructive nephropathy describes any functional or pathologic changes in the kidney that result from urinary tract obstruction.
- Obstruction is considered upper tract if it is located above the ureterovesical junction and lower tract if located below it.
- The degree of obstruction is either complete or partial.
- The common causes of obstruction are noted in Tables 7-8 to 7-10.

Etiology

- Obstructive uropathy may be the result of anatomic or functional abnormalities anywhere in the urinary tract. These abnormalities are either congenital (Table 7-8) or acquired (Tables 7-9 and 7-10). The etiology varies depending on the age and sex of the patient.
- In children, obstruction is due mainly to anatomic abnormalities, including urethral valves or stricture and stenosis at the ureterovesical or ureteropelvic junction.

TABLE 7-8 CONGENITAL CAUSES OF OBSTRUCTIVE UROPATHY

Ureter	Bladder
Ureteropelvic junction obstruction	Myelodysplasias (e.g., meningomyelocele)
Ureteroceles	Bladder diverticula
Ectopic ureter	**Urethra**
Ureteral valves	Prune-belly syndrome
	Urethral diverticula
	Posterior urethral valves

TABLE 7-9 ACQUIRED INTRINSIC CAUSES OF OBSTRUCTIVE UROPATHY

Intraluminal	Intramural
Intrarenal	**Anatomic**
Tubular precipitation of proteins: Bence Jones proteins	Tumors (renal pelvis, ureter, bladder, urethra)
Tubular precipitation of crystals: uric acid, medications (e.g., acyclovir, indinavir, sulfonamides)	Strictures (ureteral or urethral) Infections Granulomatous disease Instrumentation or trauma Radiation therapy
Extrarenal	**Functional Disorders of the Bladder**
Nephrolithiasis	Diabetes mellitus with autonomic bladder
Blood clots	Multiple sclerosis
Papillary necrosis	Spinal cord injury
Fungus balls	Anticholinergic agents

TABLE 7-10 ACQUIRED EXTRINSIC CAUSES OF OBSTRUCTIVE UROPATHY

Reproductive and Urologic
Uterus (pregnancy, prolapse, tumors)
Ovary (abscess, cysts, tumors)
Fallopian tubes (pelvic inflammatory disease)
Prostate (benign hyperplasia, adenocarcinoma)

Gastrointestinal
Crohn disease with abscess or colovesical fistula
Diverticulitis with abscess or colovesical fistula
Colorectal carcinoma

Vascular Disorders
Aneurysms (abdominal aortic, iliac)
Venous (ovarian vein thrombophlebitis, retrocaval ureter)

Retroperitoneal Disorders
Fibrosis (idiopathic, drug related, inflammatory, malignancy)
Infection/abscess
Radiation therapy
Tumor and/or lymphadenopathy (primary or metastatic)
Iatrogenic complication of surgery

- Nephrolithiasis is the most common cause of obstructive uropathy in young adults.
- In females, pregnancy (due to the effects of progesterone and mechanical pressure by the gravid uterus) and gynecologic tumors account for most of the cases.
- In the older adults, the most common causes are BPH or prostate cancer, retroperitoneal or pelvic tumors, and stones.

Pathophysiology

- Obstruction to the urinary flow affects the kidney through a variety of factors with complex interactions that alter both glomerular hemodynamics and tubular function.
- The GFR drops after the onset of obstruction, because of a decrease in net hydrostatic pressure across the glomerular capillary wall. Initially, this is due to an increase in intratubular pressure, but in the latter stages of obstruction, it is secondary to a fall in intraglomerular pressure. This reduction in intraglomerular pressure is a manifestation of decreased RBF, caused by AII- and thromboxane A2-mediated vasoconstriction.
- Obstructive nephropathy is also associated with several abnormalities of tubular function believed to be caused by increased pressure within the tubules, leading to altered transport of sodium, water, and several other ions and solutes.
- In long-standing obstruction, the parenchyma atrophies, and fibrosis and scarring of the tubulointerstitium follow.

DIAGNOSIS

Clinical Presentation

- Obstructive (hesitancy, weak stream, intermittency) and irritative (frequency, nocturia, urgency) symptoms are important to obtain, given that prostatic disease is the most common cause of lower tract obstruction. Hematuria may also relate to many other potential pathologic conditions causing obstruction.
- Pain in the flank or suprapubic region, with specific radiation patterns, is suggestive of obstruction.
- A history of urinary tract infections, stones, diabetes, or neurologic disease that could make bladder evacuation difficult is also important to determine.
- Recent surgery or history of tumors or radiation to the pelvis may provide clues to the etiology.
- Medication history must be carefully explored to assess functional causes of obstruction, such as anticholinergic medications.

Diagnostic Testing

Laboratories

- Urinalysis is expected to be bland in uncomplicated urinary tract obstruction (UTO).
- Clues to underlying etiologies may be provided by abnormalities in the urine.
- Hematuria may suggest the presence of stones, infection, or tumor.
- Crystals on urine microscopy may be seen with metabolic abnormalities and certain medications. The type of crystal seen provides information on not only the presence of a stone but possibly also the type of stone causing obstruction.

Imaging

- US is the initial imaging test of choice in most patients. It is readily available, noninvasive, inexpensive, and avoids contrast exposure. US can determine renal size and may reveal dilatation of the collecting system (hydronephrosis), which is suggestive of postrenal AKI. Figure 7-2 shows a US image of obstruction with preserved renal cortex.
- If the renal cortex is extremely thinned out, then chances are that the obstruction was long standing and relieving it will not improve renal function.

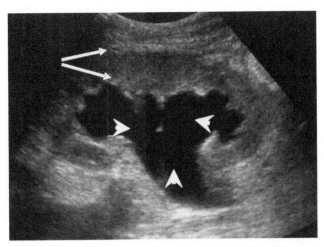

FIGURE 7-2. Ultrasound image of the kidney demonstrating the dilated calyces (*arrowheads*) with preserved renal cortex (between *arrows*). (Courtesy of William D. Middleton, MD, Washington University School of Medicine, St. Louis, MO.)

- False-positive results can be seen in cases of extrarenal pelvis, congenital megacalyces, renal cysts, calcyceal diverticula, and diuresis. A dilated collecting system without obstruction can be seen in cases of ileal conduits, vesicoureteral reflux, primary megaureter, and acute pyelonephritis.
- Absence of hydronephrosis (and false-negative results) can occur with severe dehydration, early or mild obstruction, staghorn calculi, or if retroperitoneal fibrosis or tumor encases the collecting system, preventing dilatation of the ureter.
- If obstruction is strongly suspected as the cause of AKI and US is inconclusive, the physician must strongly consider seeking a urology consultation for cystoscopy.
- Unenhanced helical CT is the modality of choice and is particularly accurate for obstruction due to ureteral calculi. It can be performed rapidly and does not require the use of intravenous contrast. The ability to evaluate the cause of obstruction affords CT an invaluable advantage.
- Antegrade or retrograde pyelography is preferred to studies that require intravenous administration of contrast agents in patients with AKI.
- Radionuclide scans can detect obstruction without use of contrast agents but require some renal function. Performed by injection of radionuclide tracer, images are then obtained with a gamma-scintillation camera and reveal delayed excretion of the tracer. Sensitivity of the test is enhanced when used in conjunction with diuresis renography. Administration of a loop diuretic (e.g., furosemide) causes a rapid washout of the tracer in cases of functional obstruction, but cannot do so if there is mechanical obstruction to urine flow. This can help to differentiate between intrinsic renal injury versus obstruction.

MANAGEMENT

- Therapy is aimed at achieving three main goals.

    1. **Elimination of any life-threatening complication of obstruction.** This involves rapid restoration of intravascular volume, treatment of severe metabolic complications (e.g., hyperkalemia, acidosis), and initiation of aggressive management of infection.

2. **Preservation of renal function.** If the problem is bilateral obstruction, immediate steps to relieve the obstruction are mandated. The longer the obstruction, the higher the risk for irreversible renal parenchymal damage. The location of the obstruction dictates the procedure of choice.
   ○ Lower obstructive uropathy may require a catheter or more proximal drainage. If a transurethral catheter cannot be placed, a urology consultation may be needed to place a suprapubic catheter.
   ○ For an upper tract obstruction, the placement of percutaneous nephrostomy tubes or ureteral catheters or stents should be requested, and performed immediately by interventional radiology or urology.
3. **Determination of the cause of obstruction and definitive treatment.** Definitive diagnosis and therapy can be planned and pursued once the patient has been stabilized and the urinary system decompressed.

   Other aspects of management include:

   ○ Once obstruction has been relieved, postobstructive diuresis may occur due to osmotic diuresis and defects in tubular concentration.
   ○ Hypovolemia may occur in the setting of severe postobstructive diuresis, if adequate volume intake is not maintained.
   ○ Volume status, urine output, and chemistry values in blood and urine need to be closely monitored to gauge fluid and electrolyte support (e.g., hypotonic vs. isotonic fluids, requirement for potassium, magnesium, and phosphorus).
   ○ It is reasonable to start with 0.45% saline and replace approximately two-thirds of the urine losses. If signs of hypo- or hypervolemia develop, the replacement rate can be adjusted accordingly. The replacement fluid rate can be gradually decreased over the course of the next few days.

REFERENCES

1. KDIGO clinical practice guideline for acute kidney injury: Section 2: AKI definition. *Kidney Int Suppl (2011)*. 2012;2:19–36.
2. Coca SG, Yusuf B, Shlipak MG, et al. Long-term risk of mortality and other adverse outcomes after acute kidney injury: a systematic review and meta-analysis. *Am J Kidney Dis*. 2009;53:961–973.
3. Zarbock A, Gomez H, Kellum JA. Sepsis-induced acute kidney injury revisited: pathophysiology, prevention and future therapies. *Curr Opin Crit Care*. 2014;20:588–595.
4. Campbell SJ, Bechara R, Islam S. Point-of-care ultrasound in the intensive care unit. *Clin Chest Med*. 2018;39:79–97.
5. Vijayan A, Faubel S, Askenazi DJ, et al. Clinical use of the urine biomarker [TIMP-2] × [IGFBP7] for acute kidney injury risk assessment. *Am J Kidney Dis*. 2016;68:19–28.
6. Koyner JL, Davison DL, Brasha-Mitchell E, et al. Furosemide stress test and biomarkers for the prediction of AKI severity. *J Am Soc Nephrol*. 2015;26:2023–2031.
7. Gaudry S, Hajage D, Dreyfuss D. Initiation of renal-replacement therapy in the intensive care unit. *N Engl J Med*. 2016;375:1901–1902.
8. Zarbock A, Kellum JA, Schmidt C, et al. Effect of early vs delayed initiation of renal replacement therapy on mortality in critically ill patients with acute kidney injury: the ELAIN randomized clinical trial. *JAMA*. 2016;315:2190–2199.

Intrinsic Causes of Acute Kidney Injury

8

Anitha Vijayan

INTRODUCTION

- The overall management of a patient with acute kidney injury (AKI), as well as pre and postrenal AKI was covered in Chapter 7.
- Once hemodynamic and postrenal causes of AKI have been excluded, acute renal dysfunction that is intrinsic to the kidneys must be considered.
- In the approach to intrinsic AKI, it is helpful to group the etiologies by the site of initial nephron pathology: the microvasculature, the glomerulus, the tubule, or the interstitium (please see Table 8-1). Although significant clinical overlap exists, a few readily attainable clinical findings might suggest the category to which a particular case of intrinsic AKI belongs, including microvascular, glomerular, tubular, and interstitial.
  - ○ Microvascular: new or accelerating hypertension with evidence of microangiopathic hemolytic anemia. This will be discussed in Chapter 11. Microvascular injury may also be caused by atheroemboli.
  - ○ Glomerular: new or accelerating hypertension and volume overload, heavy proteinuria, and/or significant hematuria, especially if red blood cell casts are present. This will be discussed in Chapters 9 and 10.
  - ○ Tubular: urinary sediment containing characteristic tubular cell casts or crystals.
  - ○ Interstitial: the presence of pyuria or white blood cell casts.
- This chapter will focus on the causes of intrinsic AKI that primarily involves the nonglomerular segments of the nephron.

Microvascular Causes of AKI

- Atheroembolic renal disease, malignant hypertension, and scleroderma renal crisis may manifest as an acute decline in renal function due to injury to the small arteries and arterioles supplying the glomeruli as the primary pathologic event.
- Special emphasis is given to atheroembolic renal disease because of its increased incidence compared with others in this category. Malignant hypertension, antiphospholipid syndrome (APS), hemolytic uremic syndrome (HUS), thrombotic thrombocytopenic purpura (TTP), preeclampsia, and hemolysis, elevated liver enzymes, and low platelets (HELLP) syndrome, are discussed in detail in Chapters 11 and 15.

Atheroembolic Renal Disease

GENERAL PRINCIPLES

- Atheroembolic renal disease refers to AKI that arises from the occlusion of the renal microvasculature from inflammation caused by deposition of lipid debris.[1]
- Three patterns of disease—acute, subacute, and chronic—may be apparent in atheroembolic renal disease.

| TABLE 8-1 | CAUSES OF INTRINSIC ACUTE KIDNEY INJURY ACCORDING TO SITE OF PRIMARY INJURY | | |

Microvasculature	Glomerulus	Tubule	Interstitium
Atheroembolic renal disease	Rapidly progressive glomerulonephritis	Crystalline nephropathy	Acute interstitial nephritis
Malignant hypertension		Myeloma kidney	Infiltrative malignancies
Scleroderma renal crisis		Acute tubular necrosis (toxic or ischemic)	Acute pyelonephritis

Antiphospholipid syndrome
Preeclampsia/HELLP syndrome
HUS/TTP

HELLP, hemolysis, elevated liver enzymes, and low platelets; HUS/TTP, hemolytic uremic syndrome/ thrombotic thrombocytopenic purpura.

- In the acute setting, there is an abrupt deterioration in renal function occurs 3 to 7 days after the inciting event, usually with multisystem organ involvement from a massive embolic shower.

Epidemiology

- Atheroembolic renal disease is most commonly a disease of the elderly white male.
- The mean age of presentation is 66 to 70 years and men are affected four times as commonly as women, paralleling the prevalence bias of atherosclerotic vascular disease.
- The incidence of clinically significant renal atheroemboli is not well defined. It occurs much more commonly with aortography and aortic surgeries.

Pathophysiology

- Although spontaneous atheroemboli may occur, more often there is an inciting event leading to plaque destabilization and distal showering of lipid debris.
- In the majority of provoked cases, plaque destabilization occurs from vascular wall trauma during either vascular surgeries or percutaneous endovascular procedures.
- The **lipid lodges in the small arterioles and incites thrombus formation,** causing distal ischemia and infarction. Within days, there may be recanalization of the thrombus and restoration of blood flow, but an inflammatory foreign body arteritis then ensues, leading to progressive fibrosis and eventual obliteration of the vessel lumen. Continued nephron ischemia thus occurs.

Prevention

- Preventive measures include **secondary prevention of atherosclerotic risk factors.**
- The possibility of using a radial, brachial, or axillary approach for endovascular procedures needs to be considered, as most atherosclerotic plaques are in the abdominal aorta.

DIAGNOSIS

- The main manifestations of atheroembolic disease are listed in Table 8-2.
- Patients usually have multiple cardiac disease risk factors, a history of cerebrovascular accidents, or an abdominal aortic aneurysm.

TABLE 8-2	CLINICAL AND LABORATORY FINDINGS IN PATIENTS WITH RENAL ATHEROEMBOLIC DISEASE		
Very Common	**Common**	**Uncommon**	
• New onset, accelerated, or labile hypertension • Skin findings: cyanotic or ulcerated digits or scrotum, livedo reticularis on back or lower extremities, nodules, and/or purpura • Elevated erythrocyte sedimentation rate or C-reactive protein • Transient peripheral blood eosinophilia	• Microscopic hematuria • Proteinuria • Mildly elevated creatinine kinase, transaminases, or amylase/lipase • Gastrointestinal symptoms: nausea, abdominal pain, and/or gastrointestinal bleeding	• Fevers • Neurologic deficits • Retinal emboli with Hollenhorst plaque visible on retinal examination • Hypocomplementemia	

- The typical patient is noted to **have blue or dark red discoloration of the toes** associated with increasing creatinine several days after a vascular procedure. Lipid embolism can occur from 3 days to 3 months after the inciting event.
  - The skin is the most commonly affected organ, but the reliance on characteristic skin findings (e.g., livedo reticularis, cyanotic changes) for diagnosis may contribute to the underrepresentation of this disease among dark-skinned races.
  - Other organ systems such as the gastrointestinal tract and central nervous system may be simultaneously involved.
  - The **multisystem disease involvement,** together with the variable occurrence of **eosinophilia** and **depressed complement levels,** may mimic a vasculitis.
- Renal histology reveals **empty clefts** in arcuate and interlobular arteries from the dissolution of lipid from these sites by the fixation process.
  - Early lesions display an inflammatory arteritis composed of eosinophils, neutrophils, and macrophages, which is later replaced by a giant cell foreign body reaction with proliferation and fibrosis of the vascular intima. Acutely, the tubules may show signs of acute tubular necrosis (ATN).
  - Late in evolution, patchy glomerular sclerosis and tubular atrophy may be visualized in areas supplied by affected vessels. Similar arteriolar inflammation or fibrosis can be found in other tissues, especially the muscle, gastrointestinal tract, and skin.

TREATMENT

- Treatment consists of **aggressive supportive care** addressing the most common mechanisms of death in the acute multivisceral forms of the disease.
- With multivisceral involvement, **further anticoagulation or intravascular manipulations should be strictly avoided,** perhaps even in the setting of recurrent cardiac ischemia.
- RAAS blockade for management of hypertension and proteinuria, and use of statins is beneficial.
- If **renal replacement therapy (RRT)** is required, hemodialysis should be performed without anticoagulation. If this is not possible, peritoneal dialysis can be employed.

OUTCOME/PROGNOSIS

- Patients with renal atheroemboli have poor overall prognosis.
- Progression to dialysis dependence occurs in approximately one-third of the patients who survive the initial insult, though a mild improvement in glomerular filtration rate can occur.
- In a large study of 354 patients, atheroembolic renal disease resulted in end-stage renal disease and death in 33% and 28% of patients, respectively, after an average follow-up of 2 years.

Other Microvascular Causes of Intrinsic AKI

GENERAL PRINCIPLES

- **Scleroderma renal crisis** refers to a clinical entity of acute and progressive renal dysfunction with worsening hypertension occurring in scleroderma patients. An incompletely understood endothelial cell dysfunction with vascular hyperresponsiveness underlies its pathogenesis, as in the other tissues that scleroderma affects Table 8-3.
- **In APS,** antibodies with specificity for anionic phospholipids or the plasma proteins that bind to them induce activation of platelets and endothelial cells, leading to a procoagulant state. If thrombosis occurs primarily in the microvasculature, this can result in an acute or chronic thrombotic microangiopathy in multiple organs, including the kidney. Macroscopic thrombosis may involve the renal arteries in APS and may mimic the microvascular forms of the disease with acute renal failure and accelerating hypertension.
  - **Catastrophic APS** is said to be present if an additional procoagulant stimulus (e.g., infection, surgery, or withdrawal of anticoagulation) initiates fulminant, predominantly microvascular thrombosis that clinically involves at least three different organ systems in a span of <1 week.
- **HUS and TTP** are syndromes of systemic thrombotic microangiopathy and prominent consumptive thrombocytopenia.
  - In HUS, drugs, infections, or toxins initiate endothelial and neutrophil activation or a deficiency in complement regulatory molecules leads to microvascular thrombosis.
  - TTP appears to result from the accumulation of large von Willebrand multimers from reduced ADAMTS13 protease activity. The large multimers then initiate platelet aggregation and activation in the small vessels.
- **Preeclampsia** is a syndrome of new or worsening hypertension with proteinuria, occurring in the late stages of pregnancy. Endothelial dysfunction seems to occur from an imbalance of placenta-derived angiogenic and antiangiogenic factors.
- **HELLP** is a more severe variant of preeclampsia in which microangiopathic anemia is more prominent and there is evidence of liver dysfunction.[2]

DIAGNOSIS

- Some of the clinical features that distinguish the diseases in this category of intrinsic AKI are discussed in Table 8-3.
- The vasculopathy in these disorders leads to glomerular ischemia, which prompts a vicious cycle of high renin- and angiotensin-induced vasoconstriction, rises in blood pressure, and further glomerular ischemia.

- ○ This is most apparent in scleroderma renal crisis, in which there is prompt reversal of the disease with the initiation of angiotensin-converting enzyme inhibition.
- The appearance of **accelerating hypertension** and worsening renal function is common to all of the diseases in this category of AKI secondary to the shared pathophysiologic mechanism of ischemia, leading to increased renin production.
  - ○ Marked hypertension may lead to signs of decompensated heart failure or angina.
  - ○ Headaches, altered mental status, seizures, or focal neurologic deficits can be evident from hypertensive encephalopathy or cerebral microvascular occlusions.
  - ○ Retinal hemorrhages, exudates, or papilledema may be observed on fundoscopic examination.
- Laboratory data may reveal findings consistent with a **microangiopathic hemolytic anemia** (schistocytosis, elevated lactate dehydrogenase, and reduced haptoglobin).
- On urinalysis, hematuria, granular casts, and worsening proteinuria may be present in varying degrees.
- Renal histology findings are remarkably similar among the diseases in this category, except that malignant hypertension and scleroderma renal crisis may involve the pre-glomerular vessels more prominently.
  - ○ Early on, **fibrinoid necrosis** with a paucity of inflammatory infiltrate is seen in the small arteries and arterioles. **Thrombi** may be visualized in glomerular capillary loops. Glomerular endotheliosis, or swelling of endothelial cells with subendothelial deposition of hyaline material, may be seen in any of these diseases, but is more prominent in preeclampsia.
  - ○ Later, the intima displays myxoid thickening and finally undergoes fibrous proliferation, resulting in the typical **concentric onion skin lesions** that may obliterate the lumen of smaller vessels. There is secondary ischemic sclerosis and dropout of supplied glomeruli and tubules.

TREATMENT

Basic principles of management are presented in Table 8-3.

Acute Tubular Injury

GENERAL PRINCIPLES

ATN refers to the AKI resulting from either **ischemic or toxic injury to the tubules.** The common etiologies of ATN are detailed in Table 8-4.

- The most commonly studied scenarios for ATN include sepsis, cardiothoracic surgery, iodine-based radiocontrast, and nephrotoxic medications. In most cases, the etiology is considered multifactorial in nature.
- Three major components that comprise the diverse pathophysiology of AKI include ischemia, inflammation, and direct tubular damage.
- The **natural history of ATN** progresses through **four phases:**
  - ○ **Initiation** refers to an early phase in which ischemia leads to cell injury.
  - ○ **Extension** refers to the phase in which tubular cell polarity is disrupted with a loss of viable and damaged cells into the urinary space, causing tubular casts with obstruction and backleak. Electrolyte transport across the tubular brush border is deranged.
  - ○ During the **maintenance** phase, the cells undergo dedifferentiation, fibroblast migration, and proliferation, and result in fully established renal failure.

TABLE 8-3	MICROVASCULAR CAUSES OF INTRINSIC ACUTE KIDNEY INJURY				
	Malignant Hypertension	Scleroderma Renal Crisis	Microvascular APS[b]	HUS/TTP	Preeclampsia/HELLP
Incidence	Most common microvascular cause of AKI at 2.6 per 100,000 patients per year	10% of patients with scleroderma, almost always within first 5 yrs after diagnosis	25% of patients with primary APS	Eleven cases per million people per year	5% of pregnancies
Risk factors	Longstanding hypertension, black race, abrupt interruption of BP medications, secondary causes of HTN	More extensive and rapidly progressive scleroderma skin involvement, cooler temperature environments, black race, initiation of corticosteroids at high dose, use of cyclosporine	Procoagulant states including a recent thrombotic event, withdrawal of anticoagulation, pregnancy, infection, surgery, and so forth	• Infection: enteritis with Shiga toxin–producing bacteria, HIV, pneumococcal infection • Drugs: quinine, contraceptives, calcineurin inhibitors, chemotherapeutic medications, thienopyridines • Peripartum	Previous preeclampsia or positive family history, primigravid, age >40 or <18, multifetal gestation, previous hypertension or renal disease, diabetes, obesity
Distinguishing clinical features[a]	Signs of scleroderma (sclerodactyly, interstitial lung disease, and so forth) are present and usually obvious. Autoantibodies (e.g., anti-Scl-70 or anti-ribonucleic acid polymerase) may be present. A total of 10% of patients may be normotensive at diagnosis		Signs of APS (previous thrombosis in an atypical vessel, infarcts in other vascular beds, livedo reticularis, and so forth) or SLE are present. Lupus anticoagulant or antiphospholipid antibody is present. Thrombocytopenia may be significant. Focal renal cortical atrophy may be evident. Course may be chronic, acute, or fulminant (i.e., catastrophic APS)	Hemolytic anemia and thrombocytopenia is prominent. Fever may be present. ADAMTS13 activity may be low in idiopathic TTP but is variable. Presence of accelerated hypertension is less consistently seen	Elevation in BP can be relatively mild. Usually occurs after 20th week of pregnancy. Evidence of fetal compromise may be evident. Reduction in GFR is usually mild. Proteinuria often becomes nephrotic in later stages. Glomerular endotheliosis is prominent early on

| **Principles of management** | • *Treatment:* Reduce BP by 25% within 2–6 hrs and toward 160/100 mm Hg by 24–48 hrs. Renal function may initially worsen slightly | • *Prevention:* Avoidance of renal ischemia from drugs or volume depletion. At-risk patients should monitor BP closely and if a sustained rise occurs, renal function should be assessed
• *Treatment:* Initiate ACEI promptly. Renal function may initially worsen, but continued therapy will allow eventual improvement, with >50% of patients able to stop dialysis | • *Prevention:* Avoidance of precipitants (see Risk factors) +/– aspirin or hydroxychloroquine
• *Treatment:* Address underlying precipitant, anticoagulation, +/– antiplatelet therapy, +/– glucocorticoids. If catastrophic APS present, initiate plasma exchange or intravenous immune globulin in addition to above | • *Treatment:* Diarrhea-associated HUS—supportive care alone
• Atypical HUS—eculizumab (discussed in Chapter 11)
• TTP—supportive care plus plasma exchange (less desirably, high-dose plasma infusion) +/– corticosteroids | • *Prevention:* Low-dose aspirin in high-risk patients
• *Treatment:* Anti-hypertensive therapy and close mother and fetal monitoring until fetal maturity. Deliver fetus if maturity is reached or severe preeclampsia occurs |

---

[a]As all may present with accelerated hypertension and worsening renal function, the clinical features that distinguish the diseases are emphasized.

[b]Antiphospholipid antibody syndrome may also present with large-artery thrombosis that may manifest similarly to the microvascular form of the disease.

ACEI, angiotensin-converting enzyme inhibitors; AKI, acute kidney injury; APS, antiphospholipid syndrome; BP, blood pressure; GFR, glomerular filtration rate; HELLP, hemolysis, elevated liver enzymes, low platelet count; HTN, hypertension; HUS, hemolytic uremic syndrome; SLE, systemic lupus erythematosus; TTP, thrombotic thrombocytopenia purpura.

TABLE 8-4	COMMON CAUSES OF ACUTE TUBULAR INJURY	
Ischemia	**Toxins**	**Drugs**
• Prolonged diuresis	• Iodinated contrast media	• Aminoglycosides
• Large vessel surgical cross-clamp	• Myoglobin (rhabdomyolysis)	• Vancomycin
	• Unbound heme fragments (intravascular hemolysis)	• Cisplatin
• Sepsis	• Ethylene glycol/methanol	• Amphotericin B
	• Tumor lysis (uric acid, phosphate)	• Intravenous bisphosphonates
	• Miscellaneous (snake venom, paraquat)	• Crystalline nephropathies (indinavir, acyclovir)

- ○ In the **recovery** phase, stem cells repopulate the tubular epithelium and cell polarity is slowly restored, allowing for an incremental capacity to shuttle solute across the brush border in a physiologic manner.
- ATN can last from days to several weeks in patients with baseline normal renal function, with the potential for renal recovery even after weeks of oliguria.
- Of the patients with ATN who required RRT, about 75% to 80% can regain sufficient renal function to discontinue dialysis.
- However, these patients are at a higher risk of developing CKD and end-stage renal disease and need to be followed closely.

Ischemic Acute Kidney Injury

- Although 25% of the cardiac output flows into the renal circulation, most of the blood flow is relegated to the cortex, and the medulla is maintained in a relative hypoxic state.
- The S_3 segment of the proximal tubule is especially vulnerable in ischemic states and most of the damage occurs in this segment.
- Overwhelming levels of angiotensin II, endothelin-1, and circulating catecholamines cause intense intrarenal vasoconstriction, overcoming the protective effects of prostaglandins and nitric oxide.

Nephrotoxic Acute Kidney Injury

- Various endogenous and exogenous toxins can lead to tubular damage and AKI. A list of some of the important toxins is presented in Table 8-4.
- Some common etiologies of toxic ATN such as rhabdomyolysis, intravenous contrast, crystalline nephropathies are described below.

Rhabdomyolysis

- Destruction of skeletal myocytes releases cytosolic contents (potassium, phosphorus, myoglobin, CK) into extracellular space and systemic circulation.
- The incidence of AKI in rhabdomyolysis is reported to be between 10% and 50%. In cases of traumatic rhabdomyolysis, the incidence of AKI is as high as 85%.
- The **common causes** include the following[3]:
  - ○ Immobilization (e.g., alcoholic patient or patient with seizures or stroke; patient found at home after a fall; or postsurgery patients with large muscle mass or obesity, or undergoing urologic or bariatric surgeries)

- ○ Trauma (e.g., gunshot wound with vascular compromise, motor vehicle accidents, crush injury following earthquakes or building collapse)
- ○ Extreme exertion (e.g., exercise in severe heat, new recruits at army camps)
- ○ Medications such as statins
- ○ Illicit drugs—cocaine, ecstasy
- ○ Electrolyte abnormalities such as hypophosphatemia occurring in alcoholics and patients with ketoacidosis during refeeding
- Vasoconstriction plays a major role in nephrotoxicity associated with unbound myoglobin. Dimeric heme proteins can have direct cytotoxic effect on tubular epithelial cells; the mechanism remains ill defined.
- Renal ischemia is believed to result from activation of endothelin receptors as well as scavenging of nitric oxide. Myoglobin is also believed to generate free radicals that can induce oxidative injury to the tubules. This may be inhibited in an alkaline pH.
- Severe hemolysis can also trigger AKI via a similar mechanism.
- Treatment:
  - ○ In rhabdomyolysis and hemolysis, early volume resuscitation is vital.
  - ○ Isotonic crystalloid solutions or NS are the recommended solutions. Bicarbonate solutions should be used with caution as it may precipitate calcium phosphate in tissues.
  - ○ Once oligoanuria occurs, intravenous (IV) fluids are of limited benefit and should be stopped.
  - ○ RRT should be initiated as per indications outlined in Chapter 7.

Contrast-Induced Nephropathy

GENERAL PRINCIPLES

Acute rise in serum creatinine or decrease in urine output based on KDIGO criteria for AKI within 48 to 72 hours after administration of intra-arterial or IV contrast media (CM).

DIAGNOSIS

- AKI from CM is characterized by a **rise in serum creatinine,** usually within the **first 24 to 48 hours after administration of the agent.**
- If serum creatinine elevation starts >72 hours after contrast exposure, then another etiology must be sought.
- The AKI is usually **nonoliguric** and patients are usually asymptomatic.
- The elevation in serum creatinine usually peaks ~3 to 5 days after exposure.
- Some patients may develop oliguric AKI, and these patients usually have severe underlying renal insufficiency or other serious comorbidities such as severe heart failure or sepsis.
- Approximately 1% of patients will require RRT because of contrast-induced nephropathy (CIN). These patients usually have a longer recovery period.
- In general, CIN is reversible, but persistent renal injury may occur in patients with significant renal insufficiency.
- CIN must be distinguished from atheroemboli where renal injury may not be manifested for several days.

Diagnostic Testing
Laboratories
- Fractional excretion of sodium is usually <1%, due to the profound vasoconstriction that happens early in the disease process. However, this is not diagnostic.

- Urine sediment is usually bland and not conclusive, but essential to evaluate other causes of AKI. Rarely, granular casts are noted.
- CM may cause significantly elevated urine specific gravity.
- Transient peripheral eosinophilia or low complement levels may suggest renal atheroembolic disease.

Imaging

Persistent contrast within the kidney on imaging, 24 hours after exposure to CM, may suggest CIN.

Diagnostic Procedures

A kidney biopsy is not recommended to evaluate for CIN, unless further evaluation for other etiologies is needed.

TREATMENT

- Prevention is key. Patients at high risk for CIN should receive adequate volume expansion with IV normal saline (NS).
- A recent multicenter study (PRESERVE) revealed that *N*-acetylcysteine did not offer any benefit over placebo in preventing CIN. The same study showed that NS was as efficacious as IV sodium bicarbonate.[4]
- IV NS is recommended at 75 mL/hr for approximately 5 to 10 hours prior to the procedure.
- Oral hydration is not effective in prevention.
- Once patients develop AKI from CM, the management strategies are similar to other causes of AKI.

Crystalline Nephropathies

GENERAL PRINCIPLES

- The crystalline nephropathies describe the AKI that results from the intratubular precipitation of various compounds.
  - The most common cause of crystalline nephropathy is tumor lysis syndrome (TLS), which includes the entities of acute uric acid nephropathy and acute phosphate nephropathy. TLS is described in detail in Chapter 19.
  - Less commonly, crystalline nephropathy may result from the precipitation of **calcium oxalate, acyclovir, sulfonamide, methotrexate, indinavir,** or **triamterene.**
  - There are rare case reports of occurrence of crystalline nephropathy with the use of ciprofloxacin, foscarnet, and ampicillin, and with plasma cell dyscrasias.

Pathophysiology

- Intratubular crystal formation and deposition is promoted by **three mechanisms:** high tubular fluid concentration of a substance, prolonged intratubular transit time, and decreased solubility.
  - The first two mechanisms occur in the setting of decreased effective circulating volume, leading to an increase in proximal tubular fluid reabsorption. This results in both high concentrations of the offending compound in the distal tubule and decreased distal flow rates.
  - Underlying chronic kidney disease is also a major risk factor for the crystalline nephropathies, because a larger amount of the compound is excreted per functioning nephron and because drugs are frequently overdosed in renal insufficiency.

○ The third mechanism, decreased solubility, is often dependent on the distal tubular fluid pH.

■ Compounds with a pKa <7, such as uric acid, calcium oxalate, sulfonamides, methotrexate, and triamterene, tend to precipitate in acidic urine, whereas compounds with a pKa >7, such as indinavir and calcium phosphate, tend to precipitate in alkaline urine.

Prevention

• The mainstay of prevention is **avoidance of the two most frequent predisposing factors: volume depletion** and **drug overdosing** (usually from failure to adjust the dose for renal impairment).

• Establishing a brisk urine output (e.g., ≥100 to 150 mL/hr) in high-risk patients is extremely important.

• For substances with pKa <7, urinary alkalinization by administering IV isotonic bicarbonate solutions or oral citrate can be considered. Urine pH should be periodically followed to ensure an appropriate level of alkalinization. Acetazolamide may be added if a metabolic alkalosis ensues.

• Attempting to acidify the urine to increase the solubility of weakly basic compounds is dangerous and not recommended.

• These preventive strategies are based on underlying pathophysiologic mechanisms and evidence for reductions in crystalline nephropathy occurrence is lacking, except perhaps in the case of high-dose methotrexate administration.

DIAGNOSIS

Clinical Presentation

• The clinical contexts in which the more common crystalline nephropathies occur are summarized in Table 8-5. The clinical manifestations of ethylene glycol intoxication are discussed later.

• Extensive crystal deposition in any of the forms of crystalline nephropathy may result in pain from distention of the renal capsule, which is similar to ureteral colic.

• **Nephrolithiasis** may coexist with intratubular crystal deposition in some cases (especially with indinavir and sulfonamides).

• Hypocalcemia due to the coprecipitation of calcium in acute phosphate nephropathy and oxalate nephropathy may result in paresthesias, lethargy, or tetany.

• High levels of acyclovir accumulating with the onset of renal failure can lead to hallucinations, delirium, and myoclonus. Similarly, toxic levels of methotrexate can also cause neurologic disturbances, as well as nausea, rash, and mucositis.

Diagnostic Testing

• A summary of the laboratory findings characteristic for the more common etiologies of crystalline nephropathy is found in Table 8-5.

• **Urine sediment findings** will often reveal **hematuria, pyuria, and mild proteinuria.**

• The offending substances have unique crystal morphologies on urine microscopy, and examining the sediment is helpful in establishing a diagnosis.

○ As the obstructed tubules may not empty urine into the collecting system, the absence of crystals does not exclude crystalline nephropathy.

○ The presence of crystals does not prove their pathogenic role, because calcium oxalate, calcium phosphate, and uric acid crystalluria can be seen in normal individuals. In addition, patients receiving typical offending medications can sometimes display crystalluria without AKI.

TABLE 8-5 CRYSTALLINE NEPHROPATHIES: CLINICAL AND LABORATORY MANIFESTATIONS AND MANAGEMENT STRATEGIES

Inciting Agent	Context of Occurrence	Laboratory Findings	Prevention and Treatment
Phosphate nephropathy	TLS—especially posttreatment form; very rarely in rhabdomyolysis and severe hemolysis; phosphosoda bowel prep	• Crystalluria with weakly birefringent, long prisms often in rosettes • Hyperphosphatemia out of proportion to renal insufficiency and hypocalcemia; in TLS, rhabdomyolysis, and hemolysis, hyperkalemia out of proportion to renal insufficiency, and high LDH • Renal biopsy: von Kossa stain–positive crystals	• *Prevention[a]*: Non–calcium-based phosphate binders; avoid treatment of hypocalcemia unless symptomatic or ECG changes present • *Treatment[a]*: Non–calcium-based phosphate binders; consider early initiation of renal replacement therapy, especially continuous modalities
Uric acid nephropathy	TLS—especially spontaneous form; very rarely in rhabdomyolysis or HGPRT deficiency	• Crystalluria with brownish, strongly birefringent, rhomboid plates, rosettes, or needles • Uric acid >15 mg/dL in absence of prerenal state, urine uric acid: urine creatinine often >1 and almost always >0.75; in TLS and rhabdomyolysis, hyperkalemia out of proportion to renal insufficiency and high LDH	• *Prevention[a]*: In those at high risk of TLS,[b] start hypouricemic therapy, usually allopurinol but may consider rasburicase in patients with multiple high-risk features, especially children • *Treatment[a]*: rasburicase

Oxalate nephropathy	EG poisoning; primary hyperoxaluria; very rarely with high-dose IV ascorbic acid, xylitol, or sorbitol infusions	• Crystalluria with birefringent monohydrate needles or dihydrate envelope shapes • Hypocalcemia; in EG poisoning osmolal gap >10 mOsm/L and detectable serum and urine EG early, with later disappearance of both and development of severe anion gap acidosis • Renal biopsy: silver nitrate/rubeanic acid stain–positive crystals	• *Prevention[a]*: Consider urine alkalinization; for high-risk EG ingestion,[b] prompt fomepizole or, less desirably, ethanol therapy; consider thiamine, magnesium, and pyridoxine in alcoholics; avoid treatment of hypocalcemia unless symptomatic or ECG changes present • *Treatment[a]*: Consider urine alkalinization; begin fomepizole or, less desirably, ethanol if EG level >20 mg/dL; consider early dialysis support, especially if EG >50 mg/dL and renal insufficiency or acidosis is present
Acyclovir	High-dose IV acyclovir bolus; very rarely with oral acyclovir or with oral valacyclovir	• Crystalluria with birefringent needles, occasionally engulfed by white cells	• *Prevention[a]*: Increase time of IV acyclovir infusion to ≥1 hr. • *Treatment[a]*: Lowering dose without stopping the drug may be sufficient in most patients
Indinavir	20% on chronic therapy develop AKI, especially with longer treatment and smaller body size	• Crystalluria with birefringent plates, fans, or starbursts • Isosthenuria common • Contrast computed tomography with wedge-shaped perfusion defects in up to 50%	• *Treatment[a]*: May require urologic consultation for concomitant indinavir stone if present

(continued)

TABLE 8-5 CRYSTALLINE NEPHROPATHIES: CLINICAL AND LABORATORY MANIFESTATIONS AND MANAGEMENT STRATEGIES (Continued)

Inciting Agent	Context of Occurrence	Laboratory Findings	Prevention and Treatment
Methotrexate	High-dose IV therapy given for some malignancies	• Crystalluria with amorphous yellow casts • High serum methotrexate level, cytopenias	• *Prevention[a]*: Urinary alkalinization to pH ≥8 • *Treatment[a]*: Urinary alkalinization to pH ≥8; leucovorin rescue ± thymidine for extrarenal toxicity until methotrexate level <0.05 μmol/L; for very high methotrexate levels, consider carboxypeptidase G2 versus daily hemodialysis with high-flux membrane
Sulfonamides	High-dose IV therapy, especially with sulfadiazine	• Crystalluria with variable shapes from shocks of wheat to spheres • Positive lignin test (orange urine on mixing with 10% hydrochloric acid)	• *Treatment[a]*: Dose reduction and urine alkalinization to pH >7.1 usually sufficient; may require urologic consultation for concomitant sulfonamide stone if present
Triamterene	Must distinguish from AIN, which is much more common	• Crystalluria with birefringent orange casts and spheres • Hyperkalemia out of proportion to renal insufficiency	• *Treatment[a]*: Urine alkalinization to pH >7.5; may require urologic consultation for the more common triamterene stone if obstructed

[a]Saline loading with concomitant diuretic use when urine output is inadequate is recommended for prevention *and* treatment of all of the crystalline nephropathies when possible.

[b]See text for definition of high-risk features.

AIN, acute interstitial nephritis; AKI, acute kidney injury; ECG, electrocardiogram; EG, ethylene glycol; HGPRT, hypoxanthine-guanine phosphoribosyl transferase; IV, intravenous; LDH, lactate; TLS, tumor lysis syndrome.

- **Renal ultrasound** may reveal **bilaterally enlarged and echogenic kidneys** and can identify concomitant macroscopic lithiasis.
- **Renal biopsy** is required to make a definitive diagnosis.
  - Light microscopy reveals **crystalline** deposits, usually in the distal tubules, with a surrounding **interstitial infiltrate** that may contain giant cells as part of a foreign body reaction. Evidence of ATN can also be present as many of the inciting agents display direct tubular cell toxicity.
  - Polarized microscopy may demonstrate birefringence depending on the offending agent.

TREATMENT

- Treatment of established AKI consists of **discontinuing the offending agent** and, if nonoliguric and not volume overloaded, applying the same principles used in prevention: **establishing brisk urine flow** with volume expansion and the judicious use of diuretics and, for weak acids, urinary alkalinization.
- Moderate-to-large doses of diuretics may be required to establish adequate urine flow, and care must be taken with bicarbonate loading to avoid severe alkalosis.
- Additionally, **early initiation of RRT** can rapidly decrease the concentration of some inciting agents (e.g., phosphate, oxalate, acyclovir).
- Evidence for improved renal outcome with the abovementioned maneuvers is lacking.
- See Table 8-5 for details on specific management strategies for the various causes of crystalline nephropathy.

Ethylene Glycol Intoxication

- Ethylene glycol is metabolized by hepatic alcohol dehydrogenase to four toxic organic compounds: glycoaldehyde, glycolic acid, glyoxylic acid, and oxalic acid.
  - Accumulation of the organic anions glycolate, glyoxylate, and oxalate leads to a **severe anion gap metabolic acidosis.**
  - These compounds, especially glycolic acid, are direct cell toxins and cause multiorgan dysfunction with heart failure, ATN, and nervous system depression.
  - Oxalate precipitates with calcium in several tissues, including the renal tubules, causing **crystalline nephropathy.**
- The clinical manifestations of ethylene glycol intoxication evolve over time as the alcohol is metabolized. This time course is prolonged in cases of ethanol coingestion due to competitive inhibition of alcohol dehydrogenase.
  - During the first 30 minutes to 12 hours, ethylene glycol causes inebriation, with progression to **seizures or coma.**
  - At 12 to 36 hours postingestion, peak concentrations of organic acid intermediates lead to profound acidosis with Kussmaul respirations and **cardiopulmonary failure.**
  - At 24 to 72 hours postingestion, the oxalate end product accumulates in the tissues, resulting in AKI.
- If patients are at high risk, then treatment is initiated to prevent end organ damage. The **criteria for initiation of treatment** are as follows: serum ethylene glycol levels >20 mg/dL; OR a known recent ethylene glycol ingestion with an osmolal gap >10 mOsm/L; OR strong suspicion of recent ingestion plus three of the following: pH <7.3, serum bicarbonate <20 mEq/L, osmolal gap >10 mOsm/L, and/or urinary oxalate crystals.
- **Management** of ethylene glycol intoxication (see Table 8-5) should be focused on decreasing the concentration of toxic metabolites in high-risk ingestions. Reductions in the levels of toxic metabolites can be achieved by:
  - Limiting further organic acid formation with competitive alcohol dehydrogenase inhibitors such as fomepizole or ethanol.

○ Increasing metabolite clearance through early initiation of RRT.
○ Conversion to less-toxic metabolites by cofactor supplementation.

OUTCOME/PROGNOSIS

- In most cases of crystalline nephropathy, the **prognosis for full renal recovery is excellent.**
- In the drug-related crystalline nephropathies, recovery of renal function is expected to occur within days to weeks after cessation or even just dose reduction of the drug.
- Phosphate nephropathy due to phosphate-containing laxatives prior to colonoscopy may have a worse prognosis, because the population affected by this entity is older and has a higher prevalence of underlying chronic kidney disease.

Acute Interstitial Nephritis

GENERAL PRINCIPLES

Definition

Acute interstitial nephritis (AIN) is a hypersensitivity reaction characterized by inflammation in the renal interstitium, sparing the glomeruli.

Epidemiology

- AIN is the predominant finding in 10% of biopsies performed in cases of AKI.
- The incidence seems to be increasing, perhaps because of more liberal prescribing practices, increased physician awareness of the disease, and the availability of new medications.

Etiology

- The major causes of AIN are drugs (70% of cases), systemic diseases, and infections (please see Table 8-6). Among drug-induced AIN, antibiotics, nonsteroidal anti-inflammatory medications, and proton pump inhibitors are some of the major culprits.[5]
- Other less-common etiologies include idiopathic causes, tubulointerstitial nephritis with uveitis syndrome, and sarcoidosis, and IgG4 disease.

Pathophysiology

- AKI results from immune-mediated tubular injury. The localization of inflammation to the interstitium may occur through several mechanisms, including molecular mimicry with tubular epitopes or deposition of immunogenic portions of the inciting agent at a specific location in the kidney.
- Similar to other hypersensitivity reactions, AIN is not dose dependent, there is recrudescence in disease activity on reexposure to compounds with similar biochemical structure, and there is often multiorgan involvement.
- Both cell-mediated and humoral immunity seem to play a role, though the former seems to play a more significant role in pathogenesis.

DIAGNOSIS

Clinical Presentation

- The presenting features of AIN can be quite variable, due in part to the multiplicity of agents that can initiate the syndrome.

| TABLE 8-6 | COMMON CAUSES OF ACUTE INTERSTITIAL NEPHRITIS | | | |

Drugs[a]	Systemic Diseases	Infections (Rare Causes of AIN)	Other
Antimicrobial agents	Light-chain deposition disease	**Bacteria**	Wasp sting
Penicillins (initial description of AIN was due to methicillin)	Sarcoidosis	*Brucella* species	Chinese herbs
	Sjögren syndrome	*Corynebacterium diphtheriae*	Idiopathic
Cephalosporins	Systemic lupus erythematosus	*Chlamydia* species	
Sulfonamides	TINU	*Legionella* species	
Ciprofloxacin	ANCA associated, and other vasculitides	*Leptospira*	
Vancomycin		*Mycoplasma tuberculosis*	
Rifampin		*Mycoplasma pneumoniae*	
NSAIDs, COX-2 inhibitors and salicylates	IgG4 disease	*Rickettsia* species	
Anticonvulsants		*Salmonella* species	
Phenytoin		*Staphylococcus* species	
Levetiracetam		*Streptococcus* species	
Diuretics		*Yersinia pseudotuberculosis*	
Furosemide		**Viruses**	
Thiazides		CMV	
Proton pump inhibitors		EBV	
Omeprazole		Hantaviruses	
Esomeprazole		HBV	
Pantaprazole		HIV	
Others		HSV	
Allopurinol		Measles	
		Polyomaviruses	
		Parasites	
		Leishmania donovani	
		Toxoplasma gondii	

[a]Due to the fact that a very large number of drugs have been associated with acute interstitial nephritis, only drug classes and the most common individual offending medicines are listed here.

CMV, cytomegalovirus; COX-2, cyclooxygenase 2; EBV, Epstein–Barr virus; HBV, hepatitis B virus; HIV, human immunodeficiency syndrome; HSV, herpes simplex virus; NSAIDs, nonsteroidal anti-inflammatory drugs; TINU, tubulointerstitial nephritis and uveitis syndrome; ANCA, antineutrophil cytoplasmic antibody; IgG, immunoglobulin G.

- The combination of AKI, urinary symptoms (e.g., flank pain, macroscopic hematuria, or oliguria), and symptoms of hypersensitivity (e.g., rash, fever, or arthralgias) should alert the clinician to the possibility of AIN.
- Signs of hypersensitivity may be absent in up to half of AIN cases, especially in those attributable to NSAIDs.
- The temporal relationship between the initiation of a new drug and the development of renal dysfunction may also aid in the diagnosis.
- Disease manifestations develop within 3 weeks of initiation of the inciting drug in about 80% of patients, with an average latency of onset of 10 days (range 1 day to >1 year).
- The duration of onset may be longer with NSAIDs, with a mean latent period of 2 to 3 months.

- In AIN related to infection or systemic diseases, the clinical features of the inciting disease often predominate.

Diagnostic Testing

- Urinalysis may reveal nonspecific findings such as hematuria and/or sterile pyuria.
- The presence of white blood cell casts is more specific, although they can also be seen in pyelonephritis and certain proliferative glomerulonephritides.
- Eosinophiluria is neither specific nor sensitive and urine eosinophils should NOT be routinely ordered.
- Mild proteinuria is common, but sometimes it may be in the nephrotic range. Heavy proteinuria is classically associated with NSAIDs, occurring in a third of cases attributable to this drug class and associated with concomitant minimal change glomerulopathy. NSAID-induced membranous nephropathy can also occur.
- Signs of multiorgan dysfunction such as elevated transaminases and hemolysis can occasionally be seen.
- Renal imaging may occasionally reveal normal-to-large kidneys with increased echogenicity. This is especially true of IgG4 disease.
- Renal biopsy is the gold standard for definitive diagnosis and reveals an edematous interstitium infiltrated mostly by T cells and macrophages. Neutrophils, eosinophils, and plasma cells can also be found and occasionally there may be granulomatous inflammation. There may be tubulitis or frank tubular necrosis in severe AIN. The glomeruli are usually normal, but electron microscopy may reveal foot process effacement in NSAID-associated AIN. In IgG4 disease, there is extensive infiltration of IgG4-positive plasma cells in the interstitium.

TREATMENT

- The most important therapeutic maneuver in AIN is prompt removal of the inciting agent. In those cases associated with infection or other systemic disease, treatment of the underlying cause is necessary.
- Corticosteroids are typically reserved for more severe cases and those with systemic diseases such as sarcoidosis and IgG4 disease. In the latter two diseases, additional immunosuppression may also be required.
- The best data supporting the use of corticosteroids comes from a small series of 14 patients, all with methicillin-induced AIN. Corticosteroids were associated with complete renal recovery more often than withdrawal of methicillin alone, and the treated group recovered more quickly.
- Positive observational data with corticosteroids in AIN from other etiologies exist, but are limited to small case series. In many reports, the most apparent effect of corticosteroids was a more rapid recovery of renal function.
- The literature is sparse regarding the use of other immunosuppressants in setting of drug-induced AIN, and often describes cases associated with unusual etiologies. Successful treatment has been described using calcineurin inhibitors, cyclophosphamide, azathioprine, and mycophenolate mofetil.
- A reasonable treatment strategy in light of these data would be to reserve corticosteroids for patients with idiopathic AIN, systemic diseases for which corticosteroids have a proven role (e.g., sarcoidosis, Sjögren syndrome, vasculitides, IgG4 disease), or cases with poor prognostic features.
- Predictors of worse prognosis include delayed onset of improvement in renal function after withdrawal of the inciting agent (>1 week), prolonged exposure to the offending agent (>2 to 3 weeks), pre-existing chronic kidney disease, and a renal histology

characterized by intense and diffuse interstitial infiltrate, granuloma formation, or significant fibrosis and tubular atrophy.
- A frequently used regimen is oral prednisone (1 mg/kg), with the duration of therapy guided by the improvement in renal function. Most patients will improve in the first 1 to 2 weeks.

OUTCOME/PROGNOSIS

- AIN has a variable clinical course and response to treatment.
  - In the initial prototype for the disease—methicillin-induced AIN—the prognosis was excellent with complete recovery of renal function noted in 90% of patients.
  - In nonmethicillin drug-induced AIN, chronic kidney disease may persist in significant number of cases.
- The prognosis for AIN may depend on the promptness of elimination of the inciting agent.
  - The etiologies associated with milder symptoms, and therefore delayed diagnosis (e.g., NSAIDs, chronic infections, or sarcoidosis), have worse prognosis than those with more acute and dramatic presentations (e.g., methicillin, rifampin, or acute bacterial or viral infections).
- Interestingly, the peak serum creatinine does not seem to correlate with the long-term renal prognosis.

Hepatorenal Syndrome

GENERAL PRINCIPLES

Definition
- Hepatorenal syndrome (HRS) is a common cause of renal dysfunction in patients with cirrhosis. HRS can also be seen in patients with acute liver failure or alcoholic hepatitis.
- Two types of HRS (type 1 and type 2) were defined by the International Club of Ascites in 1996, and definitions were updated in 2007 and 2015.[6] In the most recent definition, it was decided that instead of a specific creatinine number, a rise in serum creatinine should be used to define HRS. In type 1 HRS, rise in serum creatinine occurs in less than 2 weeks, while HRS type 2 displays a slowly progressive course over several weeks.
- Elevation in serum creatinine is not as high as that seen in noncirrhotic patients who have AKI, because of reduced muscle mass and low endogenous production of creatinine in cirrhosis.
- Even though urine output is not mentioned as a diagnostic criterion, if a patient remains oliguric despite adequate volume resuscitation, this should be considered as an early indication of HRS since changes in serum creatinine may be delayed by 24 to 48 hours after renal injury.
- **The diagnostic criteria for HRS** are outlined in Table 8-7.

Pathophysiology
- Renal vasoconstriction is the main hemodynamic derangement that defines HRS.
- The main variable responsible for these hemodynamic changes is portal hypertension in the setting of cirrhosis, causing a splanchnic arterial vasodilation. This vasodilation occurs mainly because of the production of nitric oxide as a consequence of endothelial stretching and possibly bacterial translocation.

TABLE 8-7	DIAGNOSTIC CRITERIA FOR HEPATORENAL SYNDROME IN CIRRHOTIC PATIENTS

Cirrhosis with ascites

Diagnosis of AKI per ICA-AKI criteria (increase in serum creatinine ≥ 0.3 mg/dL within 48 hrs or % serum creatinine increase of ≥ from baseline over 7 days)

> No improvement after at least 2 days with diuretic withdrawal and volume expansion with albumin. The recommended dose of albumin is 1 g/kg of body weight per day up to a maximum of 100 g/day

> Absence of shock

> No current or recent treatment with nephrotoxic drugs

> Absence of parenchymal kidney disease as indicated by proteinuria >500 mg/day, microhematuria (>50 red blood cells per high-power field) and/or abnormal renal ultrasonography

AKI, acute kidney injury; ICA-AKI, International Club of Ascites–acute kidney injury.
Adapted from Angeli P, Gines P, Wong F, et al. Diagnosis and management of acute kidney injury in patients with cirrhosis: revised consensus recommendations of the International Club of Ascites. *J Hepatol.* 2015;62:(4)968–974.

- The accumulation of plasma volume in the splanchnic bed causes a compensatory response because of decreased central blood volume with activation of systemic vasoconstrictor and antinatriuretic systems (RAAS, sympathetic system, ADH). This accounts for the sodium and water retention, as well as renal vasoconstriction, as the kidney senses a relative hypovolemic state.
- Individuals who develop HRS most often exhibit clinical features of advanced cirrhosis along with low arterial blood pressure, low urine volume, and severe urinary sodium retention (urine sodium <10 mEq/L). Dilutional hyponatremia is almost universally found.

TREATMENT

- The only **definitive cure** for HRS is **liver transplantation** or **spontaneous recovery** of hepatic function in setting of acute failure.
- **Temporizing measures** can provide a bridge to liver transplantation or recovery. Commonly used regimens include an infusion of **albumin** in addition to a **vasoconstricting agent:**
  - ○ Octreotide (a subcutaneous medication that causes splanchnic vasoconstriction) + midodrine (an oral medication that causes renal vasodilation)
  - ○ Terlipressin (an oral vasopressin analog, available in Europe but not in the United States)
  - ○ Norepinephrine or vasopressin (IV vasoactive medications) have been found to induce similar rates of reversal of HRS as terlipressin but are usually reserved for ICU patients as they require central IV access
- **Transjugular intrahepatic portosystemic shunt** (TIPS) is an option for patients who do not respond to the above temporizing measures.
- Use of RRT in HRS should be decided on a case-by-case basis unless patient has an excellent chance for recovery from acute liver injury or they are candidates for liver

transplantation. In the absence of these possibilities, dialysis adds little to overall survival in this condition.[7]

Cardiorenal Syndrome

GENERAL PRINCIPLES

- The coexistence of renal and cardiac dysfunction in which acute or chronic dysfunction in one organ may induce acute or chronic dysfunction in the other organ has been termed as cardiorenal syndrome (CRS).
- A classification of CRS with five subtypes has been proposed that reflects the bidirectional nature of the heart and kidney interaction, the timeframe, and the pathophysiology.[8]
  - **CRS type 1 is rapid worsening of cardiac function that results in AKI** and is the classical CRS type seen in the hospital setting
  - CRS type 2: chronic worsening of cardiac function causes progressive CKD
  - CRS type 3: abrupt and primary worsening of renal function (e.g., AKI, ischemia, glomerulonephritis) leads to acute cardiac dysfunction (e.g., CHF, arrhythmia, ischemia)
  - CRS type 4: primary CKD contributes to cardiac dysfunction (e.g., ventricular hypertrophy, diastolic dysfunction, increased risk of adverse cardiovascular events)
  - CRS type 5: acute or chronic systemic disorders cause both cardiac and renal dysfunction
- **Features of CRS type 1** include low systolic blood pressure, tendency for hyperkalemia, diuretic resistance, and anemia. Pre-existing renal dysfunction as well as other risk factors such as hypertension and diabetes mellitus may contribute to worsening renal failure and poor outcome associated with decompensated cardiac disease.

TREATMENT

- **The management of the CRS** remains a challenge in spite of advances in medical therapy.
- In the setting of overt volume overload, **large doses of loop diuretics** (e.g., furosemide 120 to 200 mg) may need to be administered IV to achieve a desirable diuresis.
- For synergy, **thiazide diuretics** or analogs (e.g., metolazone) should be added, to block sodium absorption in the distal convoluted tubule and increase natriuresis.
- Diuretic therapy may be associated with rise in serum creatinine, but this may be a hemodynamic response to volume contraction, rather than renal injury. Small rise in serum creatinine should not deter from continuing diuretic therapy.
- Small studies have shown that nitrates allow for decreased doses of diuretics.
- Inotropic agents have been used successfully in the cardiogenic shock stage but are not proven to be effective in lesser degrees of cardiac failure.
- Ultrafiltration, though shown to be beneficial in achieving faster fluid removal in small trials, is invasive and expensive. A randomized controlled trial showed worse renal function and an increased risk in serious adverse events with ultrafiltration, when compared to a stepped pharmacologic therapy.[9]
- If patients are not responding appropriately to diuretic therapy, then RRT can be considered. It should be kept in mind that some patients may require chronic RRT for management of volume overload, especially in setting of significant underlying CKD and this should be kept in mind when offering RRT.

REFERENCES

1. Agrawal A, Ziccardi MR, Witzke C, et al. Cholesterol embolization syndrome: an under-recognized entity in cardiovascular interventions. *J Interv Cardiol.* 2018;31(3):407–415.
2. George JN, Nester CM. Syndromes of thrombotic microangiopathy. *N Engl J Med.* 2014; 371(7):654–666.
3. Bosch X, Poch E, Grau JM. Rhabdomyolysis and acute kidney injury. *N Engl J Med.* 2009; 361(1):62–72.
4. Weisbord SD, Gallagher M, Jneid H, et al. Outcomes after angiography with sodium bicarbonate and acetylcysteine. *N Engl J Med.* 2018;378(7):603–614.
5. Muriithi AK, Leung N, Valeri AM, et al. Biopsy-proven acute interstitial nephritis, 1993–2011: a case series. *Am J Kidney Dis.* 2014;64(4):558–566.
6. Angeli P, Gines P, Wong F, et al. Diagnosis and management of acute kidney injury in patients with cirrhosis: revised consensus recommendations of the International Club of Ascites. *J Hepatol.* 2015;62(4):968–974.
7. Allegretti AS, Parada XV, Eneanya ND, et al. Prognosis of patients with cirrhosis and AKI who initiate RRT. *Clin J Am Soc Nephrol.* 2018;13(1):16–25.
8. Ronco C, Bellasi A, DiLuollo L. Cardiorenal syndrome: an overview. *Adv Chronic Kidney Dis.* 2018;25(5):382–390.
9. Bart BA, Goldsmith SR, Lee KL, et al. Ultrafiltration in decompensated heart failure with cardiorenal syndrome. *N Engl J Med.* 2012;367(24):2296–2304.

Primary Glomerulopathies

Ying Chen

9

GENERAL PRINCIPLES

Primary glomerular diseases are a group of disorders in which the main manifestations of disease are directly related to kidney involvement rather than as part of a systemic disease process. Systemic diseases associated with glomerular disease are discussed in a separate chapter.

- Primary glomerular diseases can present with **nephrotic syndrome, asymptomatic proteinuria,** isolated **hematuria,** or **a nephritic picture.** In many cases, they are described as being idiopathic without known association or cause. For each of the primary glomerulopathies, secondary causes are also discussed. For instance, medications, infections, and malignancies are all associated with glomerular pathology that is otherwise indistinguishable from the idiopathic forms.
- Proper diagnosis and management of the primary glomerulopathies requires an understanding of patient characteristics, risk of progressive kidney disease, and safe use of immunosuppressive agents.

Focal Segmental Glomerulosclerosis

- Focal segmental glomerulosclerosis (FSGS) has become **the most important form of primary glomerular disease,** both because of increasing incidence and because of its contribution to the growth of end-stage renal disease (ESRD).
- In the United States, FSGS is the **most common cause of idiopathic nephrotic syndrome** in adult African Americans. Idiopathic FSGS is also the most common primary glomerular disease detected on renal biopsy that leads to ESRD in all races.
- FSGS is a group of disorders that shares several histologic features. Renal biopsy shows some glomeruli (focal) with sclerosis in part of the glomerular tuft (segmental). Patients with these abnormalities often present with nephrotic syndrome, but may also have asymptomatic proteinuria.
- Several means of **categorizing FSGS** are in use.
  - **FSGS can be described as a primary or secondary disorder** associated with a range of causes and potential differences in treatment. For instance, primary FSGS is usually treated with corticosteroids or immunosuppressive regimens, whereas secondary disease typically does not respond to this regimen.
  - **Histologic variants** have been described that take into account subglomerular localization of the sclerotic lesion, presence of proliferation, and presence of glomerular capillary collapse. The value of this system is thought to arise from better prediction of causation and outcomes.
    - **The collapsing FSGS variant** is associated with human immunodeficiency virus (HIV) and some drug-associated diseases. Of all the histologic variants, collapsing FSGS is **notable for a poor renal prognosis.**
    - Patients with the tip lesion pattern of FSGS have the most favorable outcome.
    - Table 9-1 summarizes the histologic variants and some of their associations.
    - In addition, a variant of FSGS has been termed **C1q nephropathy.**

TABLE 9-1 HISTOLOGIC VARIANTS OF FOCAL SEGMENTAL GLOMERULOSCLEROSIS

Name	Histology	Comments
FSGS (not otherwise specified)	At least one glomerulus with segmental increase in matrix obliterating capillary loop. Excludes other variants	Most common form
Perihilar variant	Perihilar hyalinosis and sclerosis in >50% of affected glomeruli	Seen in primary and secondary FSGS
Cellular variant	Endocapillary proliferation involving at least 25% of the tuft and occluding the lumen	Fairly responsive to immunosuppressive therapy
Collapsing variant	At least one glomerulus with segmental or global collapse and overlying podocyte hyperplasia	More aggressive with rapid progression to ESRD. Associated with secondary FSGS
Tip variant	At least one segmental lesion involving the outer 25% of the glomerulus next to the origin of the proximal tubule	May correlate with better prognosis and increased responsiveness to steroids

FSGS, focal segmental glomerulosclerosis; ESRD, end-stage renal disease.

Primary Idiopathic FSGS

GENERAL PRINCIPLES

- FSGS is responsible for 7% to 20% of idiopathic NS in children and 40% in adults.
- The disease is markedly **more common in African Americans** and the mean age of onset in adults is 40 years.
- Proteinuria is typically nonselective.
- Secondary forms of FSGS typically have lower levels of proteinuria than classic idiopathic FSGS.
- Other **common features on presentation** are **hypertension (30% to 50%), microscopic hematuria (25% to 75%), and renal insufficiency (20% to 30%).**
- Serologic testing and complement levels should be normal.

TREATMENT

- There is still considerable debate over the appropriate treatment for patients with FSGS.
- **Corticosteroid and immunosuppressive therapy should be considered only in idiopathic FSGS associated with clinical features of the nephrotic syndrome.**
- **Standard therapy** is initiated with **high-dose daily corticosteroids** (prednisone, 1 mg/kg of ideal body weight per day to maximum dose of 80 mg/d or 2 mg/kg alternate-day treatment).

○ The initial high dose of corticosteroids should be given for a minimum of 4 weeks up to a maximum of 16 weeks, as tolerated, or until complete remission has been achieved, whichever is earlier.

○ The median duration of steroid treatment to achieve complete remission is **3 to 4 months.** However, potential morbidities associated with steroid-related side effects need to be considered if this approach is planned.

○ If remission occurs, the steroids may be tapered slowly. Longer courses may be used in patients who achieve only partial remission or who relapse with steroid tapering.

• **Calcineurin inhibitors (CNIs) are considered first-line therapy for patients with relative contraindications or intolerance to high-dose corticosteroids** (e.g., uncontrolled diabetes, psychiatric conditions, or severe osteoporosis). **Cyclosporine** (3 to 5 mg/kg ideal body weight per day in two divided doses) **for steroid-resistant FSGS.** If there is a partial or complete remission, continue CSA treatment for at least 12 months, followed by a slow taper.

• **Mycophenolate mofetil (MMF)** has been investigated in a large multicenter National Institutes of Health trial (FSGS-CT) in the United States comparing cyclosporine and a regimen of oral MMF plus dexamethasone for **steroid-resistant FSGS patients.** There was no statistical difference in the primary or main secondary outcomes between the two therapies. However, there are limitations in this study.

• Recurrence of FSGS after renal transplantation is common (up to 30%) and is associated with decreased graft survival. **Plasmapheresis** has been used with limited success in the management of posttransplant FSGS recurrence.[1]

OUTCOME/PROGNOSIS

• Spontaneous remission of proteinuria is unusual.

• **Poor prognostic indicators** are nephrotic range proteinuria or massive proteinuria, elevated serum creatinine, greater degree of tubulointerstitial fibrosis, and presence of collapsing lesions at the time of biopsy, African American, and failure to achieve partial or complete remission.

• FSGS has a **significant risk of progression to ESRD,** with 5- and 10-year renal survival rates of 76% and 57% in those initially presenting with nephrotic syndrome.[2]

• Nonnephrotic proteinuria is associated with >90% 10-year kidney survival.

Secondary FSGS

GENERAL PRINCIPLES

FSGS represents a common phenotypic expression of diverse clinicopathologic syndromes with distinct etiologies.

• **Genetic causes of FSGS:**

○ Mutations in more than 30 podocyte genes can cause FSGS. Most have been related to defects in structural proteins of podocytes and slit diaphragms.

○ Mutations in the *NPHS1* gene, which codes for nephrin, are responsible for the autosomal recessive congenital nephrotic syndrome of the Finnish type. Compound heterozygous mutations in small numbers of tested adults have been linked to steroid-resistant FSGS.[3]

○ Mutations in the *NPHS2* gene, which codes for podocin, are responsible for autosomal recessive steroid-resistant FSGS in children and rarely in adults.

- ○ Autosomal dominant FSGS in children or adults is caused by mutations in *INF2* encoding inverted formin 2, *ACTN4* encoding podocyte cytoplasmic protein α-actinin-4, as well as *TRPC6* encoding transient receptor potential cation 6 channel.[4]
- **Viral infection:**
  - ○ **HIV-associated nephropathy** may occur at any time during the course of HIV infection, although it is usually diagnosed when CD4 count falls below 200.
    - The glomerular disease appears to result from **direct infection of podocytes,** leading to podocyte proliferation and dedifferentiation.
    - Up to 95% of HIV-associated nephropathy cases occur in **young African-American men** with HIV infection contracted by any route (mean age, 33 years; male-to-female ratio, 10:1).
    - The clinical presentation includes nephrotic or nonnephrotic proteinuria, progressive azotemia, and the relative rarity of hypertension.
    - Laboratory evaluation reveals HIV seropositivity, normal C3, normal C4, and CD4 count usually <200.
    - **Renal ultrasound** typically **shows enlarged kidneys** with increased echogenicity.
    - The pathology of HIV-associated nephropathy includes collapsing FSGS, mesangial proliferation, hypertrophied podocytes with protein resorption droplets, microcystic dilated tubules, and endothelial cell tubuloreticular inclusions.
  - ○ **Parvovirus B19** infection has also been associated with collapsing FSGS.
- **Drugs:**
  - ○ Drugs associated with FSGS include pamidronate, heroin, lithium, and interferon-α.
  - ○ **Pamidronate** has been associated with the collapsing form.
  - ○ Secondary FSGS was attributed to heroin use in older studies. These cases presented with nephrotic syndrome and with rapid progression to ESRD. More recent studies have shown that the incidence of heroin-associated disease has declined markedly.
- **Sickle cell nephropathy:**
  - ○ Kidney disease can occur in persons with sickle cell disease.
  - ○ The prevalence of proteinuria was 26% in one series.
  - ○ Chronic kidney disease has been seen in 7% to 30% of patients with long-term follow-up.
  - ○ Hyperfiltration and increased glomerular pressure are thought to be the mechanism for injury.
  - ○ The most common lesion on kidney biopsy is FSGS, although other histology can sometimes be found (e.g., membranoproliferative glomerulonephritis [MPGN]).
- **Other:**
  - ○ **Reduced renal mass** (unilateral renal agenesis, surgical renal ablation, chronic allograft nephropathy, and chronic vesicoureteral reflux).
  - ○ Secondary FSGS may also be seen in the setting of **chronic hypoperfusion and ischemia to the kidney.** Some examples are hypertension, morbid obesity, congenital cyanotic heart disease, obstructive sleep apnea (OSA), and atheroemboli.

TREATMENT

- **Therapy for the underlying disorder** is first-line management. Lesions of FSGS may regress with management of the underlying condition (e.g., treatment of obesity with bariatric surgery or continuous positive airway pressure for OSA).
- Nonspecific therapy to reduce edema and proteinuria with diuretics, dietary sodium restriction, and angiotensin-converting enzyme **(ACE) inhibitor/angiotensin receptor blocker (ARB) therapy** should be aggressively pursued.
- Steroid treatment as for idiopathic FSGS can be considered in refractory cases, but limited data do not support the use of aggressive immunosuppressive or cytotoxic agents.

OTHER FSGS VARIANTS: C1Q NEPHROPATHY

- Distinctive features of C1q nephropathy are a predominance of **C1q staining in the glomerulus and mesangial electron-dense deposits.**
- It is predominant in males and African Americans are commonly affected.
- Proteinuria is usually in the nephrotic range and hematuria is present in ~20% of the patients.
- The best treatment for this lesion is unclear but should include antiproteinuric strategies, such as ACE inhibitors.

Minimal Change Disease

GENERAL PRINCIPLES

- Minimal change disease (MCD) is the **most common cause of nephrotic syndrome in children** (~65%) and in up to 10% to 15% of cases of adult nephrotic syndrome. The peak incidence of MCD is in children aged 2 to 7 years, but the disease may occur at any age.
- The typical presentation of MCD is **nephrotic syndrome.** Clinical presentation is usually characterized by rapid onset of edema, often with periorbital edema, marked weight gain, pleural effusions, and ascites.
- **Children** presenting with typical features of nephrotic syndrome usually **undergo empiric steroid therapy** without a definitive diagnosis by renal biopsy. Steroid responsiveness in this group is equated with a diagnosis of MCD.
- **Acute kidney injury can occur in up to 20% to 25% of adults.** Major risk factors for this presentation are male, older and hypertensive with lower serum albumin and more proteinuria.
- **Other complications** of MCD include sepsis, peritonitis in ascitic fluid, and thromboembolism.
- The pathogenesis remains unknown but may be related to a disorder of T or B lymphocytes. There is a postulated circulating factor acting on podocytes. The majority of cases are idiopathic.
- Secondary causes of MCD:
  - **Drugs** can cause MCD, with the most common culprit being nonsteroidal antiinflammatory drugs (**NSAIDs**).
  - Hematologic malignancies, most notably Hodgkin disease, can present with MCD and this should be kept in mind in the older age group. However, it is not recommended to screen these patients extensively for malignancy.
  - Heavy metals (mercury, lead) are rare causes of MCD.
  - Systemic allergic reactions to environmental allergens or vaccines may rarely trigger MCD.

DIAGNOSIS

- **Hypoalbuminemia** and **elevated cholesterol** are frequently noted.
- In children, the **urine sediment** may show **Maltese-cross oval fat bodies** under polarized light.
- In adults, **microscopic hematuria** is common.
- Complement levels and other serologic markers are normal.
- A urine protein electrophoresis will show that the negatively charged protein albumin predominates. This has been termed **selective proteinuria.**

- **Renal biopsy** is required for diagnosis in children unresponsive to steroids and in all adults presenting with nephrotic syndrome.
- Light microscopy is typically normal, although mild mesangial hypercellularity may be found. Tubular and interstitial structures are normal.
- Electron microscopy (EM) reveals **diffuse podocyte foot process fusion,** but this is a nonspecific finding.

TREATMENT

- The initial treatment of **adults** with MCD is **corticosteroids.**
  - Typical regimens are daily dosing with **prednisone** 1 mg/kg (to a maximum of 80 mg/d) or alternate-day dosing with 2 mg/kg every other day. These approaches appear to have similar initial response rates.
  - Treat for not less than 12 to 16 weeks at first presentation. Seventy-five percent to 80% of adults achieve remission by 12 to 16 weeks of therapy.
  - Adults who initially respond to corticosteroids will experience at least one relapse around 70% of the time. Relapses are usually treated with a second course of corticosteroids.
- **Frequent relapsing** (three or more relapses within 1 year), **steroid-dependent** (relapse upon tapering steroid therapy or within 2 weeks of discontinuing steroids and need for long-term maintenance steroids), or **steroid-resistant** (failure to reach remission within 4 months of steroid treatment) patients should be treated with second-line agents. Options for management include:
  - Oral **cyclophosphamide** (2 to 2.5 mg/kg per day) for 8 weeks with tapering dose of prednisone.
  - For patients who relapse after cyclophosphamide treatment, **cyclosporine** 3 to 5 mg/kg/d or tacrolimus 0.05 to 0.1 mg/kg/d in divided doses for 1 to 2 years is also effective.
  - **MMF** has been used as an effective alternative therapy in small case series.
- A small percentage of adults initially thought to have MCD will progress to ESRD. Repeat histology will typically reveal FSGS in these patients.

MCD VARIANT: IgM NEPHROPATHY

- The term **IgM nephropathy** is used to describe patients presenting with nephrotic syndrome and with the findings of mesangial deposits of IgM, often with a minor degree of mesangial hypercellularity on renal biopsy.
- Controversy exists regarding whether to include this constellation of findings as a variant of minimal disease or FSGS or as part of a continuum related to both entities.
- Patients are less likely to respond to corticosteroids. In the largest series to date, the probability of developing ESRD was approximately 23% at 15 years.

Membranous Nephropathy

GENERAL PRINCIPLES

Epidemiology

- Membranous nephropathy (MN) is among the most common causes of the nephrotic syndrome in nondiabetic adults.
- It is more common in white males aged >40 years.

- It is uncommon in children and adolescents.
- Most cases (two-thirds) are idiopathic.

Pathogenesis

- The pathogenesis of MN is still not completely known. It is thought to be due to auto-immunity via specific nephritogenic autoantibodies.
- Heymann nephritis is a rat model of MN that is induced by inoculation with megalin, a large (516 kDa) glycoprotein extracted from rat cortical nephrons. Formation of antigen–antibody complexes are seen at the podocyte level, with complement activation and formation of the membrane attack complex (C5b–9). This leads to destruction of the glomerular base membrane (GBM) and shedding of the immune complexes to form the characteristic subepithelial deposits. However, megalin is not expressed in human glomerulus.
- Recent experimental studies have advanced understanding of the pathogenesis of human membranous glomerulonephritis.
  - Identification of neutral endopeptidase (NEP) as the target antigen on the glomerular podocyte in alloimmune MN resulting from fetomaternal immunization in NEP-deficient mothers.[5]
  - About 70% to 80% of idiopathic MN patients exhibit circulating antibodies of IgG4 subtype against the **M-type phospholipase A2 receptor (PLA2R)**, a transmembrane protein located on podocytes.[6]
  - **Thrombospondin type-1 domain-containing 7A (THSD7A)** is, like PLA2R, a transmembrane protein expressed on podocytes. THSD7A may be the responsible antigen in approximately 10% of patients with idiopathic MN who are negative for anti-PLA2R antibodies. THSD7A may also be involved in the pathogenesis of some cases of malignancy-associated MN.

DIAGNOSIS

Clinical Presentation

- MN presents as **nephrotic syndrome in 80% of patients.**
- **Microscopic hematuria** may be found in up to 50% of cases, but red blood cell casts are unusual.
- As with the other causes of nephrotic syndrome, a renal biopsy is necessary to make the diagnosis.
- Plasma complement levels are normal in the idiopathic form. Decreased C3 or C4 should prompt further evaluation for systemic lupus erythematosus (SLE) or other systemic disorders associated with hypocomplementemia.
- There is an increased incidence of **thromboembolism,** especially **renal vein thrombosis.** Thromboembolism has been reported in up to 30% of patients with MN.
- MN is characterized by **slow progression of renal insufficiency** (<20% of patients have renal insufficiency at time of presentation).
- **Hypertension** develops only with advancing renal insufficiency and is usually not characteristic of MN at earlier stages.
- A diagnosis of MN should prompt a thorough evaluation for other related diseases. It is associated with a variety of autoimmune, infectious, and malignant diseases, as well as with toxic or drug exposures.
  - **Autoimmune diseases** associated with MN include SLE (WHO class V), type 1 diabetes mellitus, rheumatoid arthritis, mixed connective tissue disease, Sjögren syndrome, Hashimoto thyroiditis, and myasthenia gravis.
  - **Associated infectious diseases** are hepatitis B, hepatitis C (HCV), syphilis, malaria, and schistosomiasis.

○ The **most common associated cancers** are those of the lung, breast, kidney, and gastrointestinal tract, but cases of MN have been reported with most forms of cancer. Nephrotic syndrome may precede clinical evidence of malignancy by 12 to 18 months.

○ **Drugs** such as NSAIDs, gold, penicillamine, hydrocarbons, mercury, formaldehyde, and captopril have been reported in association with MN.

Diagnostic Testing

* **Light microscopy:**
  ○ Normal at early stages and later progresses to thickened glomerular capillary wall with **epithelial "spikes"** seen by methenamine silver staining.
  ○ Absence of leukocyte infiltration with no evidence of hypercellularity or proliferative lesions. **The presence of significant mesangial hypercellularity** suggests immune deposit formation in the mesangium and is more consistent with a secondary MN such as class V lupus nephritis.

* **Immunofluorescence:**
  ○ Characteristic IgG granular subepithelial staining in all portions of the glomerular capillary loop. In idiopathic MN, staining is exclusively IgG. The predominant IgG subclass in idiopathic MN is IgG4. Presence of IgM or IgA staining, particularly in the mesangium, as well as tubuloreticular structures seen in glomerular endothelial cells by EM suggests class V lupus nephritis.
  ○ Complement C3 and light chains are also present with similar localization to IgG in ~50% of cases.

* **EM** demonstrates the **diagnostic subepithelial electron-dense deposits** in stages:
  ○ **Stage I:** Subepithelial dense deposits without adjacent projections of GBM; normal light microscopy.
  ○ **Stage II:** Adjacent GBM projections forming spikes around immune deposits.
  ○ **Stage III:** GBM projections surrounding deposits completely.
  ○ **Stage IV:** Markedly thickened GBM with electron-lucent zones replacing the dense deposits.
  ○ These stages reflect the severity and duration of disease but do not correlate well with prognosis. The finding of **extensive mesangial electron-dense deposits should prompt consideration of MN secondary to lupus.**

TREATMENT

* All patients with MN should be managed with **blood pressure control** (goal, <130/80 mm Hg), **dietary sodium restriction, ACE inhibition or angiotensin receptor blockade,** and **lipid-lowering therapy.**

* Patients with documented renal vein or other venous thrombosis should be **anticoagulated** with warfarin.
  ○ At present, there is no consensus for anticoagulation for primary prevention, although patients with hypoalbuminemia of <2.5 g/dL are considered to be at high risk for thrombosis and may be considered for anticoagulation as primary prevention.
  ○ Once anticoagulation is started for a thrombotic event, the patient should remain on therapy until nephrotic syndrome has resolved and should be restarted if there is recurrence.

* **Aggressive cytotoxic therapy is reserved for patients considered to be at higher risk for kidney disease progression,** as the natural history can be relatively benign in up to one-half of affected patients. The higher-risk group has decreased kidney function and/or has proteinuria in excess of 8 g/d for >6 months despite maximal therapy to reduce proteinuria.
  ○ **Ponticelli protocol** for the treatment of MN (10-year follow-up study by Italian group):

- **Months 1, 3, and 5:** Methylprednisolone, 1 g given intravenously for 3 days, followed by prednisone, 0.5 mg per kg of ideal body weight PO daily for the remainder of the 4 weeks.
- **Months 2, 4, and 6:** Chlorambucil, 0.2 mg per kg of ideal body weight PO daily for 4 weeks.
- At 10-year follow-up, 88% of patients treated with this protocol had partial or complete remission compared with 47% of controls. The original study reported using chlorambucil (0.2 mg/kg). However, these doses are limited by bone marrow toxicity of chlorambucil and lower doses may be a more prudent course.
  - ○ In the United States, a more popular protocol has been **cyclophosphamide and corticosteroids.** Cyclophosphamide, 1.5 to 2 mg/kg of ideal body weight per day PO daily, plus prednisone, 0.5 mg/kg of ideal body weight per day PO daily, can be given for 3 to 6 months. This regimen has been found to be comparable to the original Ponticelli protocol in smaller studies.
  - ○ In both regimens, **white blood cell (WBC) counts should be carefully monitored.** Typically, the WBCs are monitored weekly with both chlorambucil and cyclophosphamide use.
  - ○ **Prophylaxis against opportunistic infections** such as cytomegalovirus, herpes zoster virus, *Pneumocystis jirovecii* should be considered in the setting of immunosuppressive medications.
  - ○ **Alternative regimens** include:
    - **Cyclosporine,** 3.5 to 5 mg/kg of ideal body weight per day (trough levels of 125 to 175 ng/mL) or tacrolimus, 0.05 mg/kg/d in two divided doses with or without low-dose prednisone, which usually requires a more prolonged course (1 to 1.5 years) to sustain remission.
    - **MMF plus steroids** had shown some promise in small case series, but a recent controlled trial **did not show any significant benefit** over conservative management with blood pressure control, use of ACE inhibitors and statins. It is not recommended in the treatment of MN.
    - **Rituximab,** a monoclonal anti-CD20 antibody, has been used with success in resistant MN.

OUTCOMES/PROGNOSIS

- **Factors associated with poor prognosis** include male gender, age >50 years, presence of hypertension, decreased glomerular filtration rate (plasma creatinine >1.2 mg/dL in women, >1.4 mg/dL in men), nephrotic syndrome of >6-month duration, focal sclerosis, and >20% interstitial fibrosis on renal biopsy specimen.
- Spontaneous, partial, or complete remission is seen in up to 50% of patients with MN within 3 to 5 years of diagnosis.
- Up to one-fourth of patients who remit may experience a relapse of nephrotic range proteinuria that may require disease-specific therapy.

Membranoproliferative Glomerulonephritis

GENERAL PRINCIPLES

Definition
MPGN is a pathologic diagnosis based on the finding of diffuse mesangial proliferation, thickening of the capillary wall, subendothelial immune deposits, and

hypercellularity. Most cases are associated with circulating immune complexes and hypocomplementemia.

Classification

- Traditionally, MPGN has been classified into three types based on electron microscopic findings. Advances in our understanding of pathophysiology have led to a newer classification scheme, based on underlying immunopathology.
- Both methods of classification are outlined below.

Classification Based on Electron Microscopy: Type I MPGN
- **Pathology:**
  - Type I MPGN is defined by **subendothelial and mesangial immune deposits** seen on EM at renal biopsy.
  - Light microscopy reveals expanded mesangium with increased matrix and cellularity, with a classic lobular appearance to the glomeruli. Using the methenamine silver stain, a double contouring of the GBM can often be appreciated ("**tram tracks**").
  - Immunofluorescence usually shows discrete, granular staining of the peripheral capillary wall for IgG and C3.
  - Type I MPGN is frequently idiopathic but is also often associated with cryoglobulinemia, chronic HCV infection, chronic hepatitis B viral infection, endocarditis, or malarial infection.
  - Cryoglobulinemic MPGN may histologically appear similar to MPGN type 1. However, intracapillary hyaline-like deposits (cryoprecipitates) can be found by light microscopy occasionally. EM may also show the highly organized tubular or finely fibrillar structures consistent with cryoglobulins.
- **Pathogenesis:**
  - Type I MPGN is most likely associated with chronic immune-complex diseases.
  - The pathogenesis includes glomerular deposition of immune complexes that preferentially localize to the mesangium and subendothelial space, with subsequent **complement activation of the classical pathway** with resultant inflammation, leukocyte infiltration, and cellular proliferation.
  - Type I MPGN can also be associated with hereditary complement deficiencies (C1q, C2, C4, or C3) or with impaired reticuloendothelial system, as occurs with liver or splenic disease.
  - C3, C4, and CH50 are reduced in most cases.

Classification Based on Electron Microscopy: Type II MPGN (Dense Deposit Disease)
- **Pathology:**
  - Type II MPGN is defined by the presence of **electron-dense deposits within the mesangium and the GBM** on EM.
  - The immunofluorescence staining is positive for C3 but is negative for both classic complement pathway components and for immunoglobulins.
  - It is now reclassified as a complement-mediated glomerular disease (**C3 glomerulopathy**).
- **Pathogenesis:**
  - Type II MPGN is associated with **C3 nephritic factor** (a circulating autoantibody that binds to C3 convertase and prevents its inactivation by factor H) or the dysfunction of a constitutive inhibitor **factor H,** which leads to constitutive **activation of the alternate pathway of complement** and damage to the GBM.
  - The condition is associated with **partial lipodystrophy** in up to 25% of pediatric patients, leading to marked reduction in subcutaneous fat tissues, especially in the face and upper body.
  - **C3 and CH_{50} are reduced** in most cases; C4 is usually normal.

Classification Based on Electron Microscopy: Type III MPGN

- **Pathology:**
  - ○ Type III MPGN is defined by diffuse **subendothelial deposits** and electron-dense **deposits within the GBM and in the subepithelial spaces.**
  - ○ The immunofluorescence pattern of MPGN type III is similar to MPGN type I.
- **Pathogenesis:**
  - ○ Type III MPGN includes activation of the classic or terminal pathway of complement activation.
  - ○ The nephritic factor of the terminal pathway may be present in this form. It activates terminal components and requires properdin.
  - ○ C3 and the terminal complement components (C5 through C9) are reduced, and C5b to C9 membrane attack complex levels are elevated.

Classification Based on Immunopathology

- **Immune complex–mediated MPGN** results from chronic antigenemia and/or circulating immune complexes and can be seen in chronic infections, autoimmune diseases, and monoclonal gammopathies.
- **Complement-mediated MPGN** is less common than immune complex–mediated MPGN and results from dysregulation and persistent activation of the **alternative complement pathway.** Immunofluorescence microscopy of kidney sections demonstrates predominantly **bright C3 staining,** but **no significant immunoglobulin staining,** in the mesangium and along the capillary walls. It may be further classified as **DDD and C3 glomerulonephritis** based upon ultrastructural features observed on EM.

DIAGNOSIS

Clinical Presentation

- Clinical presentation of patients with MPGN types 1 and 2 can range from **nephrotic syndrome** and **microscopic or gross hematuria** to **acute nephritic syndrome** with rapid decline of kidney function.
- MPGN type I is frequently associated with **cryoglobulinemia and HCV** infection in older adults (aged >30 years). MPGN type II is most often seen in children.
- Hypertension is present in a majority of cases.
- Diagnosis of MPGN should prompt investigation for underlying causes, including blood cultures to rule out infective endocarditis; serologies for hepatitis B, HCV, and HIV; evaluation for malignancy; chronic liver disease; or SLE.

Diagnostic Testing

- **Type I and cryoglobulinemic MPGN:** Low C3, low C4, low CH_{50}
- **Type II:** Low C3, normal C4, low CH_{50}, C3 nephritic factor present in ~60% of cases
- **Type III:** Low C3, low C5 to C9
- **Cryoglobulinemia:**
  - ○ Cryoglobulins are immunoglobulins that precipitate in the cold.
  - ○ **Type 1 cryoglobulinemia** is a monoclonal immunoglobulin (IgG, IgM, or IgA), associated with lymphoproliferative disease (multiple myeloma, chronic lymphocytic leukemia, Waldenström macroglobulinemia).
  - ○ **Type II (mixed essential cryoglobulinemia)** is a mixture of polyclonal immunoglobulin in association with a monoclonal immunoglobulin typically IgM or IgA, with **rheumatic factor** activity.
  - ○ **Type III** is polyclonal immunoglobulin without a monoclonal immunoglobulin component. Types II and III are most commonly associated with MPGN. They have also been strongly related to **chronic HCV infection.**

○ **Systemic cryoglobulinemia** in patients who usually have chronic HCV infection may present with the **triad of weakness, arthralgias, and painless, palpable, nonpruritic purpura.** The vasculitic lesions classically involve the lower extremities and buttocks. Other manifestations may include Raynaud phenomenon, digital necrosis, peripheral neuropathy, and hepatomegaly.

TREATMENT

- Always **exclude causes of secondary MPGN** before planning treatment.
- General measures to reduce proteinuria, control blood pressure, and treat dyslipidemia are indicated for all types.
- **For patients with normal renal function and asymptomatic nonnephrotic range proteinuria, no specific therapy is necessary.** Close follow-up every 3 to 4 months is recommended.
- In patients with nephrotic syndrome or progressive renal failure, **corticosteroids** (tapering prednisone started at 1 mg/kg/d) **with or without cytotoxic agents** may be prescribed.
- Treatment with **cyclosporine, tacrolimus, or MMF** can be considered if there is no response to steroids within 3 to 4 months.
- **HCV-associated cryoglobulinemia** has been successfully treated with pegylated interferon-α plus ribavirin in the setting of stable renal function. If renal function is rapidly deteriorating (commonly termed **fulminant cryoglobulinemia**), high-dose steroid therapy is indicated, with or without cytotoxic therapy and plasma exchange.

OUTCOMES/PROGNOSIS

- Untreated MPGN progresses to death or ESRD in 50% of adults within 5 years and up to 90% in 20 years.
- The factors associated with poor outcome include nephrotic syndrome, an elevated serum creatinine, hypertension (or blood pressure well above the patient's previous baseline), and crescents on renal biopsy.
- The disease can recur after renal transplantation. Immune complex–mediated MPGN secondary to infection or autoimmune disease is less likely to recur than MPGN due to a monoclonal gammopathy or complement-mediated disease.

IGA Nephropathy and Henoch–Schönlein Purpura

GENERAL PRINCIPLES

- IgA nephropathy (also known as **Berger disease**) is the **most common form of glomerular disease diagnosed worldwide.**
- The incidence in the United States and Canada is substantially lower than that in Europe and Asia. This discrepancy may be due to rates of routine urinalysis in the United States compared with Asian countries and due to attitudes toward doing kidney biopsies in patients with asymptomatic hematuria.
- In populations of Caucasian descent, the male-to-female ratio is 3:1, whereas the ratio approaches 1:1 in most Asian populations.
- **Henoch–Schönlein purpura** is a syndrome associated with IgA deposition in the kidney with other systemic features. This disorder is seen predominantly in children and adolescents.

DIAGNOSIS

- **Microscopic or gross hematuria** is almost always part of the initial presentation of IgA nephropathy.
  - Asymptomatic microscopic hematuria with variable degrees of proteinuria is found in 30% to 40% of cases.
  - Acute macroscopic hematuria concurrent with upper respiratory tract infection is seen in roughly 50% of patients. The timing of the hematuria after the infection is usually **within 1 to 2 days.** This is in **contrast to poststreptococcal glomerulonephritis,** in which the hematuria (often associated with nephritic syndrome) **occurs 10 to 14 days** after pharyngitis.
- Occasionally, patients will present with nephrotic syndrome, acute kidney injury, or rapid progressive course with glomerular epithelial crescents on biopsy (<10%).
- Progressive renal insufficiency and hypertension are seen in a minority of patients.
- Laboratory evaluation demonstrates normal complement levels. Plasma polymeric IgA1 levels are elevated in 30% to 50% of cases, but this suggestive finding is not sufficiently specific to establish the diagnosis.
- Diagnosis is made by renal biopsy.
- **Henoch–Schönlein purpura** is a syndrome with IgA nephropathy associated with systemic vasculitis caused by IgA deposition. It is usually seen in children and adolescents and presents with arthralgia, purpuric skin rash (buttocks, abdomen, lower extremities), abdominal pain, ileus, or gastrointestinal bleeding. Renal involvement may be transient.

Differential Diagnosis

IgA deposition associated with mesangial cell proliferation can appear **secondary to systemic diseases** associated with decreased IgA clearance or increased IgA production.

- Celiac sprue
- Cirrhosis
- Inflammatory bowel disease
- Ankylosing spondylitis
- Dermatitis herpetiformis
- IgA monoclonal gammopathy
- HIV

Diagnostic Testing

- Light microscopy reveals global or segmental **mesangial hypercellularity** with normal-appearing peripheral GBMs.
- Immunofluorescence demonstrates mesangial IgA deposition, codeposition of C3, and, less commonly, IgG and IgM codeposition.
- EM shows electron-dense deposits that are primarily limited to the mesangium, but may also occur in the subendothelial and subepithelial spaces. Some patients have coexisting diffuse thinning of the GBM that is indistinguishable from thin basement membrane nephropathy.

Treatment

- Little controversy exists in the general management of patients with IgA nephropathy.
- **If proteinuria is <0.5 g/d, no specific treatment is indicated.**
- The treatment of IgA nephropathy with **proteinuria >0.5 g/d** remains controversial.
  - Blood pressure control with **ACE inhibitor or ARB** treatment when proteinuria is >0.5 g/d, with up-titration of the drug depending on blood pressure.
  - **Fish oil** is suggested in the treatment of IgA nephropathy with persistent proteinuria ≥1 g/d, despite 3 to 6 months of optimized supportive care (including ACE inhibitor or ARB and blood pressure control).

○ **Immunosuppressive therapy:**
  - If proteinuria is still >1 g/d on maximal supportive therapy and glomerular filtration rate (GFR) >50 mL/min per 1.73 m^2, consider a trial of steroids for 6 months.
  - In IgA nephropathy, when MCD with nephrotic syndrome coincides, a trial of high-dose corticosteroid therapy is justified.
  - If there is crescentic IgA nephropathy, treat aggressively to save renal function with steroids and cyclophosphamide.
- Mesangial IgA deposition occurs in up to 60% of patients receiving a renal transplant for ESRD secondary to primary IgA nephropathy, but the majority of recurrences do not worsen graft outcome and have a benign course.

OUTCOMES/PROGNOSIS

- The majority of patients with IgA nephropathy do not progress to ESRD and experience a benign disease course.
- Several **markers predicting a better outcome** are minimal proteinuria, normal blood pressure, and normal renal function on presentation. In addition, lack of fibrosis in glomeruli and tubulointerstitium is a good prognostic sign.
- Approximately 30% of patients with IgA nephropathy will experience progressive disease. These patients often have **poor prognostic features** including poorly controlled hypertension, older age at diagnosis, persistent proteinuria >1 g/d, reduced renal function at diagnosis, and tubulointerstitial fibrosis or more advanced glomerular lesions on renal biopsy.

REFERENCES

1. Matalon A, Markowitz GS, Joseph RE, et al. Plasmapheresis treatment of recurrent FSGS in adult renal transplant recipients. *Clin Nephrol.* 2001;56(4):271–278.
2. Rydel JJ, Korbet SM, Borok RZ, et al. Focal segmental glomerular sclerosis in adults: presentation, course, and response to treatment. *Am J Kidney Dis.* 1995;25(4):534–542.
3. Weber S, Gribouval O, Esquivel EL, et al. NPHS2 mutation analysis shows genetic heterogeneity of steroid-resistant nephrotic syndrome and low post-transplant recurrence. *Kidney Int.* 2004;66(2):571–579.
4. Winn MP, Conlon PJ, Lynn KL, et al. A mutation in the TRPC6 cation channel causes familial focal segmental glomerulosclerosis. *Science.* 2005;308(5729):1801–1804.
5. Debiec H, Guigonis V, Mougenot B, et al. Antenatal membranous glomerulonephritis due to anti-neutral endopeptidase antibodies. *N Engl J Med.* 2002;346(26):2053–2060.
6. Beck LH Jr, Bonegio RG, Lambeau G, et al. M-type phospholipase a2 receptor as target antigen in idiopathic membranous nephropathy. *N Engl J Med.* 2009;361(1):11–21.

Secondary Glomerular Disease

Tingting Li

10

Renal Diseases in Systemic Lupus Erythematosus

GENERAL PRINCIPLES

- Systemic lupus erythematosus (SLE) is a complex, often debilitating, and potentially life-threatening chronic autoimmune disorder that can affect any organ.
- Lupus nephritis is a common and severe manifestation of SLE that can lead to significant morbidity and mortality.
- Renal involvement is extremely diverse, ranging from asymptomatic urinary findings to fulminant renal failure or florid nephrotic syndrome.
- Renal manifestations may be the initial presentation of SLE, or may emerge later in the disease course.
- The incidence and prevalence of SLE vary with age (more common in those <55), gender (female >> male), and ethnicity (blacks and Hispanics > Caucasians).
- Approximately 20% to 50% of patients with SLE will develop clinically evident lupus nephritis.
- The risk of nephritis is the greatest during the first 2 years following SLE diagnosis and the incidence is significantly higher in Asians, blacks, and Hispanics compared to Caucasians. Male gender and younger age at SLE diagnosis are also risk factors for development of lupus nephritis.
- Up to 30% of patients with proliferative lupus nephritis will develop end-stage renal disease (ESRD) within 15 years of diagnosis.
- Patients with lupus nephritis have increased risk of cardiovascular mortality and all-cause mortality.

DIAGNOSIS

Clinical Presentation

- Lupus nephritis is often accompanied by extrarenal manifestations of SLE.
- Proteinuria is present in virtually every patient with renal involvement. Nephrotic-range proteinuria and/or nephrotic syndrome occur in approximately 50% of patients with proteinuria.
- Microscopic hematuria is present in the majority of patients with lupus nephritis and both red blood cell casts and white blood cell casts can be seen on urine microscopy.
- Reduced renal function can occur in >50% of patients with lupus nephritis although rapidly progressive glomerulonephritis (RPGN) is uncommon.
- Hypertension can be present, especially in those with severe nephritis.
- Renal tubular dysfunction (type I and IV renal tubular acidosis) can also occur and may be associated with hypokalemia or hyperkalemia.

TABLE 10-1	ABBREVIATED INTERNATIONAL SOCIETY OF NEPHROLOGY/RENAL PATHOLOGY SOCIETY 2003 CLASSIFICATION OF LUPUS NEPHRITIS
I	Minimal mesangial lupus nephritis
II	Mesangial proliferative lupus nephritis
III	Focal lupus nephritis (<50% of glomeruli involved)
IV	Diffuse segmental (IV-S) or global (IV-G) lupus nephritis (≥50% of glomeruli involved)
V	Membranous lupus nephritis
VI	Advanced sclerosing lupus nephritis (≥90% glomeruli globally)

From Weening JJ, D'Agati VD, Schwartz MM, et al. The classification of glomerulonephritis in systemic lupus erythematosus revisited. *J Am Soc Nephrol.* 2004;15(2):241–250.

Diagnostic Testing

- Lupus nephritis is usually suspected based on abnormal urinary findings and elevated serum creatinine in a patient with known SLE or suspected SLE.
- Although certain clinical features may suggest a particular class of lupus nephritis, clinical presentation does not necessarily correlate with histologic findings. Therefore, renal biopsy is necessary for definitive diagnosis. Renal pathology can also inform prognosis and guide treatment.
- Renal biopsy is usually recommended in all patients with SLE who have proteinuria (usually >500 mg/day), active urinary sediment, and/or reduced renal function, unless there is a contraindication for the biopsy procedure.
- All compartments, including the glomeruli, tubules, interstitium, and vasculature, can be affected.
- The 2003 International Society of Nephrology/Renal Pathology Society classification of lupus nephritis is a modification of the older World Health Organization classification scheme.[1] It focuses on glomerular lesions and divides them into six patterns based on light microscopy, immunofluorescence (IF), and electron microscopy (EM) (please see Table 10-1).
- On IF microscopy, IgG is the predominant immunoglobulin in the glomerular deposits. Complements are usually present. The presence of IgG, IgA, IgM, C3, and C1q, also known as "full-house" staining pattern, is highly suspicious for lupus nephritis.

TREATMENT

- Significant advances have been made over the last few decades in the diagnosis and treatment of lupus nephritis, leading to considerable improvement in patient survival.
- However, the number of patients reaching ESRD has not changed significantly in the last decade, reflecting limitations in our management strategies.
- In addition, adverse effects of therapy remain an important contributor to morbidity and mortality.
- The goal of lupus nephritis treatment is to prevent ESRD and death by inducing remission of nephritis, preventing relapse, and minimizing therapy-related complications.
- In all classes of lupus nephritis, blockade of renin–angiotensin–aldosterone system and treatment of dyslipidemia should be implemented. Blood pressure needs to be well controlled.

- Antimalarial therapy (hydroxychloroquine or chloroquine) has been shown to decrease lupus flares and possibly reduce the incidence of ESRD and should be used in all patients with lupus nephritis in the absence of contraindications. Routine monitoring for ocular toxicity is mandatory.
- **Class I and II:**
  - ○ Patients with mesangial lupus nephritis have an excellent renal prognosis and immunosuppressive therapy is not indicated (unless needed for extrarenal manifestations of lupus). Conservative management should include optimal blood pressure control and blockade of the renin–angiotensin–aldosterone system, as well as addition of antimalarial therapy.
  - ○ One should be aware that transformation to a different class of lupus nephritis can occur and close monitoring of renal function and proteinuria/hematuria is crucial.
- **Class III and IV:**
  - ○ Immunosuppressive therapy is necessary and should be given promptly when active proliferative lupus nephritis is present as the risk for progressive renal failure is high if treatment is inappropriate or is delayed.
  - ○ **Induction therapy** usually consists of glucocorticoids (methylprednisolone 500–1000 mg IV daily for 3 days, followed by prednisone 1.0 mg/kg/day with tapering over 6 to 12 months) and either cyclophosphamide or mycophenolate mofetil (MMF). Other agents have been less well studied and are not recommended as first-line induction therapy.
    - ■ **Cyclophosphamide:** Both oral and intravenous forms have been used for induction and have been shown to have similar efficacy. The cumulative dose is usually higher with oral cyclophosphamide and this may have implications in long-term toxicity (risk of malignancy and infertility). The choice of oral versus intravenous cyclophosphamide is often center dependent and may also be influenced by other factors such as cost, medical adherence of the patient, and previous exposure to cyclophosphamide. The following regimens have been used:
      - □ Cyclophosphamide 0.5 to 1 g/m^2 IV monthly for 6 months, followed by maintenance therapy (see below). This is the National Institute of Health (NIH) protocol.
      - □ Cyclophosphamide 500 mg IV every 2 weeks, for a total of 6 doses, followed by maintenance therapy. This is the Euro-Lupus Nephritis Trial regimen which was shown in a European cohort to be as effective as the NIH protocol but with fewer side effects. More recently, this regimen has been used effectively in an Asian Indian population and a North American cohort.
      - □ Cyclophosphamide 1.0 to 1.5 mg/kg PO daily (maximum dose 150 mg/day) for 2 to 4 months, followed by maintenance therapy.
      - □ If response to cyclophosphamide is inadequate in 3 to 6 months, it should be switched to MMF.
      - □ Adverse effects of cyclophosphamide include cytopenias, infections, bladder toxicity, gonadal toxicity, cardiac toxicity, and long-term risks of malignancy. Most of these complications are dose dependent, therefore cyclophosphamide should be used at the lowest effective dose and with the shortest duration possible. Dose adjustment should be made based on white blood cell count, age, and renal function.
    - ■ **MMF** 2 to 3 g PO daily for 6 months followed by maintenance therapy. We start with a lower dose of 500 mg bid for the first week, and increase to 1000 mg bid in the second week. If response is inadequate with 1000 mg bid and MMF is well tolerated, we then increase the dose to 1500 mg bid (or 1000 mg tid, which may be better tolerated from the GI standpoint).
      - □ As induction therapy, MMF has been demonstrated to be equally efficacious as cyclophosphamide. Adverse events were also found to be similar.

□ Limited data have suggested that MMF may be more effective in blacks and the Hispanic population.

□ In our opinion, MMF should be the preferred induction agent if a patient has had repeated exposures to cyclophosphamide therapy previously.

□ If response to MMF is inadequate in 3 to 6 months, it should be changed to cyclophosphamide. If cyclophosphamide were not an acceptable therapy for any reason, our next option would be rituximab (see below).

□ As MMF has not been tested vigorously in patients with severe lupus nephritis, it is unknown at this time whether MMF should be used as the first-line induction agent for severe lupus nephritis. In addition, data on long-term outcomes in patients treated with MMF are lacking.

□ Adverse effects include GI intolerance (nausea, vomiting, diarrhea, dyspepsia, and abdominal pain), infections, and cytopenias are most common. Dose adjustment should be made in decreased renal function.

□ In the case of severe GI side effects, consideration can be made to switch MMF to enteric-coated mycophenolate sodium although the latter has not been adequately studied in lupus nephritis patients.

- **Calcineurin inhibitors** (cyclosporine and tacrolimus) have been shown to be as effective as cyclophosphamide or MMF in small studies (mostly in the Asian population). They are not recommended as first-line induction therapies at this time. However, they can be considered in patients who do not respond to standard-of-care induction therapies. An ongoing multinational clinical trial is evaluating the efficacy of voclosporin in patients with lupus nephritis and receiving background therapy with MMF.

- **Rituximab,** a monoclonal antibody directed against the CD20 antigen on B cells, has not been proven to be efficacious as initial induction therapy in lupus nephritis but it may have a role in the management of patients with refractory lupus nephritis.

- **Azathioprine** is no better than prednisone alone and may have a higher relapse rate than IV cyclophosphamide based on previous studies. It is not recommended as an induction agent in lupus nephritis but its use can be considered in pregnant patients with active lupus nephritis.

- There is no role for the use of plasma exchange in the treatment of lupus nephritis.

○ **Maintenance therapy**

- Up to 35% of patients with lupus nephritis will have a renal relapse after achieving initial remission. Maintenance therapy provides a lower-intensity immunosuppression and aims to prevent relapse.

- After achieving remission (usually after 3 to 6 months of induction therapy), MMF (1 to 2 g/day PO) or azathioprine (1.5 to 2.5 mg/kg/day PO) along with low-dose prednisone is generally prescribed. Both MMF and azathioprine have been shown to be safer and perhaps more effective than cyclophosphamide in the maintenance phase.

- MMF and azathioprine were found to be equally effective as maintenance therapy in a European cohort but MMF was superior to azathioprine in a diverse international cohort of lupus nephritis patients.[2,3] These two agents appeared to have similar side-effect profiles in these studies.

- Factors that determine the choice between MMF and azathioprine may include patient race/ethnicity, cost, and side effects. Azathioprine can be used relatively safely in pregnancy for maintenance whereas MMF is contraindicated in pregnancy.

- If a patient is unable to tolerate MMF or azathioprine, a calcineurin inhibitor can be used although there is less evidence supporting the use of this class of drugs for maintenance.

- The optimal duration of maintenance therapy is unknown. Most centers recommend at least 1 year. A repeat renal biopsy may help confirm histologic remission but this is rarely performed for this indication. In patients with frequent relapses or severe renal disease, maintenance therapy may need to be continued indefinitely.

- **Class V (lupus membranous nephropathy)**
  - Although patients with class V lupus nephritis have a better renal prognosis than those with proliferative lupus nephritis, up to 20% of patients progress to ESRD within 10 years.
  - Class V lupus nephritis can coexist with proliferative lupus nephritis or transform from a membranous pattern to a proliferative one.
  - Most nephrologists agree that immunosuppressive therapy should be offered to class V patients with nephrotic-range proteinuria/nephrotic syndrome and/or declining renal function, and to those with combined membranous and proliferative features on renal pathology.
  - There is no well-defined treatment strategy for those with subnephrotic proteinuria and normal renal function. Some advocate for close monitoring with conservative management while others recommend treatment with immunosuppressive therapy.
  - In patients with pure class V lupus nephritis, MMF, cyclosporine, IV cyclophosphamide, and azathioprine along with corticosteroid therapy have all shown efficacy. MMF was noted to be as effective as IV cyclophosphamide in a pooled analysis of 65 pure class V patients from two large randomized trials of lupus nephritis.[4] In a smaller randomized trial of 42 pure class V patients, cyclosporine and IV cyclophosphamide achieved similar rates of remission but relapse rate was higher in the cyclosporine group.[5]
  - The choice of induction therapy may be dependent upon cost, side effects, desire for fertility, and degree of renal dysfunction (caution with cyclosporine in patients with moderate to severe renal dysfunction). Induction therapy should be continued for 6 to 12 months before switching to maintenance therapy (with MMF or azathioprine).
  - Patients with concurrent proliferative features have worse long-term renal outcomes and should be treated based on the proliferative component of the disease. There is also some evidence supporting the use of combination therapy with MMF and tacrolimus as induction therapy in this subgroup of patients (multitarget therapy).

COMPLICATIONS

- **Lupus podocytopathy:** A distinct clinical entity in patients with SLE that is characterized by the presence of nephrotic syndrome and histologic findings that are similar to that of minimal change disease (MCD) or focal segmental glomerulosclerosis (FSGS), with severe podocyte foot process effacement and absence of immune deposits in the glomerular capillary wall. Patients may have concurrent class I or II lupus nephritis. Treatment with a course of high-dose corticosteroids usually results in rapid resolution of nephrotic syndrome in those whose pathology findings are similar to MCD. Response to corticosteroids in those with FSGS is variable.

- **Collapsing glomerulopathy** (also known as collapsing FSGS): Patients with this rare diagnosis usually present with nephrotic syndrome and renal insufficiency, and often progress to ESRD within months. It is seen more commonly in blacks and APOL1 risk alleles may be a predisposing factor. There is no proven therapy for collapsing glomerulopathy. Response to various immunosuppressive therapies is generally poor.

- **Thrombotic microangiopathy:** This usually occurs in association with antiphospholipid antibodies and can coexist with lupus nephritis. Patients with glomerular thrombotic microangiopathy frequently have other systemic manifestations of antiphospholipid syndrome. Treatment consists of long-term anticoagulation.

Pauci-Immune Glomerulonephritis

GENERAL PRINCIPLES

- **Pauci-immune GN** is characterized by necrotizing GN with minimal or no immune deposits in the glomerular capillary wall.
- It is a common manifestation of a spectrum of necrotizing small-vessel vasculitides that includes granulomatosis with polyangiitis (GPA), microscopic polyangiitis (MPA), renal-limited vasculitis (RLV), and rarely eosinophilic granulomatosis with polyangiitis (EGPA).
- These small-vessel vasculitides are strongly associated with the presence of circulating antineutrophil cytoplasmic antibodies (ANCA). Together, they are referred to as ANCA-associated vasculitis (AAV), for their clinical and histologic similarities, and the potential role of ANCA in the disease pathogenesis.
- ANCA is positive in 80% to 90% of patients with GPA, MPA, and RLV.
- The incidence and prevalence of AAV vary with the geographic region and are estimated at 20 patients/million and 100 to 250 patients/million, respectively.
- AAV is more common in men and in those >60 years of age, and there appears to be a Caucasian predominance.
- AAV is the most common cause of RPGN in adults. The disease is limited to the kidney in one-third of the patients.
- In GPA and MPA, renal involvement is seen in 18% to 50% of patients at presentation and increases to >80% to 90% during the course of their disease.

DIAGNOSIS

Clinical Presentation

- The clinical presentation of GPA and MPA can be quite diverse and the extent of systemic organ involvement may differ. Generalized, nonspecific signs and symptoms of systemic inflammation are common (malaise, anorexia, weight loss, fever, arthralgia, myalgia, etc.).
- GPA is characterized by necrotizing, granulomatous inflammation that typically involves the upper and lower respiratory tracts and the kidneys, although almost any other organ can be involved.
- MPA is also a multisystem disease. Similar to GPA, the kidneys and lungs are major target organs. However, the upper airway is less frequently involved.
- Renal involvement can develop in 80% to 90% of patients with GPA and over 90% to 95% of patients with MPA. Patients typically present with nephritic urine sediment, varying degrees of proteinuria, hypertension, and often a rapid decline in renal function (over days to weeks). Some patients, however, follow a more indolent renal course.

Diagnostic Testing

- The diagnosis of AAV should be made promptly so appropriate therapy can be initiated in a timely fashion. Clinical presentation and urinalysis are often suggestive. High index of suspicion is required in many cases.
- ANCA is a useful diagnostic marker and should be obtained if there is pretest suspicion for ANCA-associated GN.
- Indirect immunofluorescence microscopy (IIF) is performed as a screening test (cANCA vs. pANCA), followed by ELISA which identifies the specific autoantigen (myeloperoxidase [MPO] vs. proteinase 3 [PR3]).

- cANCA most often has specificity for proteinase 3, and pANCA most often has specificity for MPO. GPA is predominantly associated with PR3-ANCA, whereas MPA and RLV are primarily associated with MPO-ANCA.
- A negative ANCA test does not exclude the diagnosis, as 10% to 20% of patients with pauci-immune vasculitis do not test positive for ANCA.
- Given the potential toxicities associated with immunosuppressive therapy, renal biopsy is often necessary for definitive diagnosis of pauci-immune GN, unless there is an absolute contraindication to the biopsy procedure. Renal pathology also has prognostic implications.
- Segmental fibrinoid necrosis, crescent formation, and a paucity or lack of immune deposition by IF or EM are the main features. Granulomatous inflammation can be present in the kidney of patients with GPA but this finding is rare.

TREATMENT

- **Induction therapy**
  - **Cyclophosphamide**
    - Cyclophosphamide is given either orally at 1.5 to 2.0 mg/kg daily, or intravenously at 15 mg/kg every 2 weeks for 3 doses followed by pulses every 3 weeks, for a duration of 3 to 6 months. The dose of cyclophosphamide should be adjusted based on age, renal function, and WBC count.
    - PO and IV forms of cyclophosphamide have similar efficacy but total drug exposure is less in the IV form, which may translate into fewer side effects. Several studies have reported higher relapse rates in patients treated with IV cyclophosphamide but there were no differences between the PO and IV groups in terms of long-term patient or renal survival.
    - Patients need to be closely monitored for adverse effects of cyclophosphamide (previously discussed). At our center, we routinely administer Mesna with IV cyclophosphamide to prevent hemorrhagic cystitis.
  - **Rituximab** has been shown to be noninferior to cyclophosphamide (PO and IV) and perhaps more effective for relapsing disease, and the side-effect profiles are similar to that of cyclophosphamide.[6]
    - It is unclear, however, if rituximab alone is effective in severe renal disease (serum creatinine >4 mg/dL) or alveolar hemorrhage requiring mechanical ventilation (such patients were excluded from the clinical trial). Concurrent use of rituximab and IV cyclophosphamide (15 mg/kg × 2 doses) has been shown to be as effective as standard IV cyclophosphamide regimen in severe renal disease.
    - Rituximab is given at a dose of 375 mg/m^2 IV weekly for 4 weeks.
    - Some have used a regimen of 1000 mg IV on day 1, followed by another 1000 mg 2 weeks later.
    - Rituximab may be preferred in relapsing disease and in younger patients (due to fertility concerns from cyclophosphamide). The choice between rituximab and cyclophosphamide may also depend on disease severity, previous exposure to cyclophosphamide, and cost.
    - Plasma exchange (if used concurrently) should not be performed for 48 hours after administration of rituximab to prevent removal of the drug.
  - **Glucocorticoid therapy** is used in conjunction with either cyclophosphamide or rituximab for induction.
    - Pulse methylprednisolone 250 to 1000 mg IV daily × 3 days is given, followed by prednisone at 1 mg/kg/day.
    - Currently, there is no consensus on the duration of glucocorticoids or the rapidity of tapering in AAV. We hope that the recently completed PEXIVAS trial (plasma exchange and glucocorticoid dosing in antineutrophil cytoplasm antibody associated

vasculitis: a randomized controlled trial) will provide some guidance in this area of uncertainty.
  - At our center, we begin prednisone taper at 3 to 4 weeks if clinical improvement is observed, with the goal of discontinuing glucocorticoids by 6 to 9 months (if no extrarenal manifestations).
- **Therapeutic plasma exchange (TPE)** is often used as an adjunctive therapy in patients with severe renal insufficiency or dialysis dependency at presentation, alveolar hemorrhage, or concomitant antiglomerular basement membrane antibodies.
  - Rationale for TPE in AAV: Removal of pathogenic ANCA and mediators of inflammation may help achieve early disease control and limit organ damage.
  - However, studies evaluating the role of TPE in patients with AAV and renal disease have been limited by their small sample size and inclusion of non-AAV patients. The long-term benefits of TPE have not been demonstrated in these studies.
  - The PEXIVAS trial is the largest, randomized controlled trial that aims to evaluate the efficacy of TPE in patients with severe AAV (moderate to severe renal insufficiency and/or diffuse alveolar hemorrhage). This trial will more definitively determine the role of TPE in AAV.
- For those patients who are dialysis dependent but do not show signs of renal recovery after 2 to 3 months of induction therapy, continued immunosuppressive therapy should be dictated by extrarenal involvement.
- **Maintenance therapy**
  - After 3 to 6 months of induction therapy, patients are switched to maintenance therapy in order to prevent disease relapse.
  - Due to concerns for significant toxicity, cyclophosphamide is no longer recommended as a maintenance agent.
  - Azathioprine (2 mg/kg PO daily) has been shown to be as effective as cyclophosphamide and is the most commonly used maintenance therapy.
  - MMF is less effective than azathioprine for maintaining disease remission but can be used if azathioprine is not tolerated.
  - Methotrexate is also a reasonable option but its use is limited to patients with eGFR >60 mL/min/1.73 m^2.
  - Rituximab may be more likely to induce sustained remission than azathioprine in PR3-positive patients and is increasingly used as maintenance therapy. The most common regimen is 500 mg IV every 6 months.
  - Glucocorticoids play very little role in the maintenance phase and should be tapered to a very low dose or tapered off.
  - The optimal duration of maintenance therapy is unknown. Most recommend 12 to 18 months to reduce the risk of relapse. Those who are at higher risk for relapse may require a longer maintenance duration.

OUTCOME/PROGNOSIS

- Without treatment, 1-year mortality in patients with AAV is about 80%. With aggressive immunosuppressive therapy, both 5-year patient survival and renal survival have increased to >80% in the recent years.
- Despite the improvement in patient survival, patients with AAV continue to have significantly higher mortality rate compared to that of the general population. Older age at disease onset, dialysis dependence, and presence of pulmonary hemorrhage are all risk factors for poor patient outcome.
- About 25% of patients progress to ESRD. The best predictors of poor renal outcome are the degree of renal dysfunction at the time of presentation and the extent of renal injury on renal pathology.

- Twenty to 50% of patients will relapse within 5 years of achieving remission. Patients with PR3-ANCA are more likely to relapse compared to those with MPO-ANCA.
- Renal transplantation remains a good option in ESRD patients who have quiescent clinical disease for at least 6 months prior to receiving a transplant. The presence of circulating ANCA without clinical disease activity is not a contraindication to renal transplantation.

Antiglomerular Basement Membrane Antibody Disease

GENERAL PRINCIPLES

- Antiglomerular basement membrane (anti-GBM) antibody disease is a small-vessel vasculitis that is characterized by necrotizing and crescentic immune-complex GN and/or alveolar hemorrhage in association with circulating antibodies against the noncollagenous 1 domain of the alpha-3 chain of type IV collagen in the glomerular and pulmonary capillaries.
- Anti-GBM antibody disease is a very rare condition, accounting for 1% to 2% of all glomerular diseases and <20% of all RPGN.
- The disease can occur at any age, but peaks usually in the second to third decade, with a smaller peak later in the sixth decade. There tends to be a male predominance in the younger patients and female predominance in the elderly patients.
- About 70% of patients have alveolar hemorrhage. Pulmonary involvement is more common in young males, whereas older patients are more likely to have isolated renal involvement. There appears to be an association between pulmonary hemorrhage and cigarette smoking.
- Up to 40% of patients with anti-GBM antibody disease have coexistent ANCA, typically MPO-ANCA (double-antibody positivity).

DIAGNOSIS

Clinical Presentation

- Renal disease typically presents as RPGN with rapid decline in renal function (over days to weeks), oliguria, and an active urinary sediment. Hypertension and edema can also be present. Rarely, patients may have a subacute course with slower decline in renal function.
- Pulmonary manifestations include hemoptysis, cough, and dyspnea with alveolar infiltrates on imaging studies.
- Patients with both anti-GBM antibody disease and AAV may have other features of a systemic vasculitis such as fever, malaise, or weight loss.

Diagnostic Testing

- Anti-GBM antibody disease is suspected when one presents with RPGN, especially in the setting of pulmonary-renal syndrome. The diagnosis is confirmed by the presence of circulating anti-GBM antibodies and findings on renal pathology.
- Serologic testing for ANCA should be done in all patients with anti-GBM disease given the high frequency of double-antibody positivity.
- One needs to keep in mind that patients with X-linked Alport syndrome can develop de novo anti-GBM antibody disease after renal transplantation, with the antibodies targeting primarily the alpha-5 chain of type IV collagen.
- On light microscopy, focal and segmental proliferative GN with areas of fibrinoid necrosis and crescent formation is typically seen.
- IF microscopy shows the classic pattern of linear IgG deposition along the glomerular basement membrane.

TREATMENT

- Standard therapy consists of TPE and cyclophosphamide/glucocorticoids.
- TPE is aimed at removal of circulating anti-GBM antibodies. It is performed daily or alternate day for 14 days or until antibody titer is at a very low level or undetectable. Please refer to TPE chapter on methods and prescription of plasma exchange.
- Cyclophosphamide (2 mg/kg/day PO for 3 months) and glucocorticoids (pulse methyl-prednisolone 500 to 1000 mg/day for 3 days, followed by prednisone 1 mg/kg/day PO, with taper over the next 6 to 9 months) are used to suppress production of anti-GBM antibodies.
- Other immunosuppressive agents such as rituximab and MMF have been used but evidence supporting the use of these therapies is lacking.
- Patients who do not have pulmonary disease and are dialysis dependent at the time of diagnosis, particularly those with crescents in all glomeruli, have a very poor renal prognosis and may not benefit from aggressive immunosuppression.
- For most patients, 2 to 3 months of therapy is adequate to induce complete remission. Clinical response and anti-GBM antibody titer should be monitored to determine the duration of therapy for the individual patient.
- Because of the low relapse rate in anti-GBM antibody disease, there is usually no need for maintenance therapy. However, maintenance therapy and close follow-up are required in those with concurrent ANCA positivity.

OUTCOME/PROGNOSIS

- Untreated patients have a fulminant course with mortality rate over 90%, emphasizing the need for a high level of suspicion for this disease, as well as early diagnosis and treatment.
- Patients who are dialysis dependent at the time of presentation have extremely poor prognosis with patient and renal survival of only 65% and 8%, respectively, at 1 year despite appropriate treatment. Patient and renal survival are significantly better if serum creatinine is <5.7 mg/dL at presentation.
- The prognosis of patients with double-antibody positivity parallels that of the anti-GBM antibody disease. As mentioned above, their relapse rates are similar to those with AAV.
- Those who reach ESRD should only undergo renal transplantation if their serum anti-GBM antibody titer remains negative for 6 months or longer.

Bacterial Infection–Related Glomerulonephritis

GENERAL PRINCIPLES

- Bacterial infections have been associated with acute immune-complex GN for many decades.
- Poststreptococcal GN (PSGN) is the prototype of infection-related GN (IRGN), which occurs following a pharyngeal or skin infection caused by certain nephritogenic strains of group A *Streptococci*.
- PSGN is primarily a disease of children and the peak incidence is in the first decade.
- The incidence of PSGN has been on the decline over the last 3 to 4 decades, especially in the developed countries. At the same time, there has been a notable increase in IRGN caused by bacterial pathogens other than Streptococci and affected patients are generally

adults, especially those whose age is >60 and immunocompromised. Diabetics are particularly at risk for IRGN.

- In the adult IRGN, the most common organism appears to be *Staphylococcus*, especially methicillin-resistant *Staphylococcus aureus* although many other gram-positive and gram-negative organisms have been identified as causative agents.
- In the adults, the infection is usually active when the acute GN is diagnosed, therefore the term "post-infectious GN" is inappropriate. The infection could be in any location of the body. Endocarditis, osteomyelitis, oral/visceral abscesses, pneumonia/empyema, skin infection, and eye infection have all been observed at our center.

DIAGNOSIS

Clinical Presentation

- In PSGN, there is typically a sudden onset of gross hematuria that is tea-colored, acute decline in renal function, varying degrees of proteinuria, hypertension, and edema that occur about 1 to 3 weeks after pharyngitis or a skin infection (latency period may be longer). Oliguria and, less commonly, anuria may occur. There is usually a recent history of streptococcal throat infection or skin infection.
- Renal manifestations are similar in adult IRGN except that renal failure tends to be more severe and a significant proportion of adults become dialysis dependent. In many cases, a concurrent infection is clinically evident.

Diagnostic Testing

- Urine sediment usually reveals dysmorphic red blood cells, red blood cell casts, granular casts, and sometimes WBC casts.
- Proteinuria is variable; nephrotic range is more common in adult IRGN.
- In PSGN, throat and skin cultures are infrequently positive as GN occurs after resolution of the infection. Anti-streptolysin O (ASO) and anti-deoxyribonuclease B (anti-DNAse B) titers are frequently elevated, the latter being more specific for skin infection. The streptozyme test (which measures antibodies to five different antigens—ASO, anti-DNAse B, anti-hyaluronidase, anti-streptokinase, and anti-NAD) is more sensitive.
- In adult IRGN, blood and/or wound cultures are frequently positive, as the infection is ongoing in most cases. When the infection is not clinically obvious, a thorough infectious workup should be pursued.
- Hypocomplementemia is common in both children and adults with IRGN. C3 is more frequently depressed than C4.
- ANCA and ANA can be positive in adult IRGN, especially in the setting of bacterial endocarditis. In patients who are ANCA positive, frequently both PR3- and MPO-ANCA are positive. Rarely, cryoglobulinemia has been found in patients with IRGN.
- The definitive diagnosis of IRGN is made based on renal pathology.
- On light microscopy, a diffuse endocapillary proliferative GN is seen. Neutrophils are abundant. Monocytic infiltrate can be present. The presence of crescents indicates a poor prognosis.
- IF microscopy reveals granular staining of C3 and IgG along the glomerular capillary walls and/or in the mesangium, frequently with codeposition of IgA and IgM, and possibly C1q. In certain cases, the glomerular staining may be C3-dominant. More recently, an IgA-dominant IRGN has been described with IgA as the dominant or co-dominant (with IgG) immunoglobulin. This is usually observed in older diabetic patients with an ongoing staphylococcal infection.
- On EM, large, dome-shaped subepithelial electron-dense deposits ("subepithelial humps") are characteristic. Smaller mesangial and subendothelial can also be seen.

TREATMENT

- In PSGN, treatment is generally supportive, including salt restriction, diuretics for edema, and blood pressure control.
- In adult IRGN, in addition to supportive management, antibiotics should be given if there is evidence of a persistent infection.
- For those patients who do not improve spontaneously (especially those with crescentic GN), glucocorticoids may be tried but the benefits are not well established. The use of more aggressive immunosuppressive therapy is not usually recommended, especially in the setting of an active infection.

OUTCOMES/PROGNOSIS

- In general, the clinical course and outcome of PSGN are favorable. Most children attain complete remission within a few weeks. In some patients, microscopic hematuria may persist for up to 6 months while mild proteinuria can be seen for years.
- In adult IRGN, complete remission is only seen in a minority of patients. At our center, 30% to 40% of patients reach ESRD, emphasizing the need for early detection and treatment of the underlying infection.

REFERENCES

1. Weening JJ, D'Agati VD, Schwartz MM, et al. The classification of glomerulonephritis in systemic lupus erythematosus revisited. *J Am Soc Nephrol.* 2004;15(2):241–250.
2. Houssiau FA, D'Cruz D, Sangle S, et al. Azathioprine versus mycophenolate mofetil for long-term immunosuppression in lupus nephritis: results of the MAINTAIN nephritis trial. *Ann Rheum Dis.* 2010;69(12):2083–2089.
3. Dooley M, Jayne D, Ginzler E, et al. Mycophenolate versus azathioprine as maintenance therapy for lupus nephritis. *N Engl J Med.* 2011;365(20):1886–1895.
4. Radhakrishnan J, Moutzouris D, Ginzler E, et al. Mycophenolate mofetil and intravenous cyclophosphamide are similar as induction therapy for class V lupus nephritis. *Kidney Int.* 2010;77(2):152–160.
5. Austin H, Illei G, Braun M, et al. Randomized, controlled trial of prednisone, cyclophosphamide, and cyclosporine in lupus membranous nephropathy. *J Am Soc Nephrol.* 2009;20(4):901–911.
6. Stone J, Merkel P, Spiera R, et al. Rituximab versus cyclophosphamide for ANCA-associated vasculitis. *N Engl J Med.* 2010;363(3):221–232.

Thrombotic Microangiopathy

Anuja Java

11

GENERAL PRINCIPLES

- Thrombotic microangiopathy (TMA) is a pathologic process caused by thrombotic occlusion of the systemic microvasculature, leading to end-organ ischemia and infarction.
- TMAs are characterized by thrombocytopenia (due to consumption), microangiopathic hemolytic anemia (MAHA; due to intravascular fragmentation), and variable degree of organ damage, with the kidney and the central nervous system being the most affected.
- The histologic lesions of a TMA are seen in several clinically diverse disorders. The major TMAs include thrombotic thrombocytopenic purpura (TTP), hemolytic uremic syndrome (HUS), and atypical hemolytic uremic syndrome (aHUS).

Definitions

The current **diagnostic criteria for TTP** include otherwise **unexplained thrombocytopenia** and **MAHA.** The classic pentad of thrombocytopenia, MAHA, fever, neurologic changes, and acute renal failure is seen in only 3% to 5% cases.

- Most cases of TTP are acquired and occur in adults (due to an autoantibody to ADAMTS-13, the 13th member of a disintegrin and metalloprotease family with thrombospondin domains).
  - Congenital TTP (Upshaw–Schulman syndrome) is a rare syndrome caused by deficiency of ADAMTS-13 due to homozygous or compound heterozygous mutations.
- **HUS** is defined by the same criteria as **TTP plus the presence of renal failure.**
  - Typical age of presentation is 1 to 5 years.
  - In the United States and Europe, 90% of cases are caused by Shiga toxin–producing *E. coli* O157:H7.
- **aHUS (complement-mediated HUS)** is a TMA resulting from an overactive complement system due to mutations in complement proteins.[1]

Pathophysiology

- **Thrombotic thrombocytopenic purpura**
  - TTP is often idiopathic but may be familial or related to pregnancy, collagen vascular diseases such as SLE, malignancy, infections (HIV, parvovirus), bone marrow transplantation, or medications. Oral contraceptives, ticlopidine (and less commonly clopidogrel), mitomycin C, gemcitabine, and multiple other chemotherapeutics, calcineurin inhibitors, interferon-α, and quinine have all been associated with TTP.
  - The pathogenesis of TTP is linked to inherited or acquired deficiencies of von Willebrand factor (vWF)-cleaving protease, which is normally responsible for cleaving and clearing large vWF multimers that promote platelet aggregation and microvascular thrombosis. An inhibitory autoantibody to vWF-cleaving protease has been found in patients with acquired TTP.
- **Hemolytic Uremic Syndrome:** Classic childhood Shiga toxin–mediated HUS, or **D+ HUS,** is caused by **certain *E. coli* strains (usually O157:H7) and Shigella.** Transmission is from contaminated food (e.g., undercooked meat) or secondary person-to-person

contact. The Shiga toxin triggers the microangiopathic process by entering the circulation via inflamed colonic tissue and causing endothelial damage and platelet activation.

- **Atypical Hemolytic Uremic Syndrome:** Mutations in genes for complement proteins are seen in ~50% to 60% of aHUS cases. These are either loss-of-function mutations in complement regulators (membrane cofactor protein [MCP], Factor H and Factor I) or gain-of-function mutations in complement proteins (C3 and Factor B). The delicate balance between complement activation and regulation is disturbed on endothelial cells, resulting in a TMA.

DIAGNOSIS

Clinical Presentation
- **Thrombotic thrombocytopenic purpura**
  - TTP occurs in adults, disproportionately affecting African-American women.
  - Clinical features are diverse (weakness, GI symptoms, and transient focal neurologic abnormalities are common). TTP is unique for rarely causing severe acute kidney injury. The diagnosis of TTP is a clinical one and the measurement of ADAMTS-13 activity level of <10% supports the clinical diagnosis.
- **Hemolytic uremic syndrome**
  - D+ HUS occurs most commonly in young children (aged <5 years) in the summer and is preceded by an acute hemorrhagic diarrheal illness. D+ HUS accounts for >90% of HUS.
  - Clinical features of HUS include abdominal pain and diarrhea, usually 3 to 4 days after consuming contaminated food. Thrombocytopenia and renal failure begin as GI symptoms resolve. Hypertension, purpuric rash, jaundice, pancreatitis, and mental status changes (lethargy, confusion, coma, and seizures) can be seen in some patients.
  - Laboratory features include schistocytes on peripheral blood smear, elevated lactate dehydrogenase, thrombocytopenia, elevated blood urea nitrogen and serum creatinine, and normal PT and PTT. Most patients have microscopic hematuria on urinalysis and proteinuria of varying degree. Evidence of *E. coli* O157:H7 infection may be present.
- **Atypical hemolytic uremic syndrome**
  - Clinical presentation includes the characteristic findings of TMA (MAHA, thrombocytopenia, and acute kidney injury). Extrarenal TMA manifestations are observed in up to 20% of patients including involvement of the central nerve system (CNS), cardiovascular system, lungs, skin, skeletal muscle, and GI tract.
  - A family history of aHUS is obtained in about 20% to 30% of patients.
  - Presentation later in life is consistent with the need of an environmental trigger (e.g., infection, pregnancy) that is thought to play a role in complement activation.

Diagnostic Testing
- ADAMTS-13 activity.
- Stool culture/serology/PCR to rule out Shiga toxin.
- Serum antigenic levels of complement proteins (C3, C4, Factor H, Factor I, Factor B) and surface expression of MCP (CD46).
- Genetic screening for mutations in complement genes.
- Renal histology in TMA reveals fibrin and platelet thrombi in glomerular capillaries, arterioles, and arteries. Arterioles and arteries demonstrate endothelial swelling and intimal thickening, causing luminal narrowing. Capillary wall double contours may be seen due to widening of the subendothelial space. Ischemic glomeruli may have wrinkled, partially collapsed capillaries. Acute cortical necrosis may occur in severe cases of disease.

- IF demonstrates diffuse fibrinogen staining in capillary and arterial walls.
- On EM, swelling of glomerular endothelial cells and widened subendothelial spaces are seen.

TREATMENT

- **Thrombotic thrombocytopenic purpura**
  - ○ **Plasma exchange is life saving and should be initiated promptly,** with consecutive daily treatments until platelet count is normal. Twice-daily exchanges may be required initially.
  - ○ Patients with normal ADAMTS-13 activity who clinically have TTP appear to benefit from plasma exchange as much as those with low ADAMTS-13 activity.
  - ○ For those with inadequate or no response to plasma exchange, **corticosteroids** can be used as an adjunctive therapy. Other therapies such as **plasma infusion, intravenous immunoglobulin infusion, rituximab, and splenectomy** have been used with variable efficacy.
  - ○ Newer therapies under development include recombinant ADAMTS-13 (for congenital TTP) and caplacizumab (a humanized monoclonal anti-VWF antibody).
  - ○ The prognosis of TTP varies with the underlying etiology. Mortality has decreased from 90% before availability of plasma exchange to 20% with plasma exchange. Relapses are rare.
- **Hemolytic uremic syndrome**
  - ○ **Treatment is supportive only** and includes attention to fluid–electrolyte imbalances, bowel rest, RBC transfusion, and renal replacement therapy if needed.
  - ○ The role of plasma exchange has not been adequately evaluated by randomized, controlled studies. Some recommend a trial of plasma exchange in severe cases.
  - ○ **Antibiotics and antimotility agents are not recommended.** In fact, there are several epidemiologic and retrospective studies showing increased incidence of HUS in patients treated with antibiotics and antimotility agents for diarrheal illnesses.
  - ○ Up to 90% have a partial recovery, although up to 40% may have reduced GFR and residual proteinuria. Adults tend to do worse than children.
- **Atypical hemolytic uremic syndrome**
  - ○ Patients with a diagnosis of aHUS should receive eculizumab (a humanized monoclonal antibody to complement C5) as the first-line treatment. The monoclonal antibody treatment should be initiated early to offer the best chance of renal recovery. However, treatment duration remains controversial.[2]
  - ○ Patients receiving eculizumab should receive vaccination against meningococcus, including type B.
  - ○ The prognosis of patients with aHUS has improved considerably with the use of eculizumab since ~65% patients treated with plasma exchange progressed to ESRD or died within 1 year.

REFERENCES

1. Java A, Atkinson J, Salmon JE. Defective complement inhibitory function predisposes to renal disease. *Annu Rev Med.* 2013;64:307–324.
2. Legendre C, Licht C, Muus P, et al. Terminal complement inhibitor eculizumab in atypical hemolytic-uremic syndrome. *N Engl J Med.* 2013;368(23):2169–2181.

Management of Chronic Kidney Disease

Nurelign Abebe and Marcos Rothstein

12

GENERAL PRINCIPLES

Definition

- Chronic kidney disease (CKD) is characterized by abnormalities of kidney structure or function, present for >3 months.
  - These abnormalities can manifest in a variety of ways, including a reduction in clearance (GFR <60 mL/min/1.73 m^2), impairment of the filtration barrier (albumin to creatinine ratio >30 mg/g), or a radiologic abnormality that reveals an underlying kidney disorder (such as polycystic kidney disease).
  - Most commonly, however, the term CKD is used to describe patients with a **GFR <60 mL/min.**
- The staging of CKD depends on the level of glomerular filtration rate (GFR).
- As patients progress through the stages of CKD, they develop complications associated with the loss of renal function, such as volume retention, electrolyte abnormalities, acid–base disorders, anemia, and mineral/bone disorders.
- The sequelae of renal disease culminate in the development of uremia, typically at a GFR of less than 15 mL/min. Preparing each patient for end-stage renal disease (ESRD) is an important part of care in the renal clinic and will be discussed in more detail later in this textbook.
- It must be kept in mind that management of CKD patients is complicated and involves close collaboration with their primary care physicians and other specialists (endocrinologists, cardiologists, vascular surgeons), as well as social workers and dieticians (please see Fig. 12-1).

Classification

- The most commonly used CKD classification is based on the Kidney Disease: Improving Global Outcomes (KDIGO) CKD Work Group and their Clinical Practice Guidelines for the Evaluation and Management of Chronic Kidney Disease (Fig. 12-2).[1]
- This classification has streamlined the management of CKD, as its terminology helps the healthcare professional, as well as the patients, to clearly understand the severity of the illness and outlines the risks for disease progression, morbidity, and mortality.

Associated Conditions

- **Electrolyte and acid–base disorders:**
  - With advancing CKD and decreasing GFR, the ability of the kidney to effectively eliminate the total acid load and potassium is reduced.
  - **Acidosis typically develops with GFR below 40 mL/min.**
  - Concomitant disorders such as diabetic nephropathy, obstructive nephropathy, sickle-cell anemia, and multiple myeloma, can cause tubular disorders which result in acidosis at earlier stages of CKD.

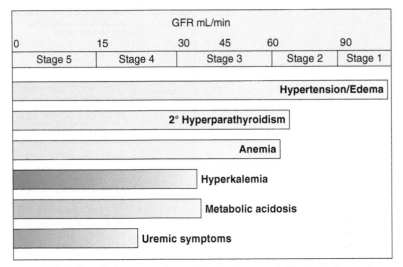

FIGURE 12-1. Onset of complications related to decreased GFR. This figure shows the complications of renal dysfunction in relation to GFR and stage of CKD. CKD, chronic kidney disease; GFR, glomerular filtration rate. (From Improving global outcomes (KDIGO) CKD work group. KDIGO 2012 clinical practice guideline for the evaluation and management of chronic kidney disease. *Kid Int Suppl.* 2013;1(3);1–150.)

- **Hypertension:**
  - The pathophysiology of hypertension is multifactorial.
  - In CKD, the retention of sodium and water, leading to extracellular volume expansion, is a significant contributor to hypertension.
  - The inappropriate secretion of renin also plays a key role in the development of hypertension in CKD.
- **Anemia:**
  - In patients with CKD, anemia is a common complication due to both impaired iron absorption and decreased secretion of erythropoietin.
  - Resistance to the action of erythropoietin also plays an important role in the development and maintenance of anemia in this patient population.
- **Mineral and bone disorders:**
  - The term renal osteodystrophy had previously been used to refer to bone disorders that resulted from CKD. However, to capture the broader implications of CKD on mineral metabolism and tissue calcification, it is now known as CKD mineral and bone disorder (CKD-MBD).
  - With reduced GFR, a complex cascade of changes begins to occur with profound impact on mineral homeostasis and bone health. These changes include the retention of phosphorus, increased levels of fibroblast growth factor 23 (FGF23), reduced activation of vitamin D, and resulting secondary hyperparathyroidism (SHPT).
- **Hyperlipidemia and cardiovascular disease:**
  - CKD is associated with increased rates of cardiovascular events, hospitalizations, and death.

				Persistent albuminuria categories Description and range		
				A1	A2	A3
		Prognosis of CKD by GFR and albuminuria categories: KDIGO 2012		Normal to mildly increased	Moderately increased	Severely increased
				<30 mg/g <3 mg/mmol	30–300 mg/g 3–30 mg/mmol	>300 mg/g >30 mg/mmol
GFR categories (mL/min per 1.73 m²) Description and range	G1	Normal or high	≥90			
	G2	Mildly decreased	60–89			
	G3a	Mildly to moderately decreased	45–59			
	G3b	Moderately to severely decreased	30–44			
	G4	Severely decreased	15–29			
	G5	Kidney failure	<15			

FIGURE 12-2. KDIGO CKD Work Group Classification of stages of CKD. Stages of CKD based on GFR (mL/min/1.73 m²); stage 1 CKD GFR >90, stage 2 CKD 60–89, stage 3 CKD 30–59, stage 4 CKD 15–29, and stage 5 CKD <15. (From Improving global outcomes (KDIGO) CKD work group. KDIGO 2012 clinical practice guideline for the evaluation and management of chronic kidney disease. *Kid Int Suppl.* 2013;1(3);1–150.)

○ It must be noted that a significantly higher number of patients with stage 3 or 4 CKD die of cardiovascular causes before reaching the need for dialysis or transplantation.
○ Modification of risk factors such as hyperlipidemia, hypertension, and bone and mineral disorders is critical in reducing mortality and morbidity from cardiovascular disease.

DIAGNOSIS

• In stable CKD, estimation of the GFR is required to appropriately stage the disease. The **MDRD** and **CKD-EPI** equations are creatinine-based estimates of GFR. Their uses and limitations are discussed more thoroughly in Chapter 1 of this book.
• **Urine protein excretion** is also a key characteristic of renal disease.
  ○ Heavy proteinuria is associated with progression of renal disease, and the amount of proteinuria serves as an indicator of the severity of disease in certain forms of glomerulonephritis.
  ○ Proteinuria can be quantified by a spot protein-to-creatinine ratio or a 24-hour urine collection for protein. Both techniques are described in Chapter 2 of this book.
• A variety of diagnostic laboratory tests can be used to help evaluate the cause of CKD.
  ○ Antinuclear antibodies (ANA), antineutrophil cytoplasmic antibody (ANCA), and complement levels (C3 and C4) are frequently sent in patients who present with

features of the nephritic syndrome. In the appropriate context, HIV and hepatitis serologies are also helpful as they may contribute to renal disease manifesting in this way.

○ In patients with nephrotic-range proteinuria, an evaluation for nephrotic syndrome includes quantification of urine protein excretion, serum albumin, and a lipid panel.

○ Older patients with concomitant back pain and/or anemia should be assessed for a monoclonal gammopathy.

  ■ **Serum free light chain ratios (FLC)** are sensitive in detecting monoclonal gammopathies and should be ordered in patients with high index of suspicion. Although this ratio is frequently elevated in CKD patients due to reduced clearance, a kappa/lambda ratio of more than 3 in CKD patients is concerning and should prompt further workup.

  ■ **Serum and urine protein electrophoresis, along with immunofixation,** are also useful diagnostic tools to evaluate for paraproteinemia and related renal disorders such as light chain deposition disease, cast nephropathy, and amyloidosis.

• **Evaluation of anemia associated with CKD**

  ○ Complete blood cell count is required at initial and subsequent office visits.

  ○ Ferritin and transferrin saturation levels are required to help guide the treatment of anemia.

  ○ The Kidney Disease Outcomes Quality Initiative (KDOQI) work group recommends a **ferritin level >100 ng/mL and a transferrin saturation >20%** in predialysis CKD patients.[2]

  ○ Some patients may respond to iron therapy even if these goals are met.

• **Evaluation of CKD-MBD**

  ○ **Parathyroid hormone (PTH), calcium, phosphorus, and 25-OH vitamin D** levels should be measured to assist in directing the management of renal osteodystrophy.

  ○ For CKD stages 3 and 4, the KDOQI work group recommends maintaining corrected calcium in the "normal" range for the laboratory used and a phosphorus value between 2.7 and 4.6 mg/dL.[3]

  ○ The same work group recommends measurement of intact PTH every 6 to 12 months.

  ■ KDOQI recommends a target PTH level between 35 and 70 pg/mL in stage 3 CKD and a target level between 70 and 110 pg/mL in stage 4 CKD.[3]

  ■ Newer recommendations by the KDIGO Clinical Practice Guidelines do not endorse the use of a specific target range.[4] Instead they suggest monitoring PTH trends and intervening if PTH levels are progressively rising.

• **Evaluation of electrolyte and acid–base disorders**

  ○ A complete panel of electrolytes should be reviewed at each visit to screen for the development of hyperkalemia.

  ○ A **total CO_2 levels of ≥22 mEq/L** is recommended for patients with a GFR <60 mL/min.

• **Evaluation of concomitant cardiovascular risk**

  ○ A **lipid panel** should be checked in all CKD patients at initial office visit and annually.

  ○ The optimal low-density lipoprotein cholesterol target has not been defined for the CKD population, but given the risk for cardiovascular disease, it is generally recommended to be <100 mg/dL.

  ○ It is generally recommended that triglyceride level be kept below 200 mg/dL.

• **Evaluation of nutritional status:** The current KDOQI Nutrition guidelines recommend checking **serum albumin** every 3 months in patients with a GFR <20 mL/min as an assessment of nutritional status. Albumin is a strong prognostic indicator in ESRD patients.

TREATMENT

- Nephrology consultation
  - Referral to a nephrologist **is almost always indicated once the GFR has fallen to <30 mL/min.**
  - However, **referral at earlier stages of CKD (i.e., GFR <60 mL/min)** is highly recommended when the progression of renal disease is anticipated or when further evaluation is necessary (e.g., diabetic nephropathy, lupus nephritis, vasculitis).
  - The nephrology clinic is often better prepared to coordinate the care of the CKD patient with anemia, difficult-to-control hypertension, significant proteinuria, or primary renal disease.
  - Late nephrology referral is associated with poorer outcomes and increased cost.
- **Hypertension**
  - Various recommendations exist regarding target blood pressure in CKD.
    - The Eighth Report of the Joint National Committee on Prevention, Detection, Evaluation, and Treatment of High Blood Pressure (JNC 8) recommends a goal BP of less than 140/90 mm Hg in patients with diabetes and/or CKD, which is the same threshold and goal for hypertensive adults and for the general hypertensive population younger than 60 years.[5]
    - KDOQI recommends a goal systolic BP of less than 130 mm Hg and diastolic of less than 80 mm Hg in patients with diabetes and/or CKD.[6]
  - While any class of antihypertensive agents can be used to achieve blood pressure goals, **angiotensin-converting enzyme (ACE) inhibitors or angiotensin receptor blockers (ARBs)** are particularly useful in CKD patients with proteinuria.
    - ACE inhibitors and ARBs classically lower intraglomerular pressure, thus protecting the kidneys from disease progression.
    - A renal function panel should be checked 1 to 2 weeks after starting treatment with ACE inhibitors or ARBs.
    - A 30% increase in creatinine is considered acceptable, although often hyperkalemia can limit the use of these medications.
    - No benefit is accrued from combined use of ACE inhibitors and ARBs.
  - Diuretics can also be extremely helpful given the importance of sodium and water retention to the development of hypertension in CKD. In addition, these agents serve additional purposes in the control edema and attenuate hyperkalemia.
- **Edema and volume overload**
  - Edema and volume overload are frequently seen in CKD, especially in the setting of nephrotic range proteinuria, congestive heart failure, pulmonary dysfunction, sleep apnea, and GFR <30 mL/min. It is important to evaluate and treat other etiologies of edema which may coexist in the CKD patient.
  - **Sodium restriction** is a critical component of fluid management. However, dietary restriction is often difficult to attain and insufficient to control edema.
  - **Diuretics** are an effective therapy in the management of hypertension and edema in CKD.
    - The effectiveness of thiazide diuretics is reduced in patients with GFR <40 mL/min.
    - Loop diuretics are useful in patients with low GFRs, but their effectiveness may be more limited in patients with a low serum albumin.
    - A reasonable starting dose for a loop diuretic in a patient with CKD is **furosemide 40 mg PO bid or bumetanide 1 mg PO bid.** A new steady state will be reached within 1 to 2 weeks.
- **Hyperkalemia**
  - Hyperkalemia is a potentially life-threatening complication of CKD.

○ Patients with CKD often have multiple risk factors which can predispose toward the development of hyperkalemia, including reduced renal potassium clearance, transcellular shift from acidemia, and concurrent use of renin–angiotensin–aldosterone inhibitors.

○ The acute and chronic management of this electrolyte disorder is discussed in detail in Chapter 4.

○ In the CKD population, the following interventions should be considered:
  ■ Restriction of dietary potassium intake
  ■ Increased kaliuresis using loop diuretics
  ■ Correction of metabolic acidosis
  ■ Use of enteric potassium-binding agents such as patiromer for persistent hyperkalemia despite the above interventions

● **Metabolic acidosis**
  ○ Metabolic acidosis can lead to decreased albumin production, increased calcium resorption from bone, and worsening of SHPT.
  ○ **Maintaining bicarbonate levels above 22 mEq/L** will help preserve bone histology and lessen the impact of acidosis on protein catabolism. There is also data suggesting that treatment of metabolic acidosis slows the rate of progression to ESRD while improving nutritional parameters in CKD patients.
  ○ The best available option for treating acidosis is **sodium bicarbonate 650 to 1300 mg PO BID–TID.** A 650-mg tablet contains 7.6 mEq of bicarbonate.

● **Hyperuricemia**
  ○ Hyperuricemia is prevalent in CKD due to decreased uric acid excretion. The use of thiazide diuretics may further decrease uric acid excretion.
  ○ Xanthine oxidase inhibitors, such as **allopurinol** or febuxostat, can be used to lower uric acid levels.
  ○ In patients who develop gout, acute flares are often treated with steroids. **Colchicine,** which undergoes renal excretion, can be used with close monitoring of side effects, such as diarrhea. Nonsteroidal anti-inflammatory medications should be used with extreme caution (if used at all) due to the potential for worsening renal function, increasing blood pressure control, and causing hyperkalemia.

● **Hyperlipidemia**
  ○ CKD patients should be considered in the highest-risk group for coronary artery disease.
  ○ The updated National Cholesterol Education Program Adult Treatment Program (NCEP ATP) III guidelines for cholesterol management recommends a low-density lipoprotein (LDL) cholesterol goal of <100 mg/dL for high-risk patients, defined as those with established CHD or coronary heart disease risk equivalents.
    ■ Lifestyle modifications are recommended for patients with LDL 100 to 130 mg/dL. Medications are recommended for those with LDL above 130 mg/dL or those failing lifestyle modifications.
    ■ Statins are first-line agents in CKD.
  ○ Hypertriglyceridemia is treated using lifestyle and dietary modifications, as well as medications with **goal of triglycerides of <200 mg/dL.**
    ■ Fibrates, such as gemfibrozil, are appropriate for use in CKD but the combination of fibrates and statins in the setting of CKD can result in increased risk of rhabdomyolysis.
    ■ Appropriate dose adjustments are necessary for the levels of renal function.
    ■ Fibrates are associated with reversible elevations of creatinine and carry a risk of interstitial nephritis.

● **Anemia and iron deficiency**
  ○ Iron deficiency should be aggressively managed in CKD patients.
    ■ Even in the absence of anemia, iron deficiency is associated with neurologic dysfunction, restless legs syndrome, fatigue, hair loss, and even worsening of cardiac dysfunction.

- If no contraindications exist, **iron replacement should begin via the oral route,** which is the preferred first line of treatment.
  - We recommend **ferrous sulfate 325 mg PO BID.**
  - Iron is best absorbed on an empty stomach and in an acidic environment.
  - Patients treated with antireflux medications will not absorb iron as efficiently as patients not taking these drugs.
- If the patient has suboptimal response to oral iron or if the patient is unable to tolerate the treatment, then **intravenous iron should** be considered.
  - The least expensive option is iron dextran. Because of risk of anaphylactic reactions, a 25-mg test dose should be administered and the patient monitored for any adverse events. If the patient tolerates the test dose without difficulty, a 500-to-1000 mg dose of iron dextran can be administered over 3 to 4 hours.
  - Iron sucrose and ferric gluconate preparations require multiple infusions of small doses.
  - Ferric carboxymaltose (Injectafer) 750 mg can be given in two doses, 1 week apart, to a maximum cumulative dose of 1500 mg per course of treatment.
  - An iron-deficient stage 3 CKD patient requires a standard anemia workup, including age-appropriate cancer screening measures to rule out malignancies.
  - Erythropoiesis-stimulating agents (ESAs) should be considered in CKD patients who remain anemic despite adequate iron stores.
    - The current Food and Drug Administration guidelines recommend that ESA should be used only to prevent blood transfusion and not to treat symptoms such as fatigue and decreased energy.
    - The risks and benefits of ESAs should be discussed with iron-replete CKD patients once hemoglobin levels fall under 10 g/dL.
    - Currently approved ESAs include **epoetin alfa, darbepoetin alfa, and the longer-acting Mircera. A typical starting dose** of epoetin alfa is 50 to 100 units/kg subcutaneously every week, darbepoetin alfa 40 mcg subcutaneously every 2 weeks, or Mircera 60 mcg SC every 2 weeks or 120 mcg every month. The subcutaneous route is preferred in stages 3 and 4 CKD patients.
    - The Food and Drug Administration also recommends an upper target hemoglobin limit of 12 g/dL.
    - Hemoglobin levels >13 g/dL during ESA therapy have been associated with increased rates of blood clots, heart attacks, strokes, and death.
    - A **complete blood cell count should be monitored at least monthly** while administering an ESA to avoid exceeding that level.
- CKD-MBD/SHPT. The management of CKD-MBD is complex and involves reduction of phosphorus in diet, use of phosphate binders, and appropriate use of vitamin D analogs.
  - Dietary restriction:
    - It is generally recommended to restrict phosphorus intake to 600 to 900 mg/day.
    - Phosphorus is naturally found in protein-rich foods such as meats, poultry, fish, dairy products, nuts, and beans.
  - Phosphorus binders:
    - Phosphorus binders reduce the enteric absorption of ingested phosphorus.
    - Calcium-based binders, such as calcium carbonate or calcium acetate, are frequently used in CKD patients. Because of concern for excessive calcium loading and vascular calcification, it is generally recommended to **limit the amount of elemental calcium to no more than 2000 mg/day.**
      - Non-calcium binders, such as **Sevelamer hydrochloride or carbonate, lanthanum carbonate, are not approved for use in predialysis CKD.**

□ Similarly, **newer phosphate binders, including sucroferric oxyhydroxide (Velphoro)** and **ferric citrate (Auryxia),** are effective iron-based phosphorus binders **but are not approved for use in predialysis patients.**

○ Vitamin D: We recommend replacement of 25-hydroxy vitamin D once levels fall to <30 ng/mL.

▪ Cholecalciferol (vitamin D3) or ergocalciferol (vitamin D2) can be used for replacement of low vitamin D levels.

▪ Vitamin D replacement should be deferred in patients who are hypercalcemic or hyperphosphatemic.

▪ Levels of 25-hydroxy vitamin D should be reassessed after 6 months of treatment.

○ **Active vitamin D and vitamin D analogs:**

▪ Active vitamin D **(1,25-dihydroxycholecalciferol also known as "calcitriol")** reduces PTH production and secretion through a feedback mechanism.

□ Calcitriol can be considered if PTH levels are persistently elevated despite tight phosphorus control and vitamin D repletion.

□ Calcitriol is typically started at a dose of 0.25 mcg PO daily.

□ Active vitamin D therapy can lead to increased calcium and phosphorus absorption. Therefore, it should be used cautiously and reserved for patients whose calcium and phosphorus are already controlled with the interventions listed above.

▪ Active vitamin D analogs, such as paricalcitol and doxercalciferol, retain the PTH-lowering effect of calcitriol with less hypercalcemia and hyperphosphatemia.

□ The typical starting dose for paricalcitol is 1 mcg PO daily or 2 mcg PO three times a week.

□ The typical starting dose for doxercalciferol it is 1 mcg/day.

□ Whether calcitriol or vitamin D analogs are initiated, serum calcium and phosphorus should be evaluated within 2 to 4 weeks of therapy initiation to check for hypercalcemia and hyperphosphatemia.

- **Prevention of acute kidney injury**

○ Prevention of additional renal insults is essential in decreasing progression to ESRD.

○ Intravenous contrast is a frequent cause of acute kidney injury (AKI) and high-risk patients should avoid any form of contrast if possible.

○ Likewise, surgeries or other procedures which may result in reduced renal perfusion can increase the risk of AKI.

○ Studies have shown that CKD patients who develop AKI progress faster to ESRD, even if they appear to recover from the acute injury.

- **Monitoring of concomitant medications**

○ CKD patients are at high risk for drug-related adverse events. Medication lists should be reviewed at every clinic visit to make sure drugs are dosed appropriately for the current estimated renal function.

○ Common medication errors in CKD patients include the following:

▪ The use of dual RAAS-blocking agents should be avoided given the risks of developing hyperkalemia.

▪ Metformin should be used with caution in CKD patients due to concerns for the development of lactic acidosis.

□ Metformin should not be initiated in patients with an eGFR of <45 mL/min/1.73 m^2, although patients who are already on the drug can continue taking it with close monitoring until their eGFR dips below 30 mL/min/1.73 m^2.

□ The FDA currently recommends against using metformin in patients with an eGFR <30 mL/min/1.73 m^2.

▪ Bisphosphonates should be avoided for eGFR <30 mL/min/1.73 m^2.

○ Gadolinium-based contrast agents should be used with caution for eGFR <30 mL/min/1.73 m^2 due to risk of nephrogenic systemic fibrosis (NSF). MRI contrast agents that contain macrocyclic chelators of gadolinium may decrease the risk of NSF in CKD patients.

SPECIAL CONSIDERATIONS

Preparation for Dialysis and Renal Transplant

Patient Education

- Lifestyle modifications are essential in decreasing cardiovascular risk and include weight loss, reduction of dietary sodium intake, regular exercise, and smoking cessation.
- Smoking is associated with increased progression to ESRD.
- A **comprehensive education program** is usually offered to all CKD patients, typically when GFR falls below 30 mL/min, to prepare them for renal replacement therapy (RRT).
  ○ The program should encompass education in all options for ESRD, including hemodialysis (HD), peritoneal dialysis (PD), transplantation, and palliative care.
  ○ The dieticians should be available to give nutritional counseling regarding low potassium and low phosphorus diets.
  ○ Patients should be encouraged to tour an HD facility and meet HD and PD patients.
  ○ Social work staff should be available to address concerns, such as insurance, medication affordability, employment, transportation to dialysis, and other costs.
- It is the **responsibility of the treating nephrologist to address the suitability of dialysis** initiation with his/her patients, and often their family members, and plan accordingly.
- Dialysis initiation **may not be appropriate** at extremely advanced age (in patients with multiple comorbid conditions) or patients in nursing homes, since dialysis has not been shown to improve quality of life or significantly prolong it.

Immunizations

The Centers for Disease Control and Prevention's February 2017 adult vaccination schedule can be found online at www.cdc.gov/vaccines/schedules/index.html.[7] The most commonly administered vaccines to CKD patients are listed below.

- ***Hepatitis B:***
  ○ Although hepatitis B immunization is not required for all patients with CKD, it is generally recommended for those expected to start dialysis, given the risk of transmission in dialysis units.
  ○ There is a three-dose regimen, with the second dose given at least 1 month later and the third given at least 2 months later, but >4 months from the first dose.
  ○ Surface antibody immunity can be checked 1 to 6 months after the vaccination has been completed. Levels of hepatitis B surface antibody should exceed >10 mIU/mL.
  ○ Booster doses are recommended for dialysis patients if levels fall below this value.
- ***Pneumococcal vaccination:***
  ○ The CDC recommends pneumococcal polysaccharide vaccination for all patients with CKD.
  ○ Current guidelines recommend a one-time revaccination 5 years after the initial vaccination for patients older than 65 years, if the initial vaccination was given when they were younger than 65 years.
- ***Influenza vaccination:***
  ○ Influenza vaccination is recommended annually for all individuals aged 50 years and older.

○ The CDC also recommends annual influenza vaccination (inactivated vaccine) for all younger patients with CKD.

Referral for Dialysis Access and Transplantation

- Patients with GFR <30 mL/min (stage 4 CKD) should be referred for vascular access if **HD** is the preferred RRT of choice.
- The KDOQI practice guidelines detail recommendations for vascular access.[8]
  ○ Early referral to a vascular surgeon is critical to ensure that preoperative studies (vein mapping) and access creation occur in a timely manner.
  ○ An **arteriovenous fistula (AVF)** is the preferred access for HD patients. An AVF should ideally be placed 6 months prior to the start of HD.
  ○ In some patients with poor vasculature, creation of an AVF may not be feasible. The next preferred access is **arteriovenous graft (AVG),** where a synthetic material is used to connect the artery to the vein. Grafts have a higher tendency to thrombose compared with fistulas, but they are preferred over tunneled HD catheters. An AVG should be placed at least 3 to 6 weeks prior to the start of HD.
  ○ The nondominant upper extremity should be protected from IV access, including peripheral IVs, peripherally inserted central catheter (PICC) lines, and subclavian lines. It may also be useful to avoid measuring blood pressures on the arm preferred for AVF placement.
- If **PD** is the initial preferred modality, a PD catheter should be placed at least 2 weeks prior to the anticipated start of PD. Before committing to this modality, several issues need to be addressed to ensure that the patient is an appropriate candidate.
  ○ Does the patient have adequate support at home?
  ○ Is the patient capable of understanding and performing the procedure at home?
  ○ Does the patient have a clean home environment?
  ○ Does the patient have a history of abdominal surgery or abdominal/ventral hernias which may need to be evaluated prior to the initiation of PD?
- **Transplantation:**
  ○ Suitable candidates with stage 4 CKD should be referred for evaluation by a multi-disciplinary kidney transplant clinic.
  ○ Typically, patients cannot be listed for transplantation until the GFR has fallen to <20 mL/min.
  ○ Not all patients are eligible for a kidney transplant. It is the treating nephrologist's responsibility to advise the patient regarding the appropriateness of transplantation as it involves major surgery and complications of immunosuppression.

Initiation of Renal Replacement Therapy

- Timing of initiation of RRT is patient-specific and often a difficult decision in the management of CKD.
- Signs and symptoms of uremia—such as poor appetite, nausea, vomiting, restless legs, severe itching, headaches, shortness of breath, volume overload refractory to diuretics, plus laboratory manifestations such as persistent hyperkalemia, metabolic acidosis, and SHPT—are good indicators to guide the timing of initiation of RRT.
- Most patients initiate dialysis when GFR <10 to 15 mL/min/1.73 m^2, although the initiation of dialysis should **not** be based on GFR level alone.
  ○ If a patient is completely asymptomatic with stable electrolytes, no symptoms of volume overload, and no reduction in functional capacity, the initiation of dialysis can be deferred even if eGFR levels are low.
  ○ In cases of severe malnutrition, diuretic resistant volume overload, or profound, resistant metabolic acidosis, RRT may need to be initiated at higher levels of GFR.

REFERENCES

1. Improving Global Outcomes (KDIGO) CKD Work Group. KDIGO 2012 clinical practice guideline for the evaluation and management of chronic kidney disease. *Kid Int Suppl.* 2013;1(3);1–150.
2. Kidney Disease Outcomes Quality Initiative (K/DOQI). Clinical practice guidelines and clinical practice recommendations for anemia in chronic kidney disease in adults. *Am J Kidney Dis.* 2006:47(S3):S16–S85.
3. Kidney Disease Outcomes Quality Initiative (K/DOQI). Bone metabolism and disease in chronic kidney disease. *Am J Kidney Dis.* 2003:42(S3):1–201.
4. Kidney Disease: Improving Global Outcomes. KDIGO 2017 clinical practice guidelines for the diagnosis, evaluation, prevention, and treatment of chronic kidney disease–mineral and bone disorder (CKD-MBD). *Kidney Int Suppl.* 2017:7(1):1–59.
5. James PA, Oparil S, Carter BL, et al. The Eighth Report of the Joint National Committee on prevention, detection, evaluation, and treatment of high blood pressure: the JNC 8 Report. *JAMA.* 2013;311(5):507–510.
6. Kidney Disease Outcomes Quality Initiative (K/DOQI). K/DOQI clinical practice guidelines on hypertension and antihypertensive agents in chronic kidney disease. *Am J Kidney Dis.* 2004:43(5):S1–S290.
7. Immunizations Schedules. 2019. Available at www.cdc.gov/vaccines/schedules/index.html (Last Accessed June 10, 2019.)
8. Kidney Disease Outcomes Quality Initiative (K/DOQI). Clinical practice guidelines for vascular access. *Am J Kidney Dis.* 2006:48(S1):S176–S247.

Diabetic Nephropathy

George Jarad

13

GENERAL PRINCIPLES

Diabetic nephropathy (DN) is the most common cause of chronic kidney disease (CKD) and end-stage renal disease (ESRD) in diabetic patients. Early recognition, diagnosis, and institution of appropriate treatment are necessary to prevent the disease or slow disease progression.

Definition

DN is a clinical syndrome characterized by progressive loss of kidney function that develops as a direct consequence of diabetes mellitus. The hallmark of DN is the development of glomerular hyperfiltration and albuminuria. Definitive diagnosis of DN requires a kidney biopsy. However, in most cases, careful analysis of patient clinical characteristics is sufficient to make the diagnosis.

Epidemiology

- DN is the most common cause of ESRD in the United States and the world.
- DN develops secondary to either type 1 or type 2 diabetes. However, most cases are secondary to type 2 diabetes considering its higher prevalence.
- The risk of DN is equivalent in both types of diabetes, although the prevalence might be higher among patients with type 1 diabetes.
- The development of DN imparts a significant increase in morbidity and mortality, before and after the development of ESRD. After starting dialysis, the mortality of diabetic patients is more than 50% higher than nondiabetic ESRD population.

Pathophysiology

The pathophysiology of DN is not fully understood, although hyperglycemia, hyperinsulinemia, and hemodynamic changes appear to play important role.

- **Hyperglycemia** plays the central role in the development of DN by mediating hemodynamic and structural changes in the kidney through multiple mechanisms.
  - Prolonged hyperglycemia might induce production or glycosylation of mesangial proteins, leading to mesangial expansion and injury to kidney epithelial cells.
  - The accompanied increase in advanced glycation end products (AGEs) has been linked to microvascular diabetic complications, including DN.
  - Hyperglycemia and AGEs induce multiple signaling pathways that are injurious to kidney cells. These include the generation of advanced glycosylation end products, reactive oxygen species, changes in cellular microRNA, stimulation of transforming growth factor-β (TGF-β), vascular endothelial growth factor (VEGF), and other proinflammatory cytokines.
- **Impaired insulin signaling in podocytes** may also play a role in podocyte injury, glomerular basement membrane (GBM) thickening, and glomerular hyperfiltration.
- **Intraglomerular hypertension and glomerular hyperfiltration** eventually lead to the development of microalbuminuria and proteinuria.
  - Albuminuria may play a direct role in the progression of DN.

Risk Factors

Modifiable Risk Factors

- **Hyperglycemia:** Among modifiable risk factors, **control of blood glucose level** is the most obvious and most important.
  - ○ DN is rare if A1C is maintained below 7.0% throughout life.
  - ○ The risk is increased for all A1C levels above the nondiabetic range, and is greatest at levels >12%.
  - ○ Large clinical studies, including the United Kingdom Prospective Diabetes Study (UKPDS) and the Diabetes Control and Complications Trial, have shown that poor glycemic control is associated with increased risk of microalbuminuria and other microvascular complications of diabetes, such as nephropathy, retinopathy, and neuropathy.[1,2]
- **Hypertension:** Hypertension may precede or follow the development of DN. Poor hypertension control plays an important role in the development and the progression of disease.
  - ○ Hyperinsulinemia and increased arterial stiffness contribute to the development of hypertension.
  - ○ The development of nephropathy exacerbates hypertension due to sodium and fluid retention.
  - ○ Blood pressures higher than 130/80 mm Hg increase the risk of development and progression of DN.
- **Obesity:** Further increases this risk, although it is uncertain whether this effect is independent of diabetic and glycemic control.

Nonmodifiable Risk Factors

- **Genetic factors:**
  - ○ The risk of developing microalbuminuria and proteinuria increases in the presence of a family history of DN.
  - ○ Variation of the gene encoding the angiotensin-converting enzyme (ACE) has been suggested as a risk factor, although this has not been confirmed.
  - ○ In African American, high-risk APOL1 genetic variants do not appear to play an important role.
- **Race:** Patients of African-American, Mexican-American, Pima Indian and Australian Aboriginal descent are at increased risk. Whether the increased risk is the result of genetic or socioeconomic factors or a combination of the two is not clear.
- **Age:** Older age and longer duration of diabetes are associated with increased risk of albuminuria in type 2 diabetes. In type 1 diabetes, the age at diagnosis is more important than duration. The development of diabetes before the age of 20 carries increased risk, however, if the diagnosis is made before 5 years of age, the risk is reduced.

Prevention

- Before the development of microalbuminuria, diabetes should be controlled with goal A1C below 7%. Tighter control of diabetes should be weighed against the increased risk of hypoglycemia.
- It is empirical to control coexisting hypertension. The use of ACE inhibitors or ARB for primary prevention of DN and microalbuminuria is controversial.
- All diabetic patients should be screened for DN at regular intervals.

Screening

- **Microalbuminuria** is the earliest sign of DN. Microalbuminuria refers to a small increase in urinary protein excretion that is not detectable using urinary dipstick (please see Table 13-1).

	24-hr Collection (mg/24 hr)	Adjusted for Urine Cr (mg/g creatinine)
Normal	<30	<30
Microalbuminuria	30–300	30–300
Albuminuria	>300	>300

TABLE 13-1 CLASSIFICATION OF PROTEINURIA

- **Albuminuria** (sometimes called macroalbuminuria) is the excretion of >300 mg of protein in a 24-hour period. Progression from microalbuminuria to proteinuria is an important event as it is the hallmark progression of the DN.
- **Tests for microalbuminuria:**
  - A 24-hour urine collection, while accurate, can be cumbersome and difficult to interpret because of improper sampling and the logistical difficulties of saving urine through 24 hours. Adequacy of the collection should be assessed by measuring creatinine excretion (15 to 20 mg/kg in females and 20 to 25 mg/kg in males per day).
  - A ratio of albumin (or protein)-to-creatinine in a random sample of urine can be used instead. The accuracy increases if the test is performed on first morning urine. This study is often called a spot microalbumin test or protein/creatinine ratio. The ratio of albumin excreted per 1 g of creatinine correlates well with albumin excretion in a 24-hour period.
- **Screening should be conducted yearly** in patients with type 2 diabetes staring at the diagnosis of the disease. Proteinuria assessment can be deferred for the first 5 years in patients with type 1 diabetes.
  - A routine urinalysis should not be the only test used to screen for DN. Quantifying proteinuria, whether the dipstick test is negative or positive is necessary.
  - If a routine urine dipstick test result is positive for protein, a spot protein/creatinine test is necessary to quantify albumin excretion, to follow the efficacy of treatment and disease progression.

DIAGNOSIS

Clinical Presentation

- The course of DN is better studied in type 1 diabetes because of the accurate correlation between the onset of disease and the time of diagnosis. The natural history and progression of kidney disease is believed to be similar in both types of diabetes.
- In type 1 diabetes, the first 5 years are characterized by normal laboratory values for serum creatinine and urinary albumin excretion. Despite normal laboratory values, hyperglycemia leads to glomerular hyperfiltration and early histopathologic changes (glomerular hypertrophy and thick GBM).
- **Microalbuminuria typically develops between 5 and 10 years from diagnosis of diabetes** in 40% of patients.
- From 15 to 20 years, proteinuria and hypertension develop, followed by decline in kidney function to ESRD after 20 years. Nephrotic range proteinuria signals the start of rapid deterioration of kidney function.
- Diabetic patients are frequently referred to nephrology clinic with albuminuria or elevations in serum creatinine levels. A detailed and complete evaluation of diabetic patients is necessary for two reasons:
  - First, it is necessary to establish whether the underlying kidney disease is consistent with DN. Even in the presence of typical history, other potential causes of kidney disease should be ruled out.

○ Second, it is crucial to identify the presence of modifiable risk factors and to establish appropriate goals of therapy.

History

- History should focus on the duration of diabetes, the level of glycemic control, and the presence of other end-organ microvascular disease associated with diabetes.
  ○ During each visit, patients should be asked about adherence to the diabetic diet, medications, and their current level of glycemic control. A log of recorded blood glucose is helpful in tracking overall trends and daily variations in glucose levels.
- **Concurrent history of retinopathy or neuropathy** supports the diagnosis of DN.
  ○ Type 1 diabetics with nephropathy almost always manifest evidence of retinopathy and/or neuropathy.
  ○ The association is less established in type 2 diabetes. The absence of retinopathy should not exclude DN in these patients.

Physical Examination

- **Blood pressure** recordings should be checked at each office visit. Hypertension is a common comorbidity among diabetics, especially type 2 with obesity, and plays an important role in both the development and progression of DN. Home blood pressure monitoring should be encouraged in all patients.
- Patient's **volume status** should also be carefully assessed, as expansion of the body's interstitial fluid compartment, manifesting as edema, may reflect sodium retention in association with hypertension or with nephrotic range proteinuria.
- Evidence of retinopathy and neuropathy may reflect concurrent microvascular disease and should be evaluated with a **funduscopic and neurologic exam.**

Differential Diagnoses

- The term "diabetic nephropathy" *specifically* refers to the glomerular disease caused by diabetes. Diabetic patients may also develop other forms of kidney diseases:
  ○ Other proteinuric kidney diseases such as **membranous nephropathy** and **focal segmental glomerulosclerosis (FSGS),** which are common in patients between the age of 20 and 60 should be included in the differential.
  ○ Proteinuria, abnormal kidney function and anemia, with or without hypercalcemia, should prompt evaluation for **myeloma kidney** in patients older than 40 years.
- **The following presentations should raise suspicion of other diagnosis:**
  ○ Development of albuminuria <5 years from the onset of type 1 diabetes.
  ○ Absence of retinopathy or neuropathy, particularly in type 1 diabetes.
  ○ Active urine sediment with dysmorphic RBC or RBC casts. The mere presence of microscopic hematuria has been reported in DN.
  ○ Extrarenal manifestation such as rash, arthritis, or hemoptysis.
  ○ Anemia out of proportion to the degree of kidney dysfunction.
  ○ Hypercalcemia.
  ○ Acute kidney injury (AKI) or rapid deterioration of kidney function.
  ○ Thrombosis associated with nephrotic syndrome.
- Diabetics are susceptible to the development of **renal vascular disease,** which may be unmasked with the initiation of an angiotensin antagonist.
- **Obstructive nephropathy** is a concern among the 40% of diabetics who develop neurogenic bladder.
- Diabetics are more prone to some infectious sequelae, such as renal papillary necrosis or renal tuberculosis.
  ○ **Papillary necrosis** may develop in individuals with frequent urinary tract infections (UTIs) who develop hematuria, pyuria, and AKI.
  ○ **Renal tuberculosis** presents with sterile pyuria, hematuria, and azotemia; the diagnosis is based on clinical suspicion and the growth of mycobacterial species in the urine.

Diagnostic Testing

Laboratory Testing

- Recent laboratory data **should be interpreted in the contexts of clinical presentation and long-term trends.** A single serum creatinine number or an isolated urine albumin should be confirmed with repeated testing, especially if the patient history suggests a transient rise in such markers (dehydration, febrile illnesses, UTIs, or new medications).
- **DN is confirmed by the persistence of albuminuria in two separate samples separated by 3 to 6 months.**
- The clinical course of DN follows a gradual but progressive course. Serum creatinine initially rises slowly, and small subtle increments are appreciated only when the trend in laboratory values is scrutinized over the preceding months and years. Sudden fluctuations in laboratory data warrant confirmation with repeat testing and consideration of alternative diagnoses.
- Evaluation for hepatitis virus infection should be performed.
- Other labs such as ANA, complement, ANCA and serum/urine immunofixation should be checked if the patient presents with constitutional symptoms.

Imaging

- A kidney ultrasound can aid the diagnosis and the staging of DN. Early in the disease course, the kidneys are large due to hyperfiltration and microalbuminuria. However, as the disease progresses, kidneys can shrink in size.
- Ultrasound is essential for the diagnosis of obstruction and papillary necrosis.

Diagnostic Procedures

- The **definitive diagnosis requires kidney biopsy;** however, biopsy is rarely performed in typical cases. Biopsy should be pursued if the diagnosis is in doubt.
- The earliest pathologic sign is thickening of the GBM by electron microscopy.
- Glomerular hypertrophy can be seen early in DN coinciding with mesangial expansion, glomerular hyperfiltration, and microalbuminuria.
- Glomerular pathology progresses to a nodular pattern of glomerulosclerosis, known as Kimmelstiel–Wilson nodules. Nodular lesions are not necessary to diagnose DN and can also be seen in association with other diseases, such as light chain nephropathy, amyloidosis and in heavy smokers.
- Beyond the glomerulus, vasculature, tubules, and interstitium might be involved:
  - Hyalinosis of afferent or efferent arterioles can be seen, especially in patients with long standing or severe hypertension.
  - Tubular changes include thickening of the tubular basement membrane, tubular cell atrophy, and the Armanni–Ebstein lesion, a specific, but rare manifestation of tubular glycogen deposition and tubular vacuolization.
  - Tubulointerstitial fibrosis might be the most predominant feature in patients with advanced DN and is suggestive of chronicity of the disease. The degree of tubulointerstitial fibrosis predicts kidney outcome better than glomerulosclerosis.

TREATMENT

The modifiable risk factors of hyperglycemia and hypertension are the primary targets of preventive and therapeutic interventions.
- **Glycemic control:**
  - Managing hyperglycemia to a **goal of A1C of under 7%** is the most important preventive strategy. Referral to an endocrinologist might be needed if diabetes is difficult to control.

○ A stricter diabetes control to an A1C <6.5% might offer further benefit, although such aggressive goal should be weighed against the risk of hypoglycemia.

  ■ Early and aggressive glycemic control results in decreased incidence of microalbuminuria as well as a decrease in the prevalence of hypertension.

  ■ In type 1 diabetics, intensive insulin therapy has also been shown to reduce the rate of progression from microalbuminuria to overt albuminuria.[3]

  ■ Pancreas transplantation might be indicated in some patients, especially in those with hypoglycemia unawareness, although it should be reserved for special cases considering its high surgical morbidity and the need for nephrotoxic immunosuppression.

○ Once patients develop overt nephropathy and albuminuria, the role of strict glycemic control becomes controversial. In advanced kidney disease, strict glycemic control should be weighed against the increased risk of clinically significant hypoglycemia.

○ Pharmacologic agents should be dosed with careful consideration for diminished renal clearances in patients who develop DN. The degree of renal insufficiency must be considered in the selection and titration of pharmacologic agents:

  ■ Insulin is preferred for diabetes control in patients with kidney disease.

  ■ Short half-life sulfonylureas (glipizide and glimepiride) can be used in patients with poor kidney function, although all sulfonylureas can cause hypoglycemia.

  ■ The clearance of the biguanide metformin is decreased in the setting of impaired renal function, predisposing patients to hypoglycemia and lactic acidosis. **Metformin is not recommended for patients with an eGFR <30 mL/min.**

  ■ Thiazolidinediones (rosiglitazone, pioglitazone) should be avoided in patients with an eGFR <45 mL/min due to increased risk of fluid retention and heart failure.

  ■ Sodium-glucose cotransporter-2 (SGLT-2) inhibitors can lead to volume depletion, AKI, and hyperkalemia in patients with preserved kidney function. They should be used with caution in patients with an eGFR <45 mL/min and should be avoided in patients with an eGFR <30 mL/min.

- **Hypertension:**

  ○ We recommend a target blood pressure of less than **130/80 mm Hg** in diabetic patients. A more aggressive goal is controversial, although it might be desirable and might be beneficial in slowing the progression of renal disease in patients with more than 1 g of proteinuria per day.

    ■ In hypertensive diabetics without proteinuria, **angiotensin inhibitors** and **thiazide diuretics** are often prescribed as first-line agents.

    ■ Inhibitors of angiotensin are known to decrease proteinuria. ACE inhibitors and ARBs may confer further benefits beyond reducing systemic blood pressure through an anti-inflammatory and antifibrotic mechanism.

    ■ If a patient requires two agents to achieve the blood pressure target, combining a diuretic and an ACE inhibitor or an ARB is ideal.

    ■ Optimal control of the blood pressure should as important as the medications used to achieve control.

  ○ After the development of microalbuminuria, hypertension control and the use of ACE inhibitors or ARBs become more crucial to prevent the progression of nephropathy, reduce cardiovascular morbidity and mortality, and decrease other diabetes complications such as retinopathy. Each 10 mm Hg reduction in systolic blood pressure is correlated with a 12% reduction in diabetic complications.[3]

  ○ The question of whether ACE inhibitors and ARBs are equivalent has not yet been answered, although in clinical practice they are used interchangeably.

    ■ Comparisons of equivalent doses of ACE inhibitors and ARBs in type 2 diabetics did not show significant difference in the decline in glomerular filtration rate, blood pressure control, albuminuria, serum creatinine, ESRD, cardiovascular end points, and death.

- The combination of ACE inhibitors and ARB may have theoretical advantage in reducing albuminuria, however, such a combination should be avoided due to increased risk of significant hyperkalemia and AKI, especially in patients with abnormal kidney function.
  - Renin inhibitors (Aliskiren) are not beneficial when used as a single agent in DN. The combination of Aliskiren and an ARB improved proteinuria in patients with DN, although this combination increases the risk of AKI and hyperkalemia.
    - The role of aldosterone antagonist is not well established. The concomitant use with ACE inhibitor or ARB carries increased risk of AKI and hyperkalemia.
- Albuminuria:
  - Albuminuria is viewed as a surrogate marker for DN progression. However, there is expanding evidence suggesting that albuminuria is an independent risk factor in disease progression.
  - Reduction in albuminuria using ACE inhibitors or ARBs in patients with DN confers improvements in both renal and cardiovascular outcomes.[4]
  - This beneficial effect of ACE inhibitors and ARBs is independent of blood pressure reduction, and has been demonstrated in trials comparing these agents to other antihypertensive medications.[5]

COMPLICATIONS

Clinical complications that may result from DN or the treatment of DN include hypoglycemia, AKI, hyperkalemia, and metabolic acidosis.

- **Hypoglycemia:**
  - Patients with advanced kidney disease are at risk for hypoglycemia due to:
    - Reduced clearance of renally excreted medications.
    - Increased half-life of endogenous and administered insulin due to reduced degradation in the kidney.
    - Reduced gluconeogenesis in the kidney, which normally account for around 30% of gluconeogenesis.
  - As CKD progress to ESRD, hyperglycemia becomes easier to control with less medication. Some patients with type 2 diabetes may become normoglycemic without any medical treatment, especially if this is associated with significant weight loss. All diabetic patients with worsening kidney disease should be advised to monitor their glucose closely to avoid life-threatening hypoglycemia. After kidney transplantation, hyperglycemia will return in patients with type 2 diabetes even if they are on a steroid-free immunosuppression regimen.
- **AKI:**
  - AKI is manifested by a sudden increase in creatinine that exceeds the predicted gradual decline of kidney function seen with DN.
  - Both pre- and postrenal etiologies are common, as diabetics are prone to intravascular depletion from osmotic diuresis and the use of diuretics and to obstruction due to neurogenic bladder.
  - An elevation in creatinine is expected after a patient starts an angiotensin-inhibiting agent.
    - These agents induce efferent arterial vasodilation that leads to a small reduction in glomerular filtration pressure, GFR and to a rise in creatinine.
    - The rise in creatinine should not exceed 30% of starting creatinine. Further increase should prompt the cessation of the medication until renal function returns to baseline.
  - The development of AKI while receiving ACE inhibitor or ARB treatment should not prohibit the use of these medications in the future. Upon reintroduction of these

medications, a slow titration of the dose and close monitoring of kidney function and potassium are necessary.

○ Angiotensin blockade predisposes patients to develop AKI in the setting of mild volume depletion. Patients receiving these medications should be instructed to temporarily withhold ACE inhibitors and ARB if they become dehydrated.

- **Hyperkalemia:**
  ○ The risk of hyperkalemia increases with poor glycemic control, angiotensin blockade, and the development of type 4 renal tubular acidosis (RTA).
  ○ Monitoring potassium is important after the initiation and titration of ACE inhibitors or ARBs.
    - Serum potassium levels under 5.5 mEq/L can be managed medically.
    - For more severe cases of hyperkalemia, a decrease or cessation of the medication might be necessary. After normalization of potassium levels, a careful reintroduction of ACE inhibitor or ARB should be attempted.
  ○ **Type 4 RTA** might develop as a complication of DN.
    - Type 4 RTA develops secondary to impaired production of renin. The resulting hyporeninemic hypoaldosteronism impairs potassium secretion and ammoniagenesis.
    - Type 4 RTA cannot be diagnosed in patients with advanced CKD and an eGFR <30 mL/min. At this stage, the predominant factor that leads to hyperkalemia and acidosis is the reduction in kidney function.
  ○ Regardless of the cause, hyperkalemia should be managed with dietary potassium restriction and loop diuretics. A dietary consultation can be essential to ensure low potassium intake.
    - Alkali therapy may also become necessary if there is concomitant acidosis.
    - Potassium-binding resins (such as patiromer and sodium zirconium cyclosilicate) can be helpful in some patients with chronic hyperkalemia. Patiromer might allow the reintroduction of ACE inhibitor or ARB if these medications were stopped because of hyperkalemia.

MONITORING/FOLLOW-UP

Patients with overt nephropathy should be followed regularly in the nephrology clinic. Achievement of glycemic goals, attainment of adequate blood pressure control, and albuminuria should be checked at each visit. In those with progressive nephropathy, management of common complications of CKD, including anemia and renal osteodystrophy, should be addressed as discussed in Chapter 12. If kidney disease continues to progress, patients should be encouraged to be listed for kidney transplantation as soon as their eGFR is below 20 mL/min, even before they start dialysis.

REFERENCES

1. Adler AI, Stevens RJ, Manley SE, et al. Development and progression of nephropathy in type 2 diabetes: the United Kingdom Prospective Diabetes Study (UKPDS 64). *Kidney Int.* 2003;63:225–232.
2. Nathan DM, Genuth S, Lachin J, et al. The effect of intensive treatment of diabetes on the development and progression of long-term complications in insulin-dependent diabetes mellitus. *N Engl J Med.* 1993;329:977–986.
3. Adler AI, Stratton IM, Neil HA, et al. Association of systolic blood pressure with macrovascular and microvascular complications of type 2 diabetes (UKPDS 36): prospective observational study. *BMJ.* 2000:321:412–419.
4. De Zeeuw D, Remuzzi G, Parving HH, et al. Albuminuria, a therapeutic target for cardiovascular protection in type 2 diabetic patients with nephropathy. *Circulation.* 2004;110:921–927.
5. Atkins RC, Briganti EM, Lewis JB, et al. Proteinuria reduction and progression to renal failure in patients with type 2 diabetes mellitus and overt nephropathy. *Am J Kidney Dis.* 2005;45:281–287.

Cystic Disease of the Kidney

14

Seth Goldberg

Polycystic Kidney Disease

GENERAL PRINCIPLES

Classification

- Polycystic kidney disease has two well-defined autosomal dominant forms (autosomal dominant polycystic kidney disease 1 [ADPKD1] and ADPKD2) as well as one with an autosomal recessive inheritance pattern (ARPKD).
- ARPKD leads to renal failure in childhood and adolescence, while both ADPKD forms can remain asymptomatic for several decades into adulthood before renal dysfunction is evident.

Epidemiology

- ADPKD has an incidence of 1 in 400 to 1000 live births, with no racial or gender predilection; 85% have a defect in the *PKD1* gene (chromosome 16), whereas 15% have a defect at the *PKD2* locus (chromosome 4).
- ARPKD has an incidence of 1 in 10,000 to 40,000 live births, with the mutation on the *PKHD1* gene on chromosome 6.

Pathophysiology

- The gene products of *PKD1* (polycystin-1) and *PKD2* (polycystin-2) localize to the primary cilium of the epithelial cell of the renal tubule, the hepatic bile duct, and pancreatic duct, and to various other tissues in the body.
- These gene products are thought to play a role in flow-mediated mechanosensation as well as cell–cell interactions, and defects lead to abnormal epithelial cell proliferation.
- In ADPKD, vasopressin signaling may be impaired and affected cells show an abnormal response to increases in cyclic adenosine monophosphate (cAMP), exhibiting a proliferative phenotype.
- Only a small percentage of tubules develop cysts, suggesting that a "second-hit" somatic mutation to the normal allele is required to initiate cystogenesis.
- As the cysts enlarge, they become separated from the rest of the collecting system; events occurring within the cyst (such as hemorrhage or infection) may not be evident in the urine.
- Enlarging cysts may impinge upon the blood flow to normal filtration units, leading to resistant hypertension and interstitial fibrosis.

DIAGNOSIS

Clinical Presentation

- Diagnosis is often delayed because the disease is **asymptomatic until late in the course.**
- It is frequently discovered on abdominal imaging performed for an alternate indication; ADPKD-specific reasons for ultrasonography include unexplained early-onset

hypertension, elevated creatinine, or pain from an expanding cyst, cyst hemorrhage, or cyst infection.

History

- The history should include an in-depth **family history,** including relatives who may have required dialysis or a transplant and the age that they reached end-stage renal disease.
- Family history of **cerebral aneurysms or sudden death of unknown etiology** must be ascertained, as this would put the patient at risk for a similar event and necessitate screening.
- A personal history of headaches or neurologic symptoms must be sought.
- Flank and abdominal pain may be suggestive of symptomatic renal or hepatic cysts.
- A history of hematuria, dysuria, and nephrolithiasis should be investigated.
- **Caffeine intake** should be quantified.
- In women, the history of **estrogen exposure** (pregnancy, contraception, hormone replacement therapy) should be assessed.

Physical Examination

- The physical examination is often normal in the early stages of ADPKD.
- The first presenting sign of an underlying problem is frequently early-onset hypertension.
- As the kidneys progressively enlarge, the cysts may be palpable on abdominal examination.
- Hepatic cysts may also be palpable and elicit epigastric tenderness.
- Cardiac auscultation may reveal the mid-systolic click of mitral valve prolapse.

Diagnostic Criteria

- The diagnosis of ADPKD is made using the combination of renal cysts, family history, and the constellation of extrarenal manifestations.
- **Ultrasound diagnostic criteria** have been established for patients at-risk for ADPKD (those with an affected parent); however, the absence of cysts in a patient under the age of 40 does not rule out the disease.[1] Please see Table 14-1.
- As computed tomography (CT) scans or magnetic resonance imaging (MRI) can detect smaller cysts, the conventional diagnostic criteria do not apply to these modalities and no guidelines have been validated.
- **Genetic testing** is available for both forms of ADPKD, with use primarily in young patients contemplating living kidney donation to an affected family member in order to rule out subclinical disease. The accuracy of the test depends on identifying the specific mutation (which differs between families) and so the utility of the genetic test is limited in patients with few or no affected relatives.
- For children of an affected parent, it is appropriate to wait until the children are 18 years old to decide for themselves if they want to undergo testing. A diagnosis may make it more difficult to obtain health or life insurance but could allow for the option of disease-modifying therapy approved for adults.
- It is prudent for at-risk relatives to obtain regular blood pressure checks, and to pursue further evaluation if indicated.

TABLE 14-1	ULTRASOUND CRITERIA FOR DIAGNOSIS OF ADPKD
Age	Number of Cysts Required in At-Risk Individual
15–39	At least three cysts between both kidneys
40–59	At least two cysts in each kidney
≥60	At least four cysts in each kidney

Differential Diagnosis

- The diagnosis of ADPKD is not difficult when there is an established family history of disease; when absent, the possibility of an alternative renal cystic disease must be excluded.
- Acquired cystic disease in the presence of renal dysfunction typically exhibits small, shrunken kidneys.
- The cysts in medullary cystic kidney disease (MCKD) are often a late manifestation, with small-to-normal–sized smooth-contoured kidneys and cysts confined to the corticomedullary junction or renal medulla.
- Medullary sponge kidney (MSK) can also be distinguished from ADPKD by the medullary location of the cysts and collecting duct dilation.
- Solid renal nodules are uncommon in ADPKD, but may be seen in tuberous sclerosis and von Hippel–Lindau (VHL) syndrome.
- The presence of extrarenal manifestations, such as hepatic cysts, can be a helpful clue to make the diagnosis of ADPKD.

TREATMENT

- In 2018, the vasopressin antagonist tolvaptan was approved in the United States to delay progression of ADPKD. Patients with ADPKD complicated by hypertension, progressive decline in renal function (but with a glomerular filtration rate >25 mL/min/1.73 m^2), or kidney lengths >16.5 cm are potential candidates for treatment. Given the risk of liver toxicity, drug prescribing is tightly regulated and requires the frequent monitoring of liver enzymes (baseline, 2 weeks, 4 weeks, every 4 weeks for 18 months, then every 3 months afterwards). Common side effects include polyuria, nocturia, and increased thirst, which may be overwhelming for some patients and thus potential treatment subjects should be counseled on this possibility, while being instructed to maintain at least 2 to 4 L of fluid intake daily. It is generally recommend to discontinue diuretics prior to initiating tolvaptan.[2,3]
- Blood pressure control remains an important cornerstone of treatment.
- Anemia is not often an early problem for these patients, as compared to other causes of chronic kidney disease, given the production of erythropoietin by cells surrounding the cysts.
- Caffeine intake should be reduced or avoided, given the theoretical risk of increasing cAMP levels and thus cyst growth; animal models and human studies have not confirmed this risk.
- Large-volume surgical cyst reduction does not affect long-term renal outcomes, although select aspiration and sclerosis of severely symptomatic renal or hepatic cysts can provide relief.

COMPLICATIONS

Renal Manifestations

- **Hematuria** is a common finding in patients with ADPKD and may represent a ruptured cyst, a cyst infection, or nephrolithiasis.
- **Cyst hemorrhage** is self-limited, lasting from several days to 1 to 2 weeks and can be very painful; as cysts may have become separated from the rest of the urinary tract, hematuria is not always present. Cyst hemorrhage is treated conservatively with oral hydration, bed rest, and analgesia.
- **Cyst infection** may present with fever, dysuria, pyuria, and flank pain; however, as with cyst hemorrhage, there may not be direct communication with the remainder of the urinary tract and so dysuria may be absent and the urine culture may be negative.

Treatment of cyst infection should include an antibiotic with good cyst penetration (ciprofloxacin, sulfamethoxazole–trimethoprim) for 3 to 4 weeks.

- **Nephrolithiasis** can occur in patients with ADPKD, with an increased frequency of uric acid stones as compared to the general population. Calcium-based stones are also common in this group. Management would be the same as for patients without ADPKD.
- **Hypertension** in this population is thought to be mediated, at least partially, through activation of the renin–angiotensin–aldosterone axis through local ischemia from external compression by enlarging cysts. The onset of hypertension is common before the age of 35, despite preserved renal filtration.
- A concentrating defect is generally mild and may be seen early in the disease course; this may be accounted for by vasopressin receptor (V_2) signaling abnormalities.

Extrarenal Manifestations

- **Liver cysts** are common and are present in up to 80% of patients with ADPKD. Progression to liver dysfunction, however, is rare.
  - Liver enlargement may lead to abdominal fullness, discomfort, or early satiety. In unusual circumstances, the pain may be severe enough as to prompt cyst drainage with sclerosis or surgical unroofing of the culprit lesion.
  - Liver cysts are more common in women with increased estrogen exposure.
- **Cerebral aneurysms** constitute the most serious extrarenal manifestation and are found to cluster within families with certain mutations.
  - When there is a family history of a cerebral aneurysm or sudden death of unknown cause, the incidence is increased to 20%. In the absence of such a family history, the risk is no greater than in the general population (1% to 2%).
  - The risk of aneurysm rupture is greater in patients with uncontrolled hypertension.
  - Patients with neurologic symptoms or those with a family history of cerebral aneurysms should undergo magnetic resonance angiography testing. Others who should be screened include patients with high-risk occupations in which loss of consciousness would put others at risk (such as commercial pilots), patients needing anticoagulation, or those undergoing a surgical intervention with potential hemodynamic instability.
  - Referral to neurosurgery is recommended when an aneurysm is discovered; smaller aneurysms (<5 to 7 mm) are typically followed serially, while those that are at higher risk of rupture should undergo repair.
  - For patients at increased risk for cerebral aneurysms but with negative scans, reimaging within 10 years should be performed to detect new lesions.
- **Colonic diverticulosis** occurs with greater frequency in patients with ADPKD with a higher risk of perforation compared to the general population.
- **Cardiac valvular disease,** particularly mitral valve prolapse, is common in ADPKD patients. Most patients are asymptomatic, although some patients may report palpitations.
- **Abdominal wall hernias** occur with increased frequency, and may worsen if peritoneal dialysis is pursued in these patients without surgical correction.

PATIENT EDUCATION

- All patients with ADPKD should be counseled regarding the mode of inheritance and the 50% risk to each offspring.
- Monitoring of blood pressure and for neurologic symptoms suggestive of cerebral aneurysm should be undertaken in at-risk family members.
- Although the specific nature of the risk has not been defined, patients should be counseled in restricting caffeine intake and avoiding estrogen-based therapies. Increasing

water intake to 2 to 4 L/day can be recommended, although no human studies have been conducted to establish the efficacy or safety of this strategy; the theoretical benefit would be in reducing endogenous vasopressin production.

OUTCOME/PROGNOSIS

- In the absence of specific therapy to slow cyst growth, the **typical outcome is progression toward end-stage renal disease.** With tolvaptan, it is estimated that the need for dialysis or transplantation can be delayed by 6 to 8 years, although no long-term follow-up is yet available to confirm this and the overall protection may diminish over time.
- In ADPKD1, approximately 50% of patients require renal replacement therapy by the age of 60; this is delayed by 15 years in ADPKD2.
- Appropriate candidates for renal transplantation should be identified and evaluated early, anticipating their need for renal replacement therapy to minimize or entirely avoid time spent on dialysis.

Simple Renal Cysts

GENERAL PRINCIPLES

Epidemiology
- Simple renal cysts are very common in the general population and can be found in healthy kidneys.
- Prevalence increases with age, with roughly one-quarter of the general population having a simple cyst on ultrasound by the age of 50.

Pathophysiology
- Simple cysts are typically solitary, but the finding of multiple cysts is not uncommon.
- They can be unilocular or multilocular.
- They are lined with a single layer of flattened epithelial cells and are confined to the renal cortex.
- The etiology of simple cyst formation is not fully understood.

DIAGNOSIS

Clinical Presentation
- Simple cysts are **almost always asymptomatic,** usually found incidentally on imaging for an alternate purpose.
- In rare circumstances, large cysts (>10 cm in diameter) can cause local symptoms such as a palpable abdominal mass or abdominal pain.
- Cyst infection, hemorrhage, or urinary obstruction (if near the renal pelvis) rarely complicate simple cysts.
- Renal function is typically preserved, although hypertension may be noted if the cyst compresses a large vessel.

Diagnostic Criteria
- Size is quite variable, and can range from <1 cm to >10 cm in diameter.
- **Ultrasonography** is the best initial modality to evaluate simple cysts.

TABLE 14-2	BOSNIAK RENAL CYST CLASSIFICATION SYSTEM
Category	Description
I	**Simple benign cyst** Hairline-thin wall Measures water density No enhancement No septa, calcifications, or solid components
II	**Benign cyst with additional features** Fine calcifications Few hairline-thin septa "Perceived" enhancement Mass <3 cm with high attenuation but no enhancement
IIF	**Cysts with minimally complicated features** Multiple hairline-thin septa or smooth thickening of wall or septa Calcifications may be thick and nodular No measurable enhancement Generally well marginated Lesions >3 cm with high attenuation
III	**"Indeterminate" cystic mass** Thickened irregular or smooth walls or septa with enhancement
IV	**Mass with high likelihood of malignancy** All criteria of category III Adjacent enhancing soft tissue components

- Typically, on ultrasound, simple cysts are (a) anechoic, (b) round in shape with smooth walls, and (c) exhibit sharp definition of the posterior wall with a strong acoustic enhancement.
- Scanning under CT can further characterize renal cysts, should the diagnosis be in question.

Differential Diagnosis

- Simple cysts can be differentiated from polycystic disease by their fewer numbers, lack of extrarenal manifestations, normal kidney size and function, and lack of family history.
- Unlike acquired cystic disease, simple cysts are generally associated with a normal creatinine level (unless another process has caused renal dysfunction).
- The primary differential is to distinguish simple cysts from malignant masses.
- If the appearance is typical for a simple cyst on ultrasonography, no further evaluation is indicated. The Bosniak classification system on CT scanning (please see Table 14-2) can help characterize the lesion if there is still concern, with categories III and IV needing surgical evaluation as the risk of malignancy is high.[4]

TREATMENT

- Almost all simple cysts are asymptomatic and require **no specific therapy.**
- Pain from a large cyst is managed conservatively.
- If clinically warranted, a painful cyst resistant to therapy can be aspirated and sclerosed by either a percutaneous or surgical route.

OUTCOME/PROGNOSIS

- Simple cysts do not cause progressive renal dysfunction.
- If there is a decline in renal function, obstruction should be ruled out and an alternative explanation sought.

Acquired Renal Cysts

GENERAL PRINCIPLES

Epidemiology

- Acquired cystic disease occurs in patients with advanced chronic kidney disease or end-stage renal disease.
- The incidence increases with time on dialysis, with up to 90% of patients affected after 10 years or more.

Pathophysiology

- Chronic uremia with compensatory hyperplasia of the nephron is believed to underlie the development of acquired cystic disease, with bilateral involvement in most cases.
- Cysts form primarily from the proximal tubules with epithelial hyperplasia.
- The overall size of the kidney tends to be small to normal, as opposed to the massive enlargement frequently seen in ADPKD.

DIAGNOSIS

Clinical Presentation

- Most often, acquired cystic disease is **asymptomatic.**
- Cyst hemorrhage can occur, presenting with flank or back pain as well as hematuria.
- Pain may arise from an enlarging cyst itself, although this is uncommon.

Diagnostic Criteria

- Ultrasonography can easily identify cysts. However, CT/MRI is recommended for evaluating symptomatic patients or those with suspicious cysts.
- Cysts tend to be multiple, with three to five cysts in each kidney, and are typically cortical.

Differential Diagnosis

- Acquired cystic disease can be distinguished from ADPKD, as the kidneys remain small to normal in size, with a smooth contour.
- Simple cysts typically appear in fewer numbers than acquired cysts.

TREATMENT

- Acquired cysts are **generally asymptomatic and require no specific treatment.**
- Cyst hemorrhage is typically a self-limited process and can be managed with bed rest, hydration, and analgesia, as well as avoiding heparin on dialysis.
- Severe bleeding episodes are unusual, but may require embolization or nephrectomy.
- Patients with a suspicious lesion on CT/MRI that is >3 cm in diameter should undergo nephrectomy.

OUTCOME/PROGNOSIS

- Approximately 2% to 7% of patients will have transformation to renal cell carcinoma, with histologic features distinct from papillary or clear cell type cancers.
- Screening for transformation into renal cell carcinoma remains controversial, given the typically reduced life expectancy in patients on dialysis. Patients who have extended life expectancies, have survived on dialysis for more than 3 years, or who are being evaluated for transplantation may benefit from screening, although formalized guidelines are not available.

Medullary Cystic Kidney Disease

GENERAL PRINCIPLES

Classification

- MCKD is a complex of disorders with cyst formation at the corticomedullary junction. Progression with interstitial fibrosis typically leads to end-stage renal disease.
- Nephronophthisis is a related childhood disorder usually diagnosed by age 15; it is an autosomal recessive disorder.
- The adult forms of MCKD have an autosomal dominant inheritance, with MCKD1 (chromosome 1) and MCKD2 (chromosome 16).

Epidemiology

- All forms of MCKD are uncommon, with an incidence of 1 in 50,000 for the adult forms.
- Although juvenile nephronophthisis has an incidence of 1 in 1,000,000, it is the most common genetic cause of end-stage renal disease under the age of 20.
- There is no racial or gender predilection for MCKD.

Pathophysiology

- The gene products of MCKD and juvenile nephronophthisis are varied and therefore may not share a similar mechanism of disease.
- MCKD2 has a mutation in the uromodulin gene (Tamm–Horsfall protein), resulting in a misfolded protein product that accumulates intracellularly. The identity of the MCKD1 gene product has been recently identified as mucin-1.
- In many forms of juvenile nephronophthisis, the gene product localizes to the renal tubular epithelial, either within the primary cilium or at the associated basal bodies and centrosomes, suggesting a pathophysiologic link to ADPKD.
- Cysts form at the corticomedullary junction and arise late in the course of disease; they are not absolutely necessary for diagnosis.

DIAGNOSIS

Clinical Presentation

- Patients with the adult forms typically present in the third and fourth decades of life.
- A family history is common given the autosomal dominant inheritance pattern, but sporadic mutations can occur.
- A **concentrating defect** in the kidney may be pronounced, with **severe sodium wasting.**
- Other defects of the distal nephron are common, such as impaired H^+ excretion, leading to a distal renal tubular acidosis (type 1 RTA).

Diagnostic Criteria

- **CT scans** may detect numerous small cysts at the corticomedullary junction, with sizes ranging from <0.5 to 2 cm in diameter.
- **Ultrasonography** can also be used to detect the larger cysts, showing small-to-normal–sized kidneys with smooth outlines.

Differential Diagnosis

- Unlike ADPKD, the kidneys in MCKD are smooth and not enlarged, whereas the cysts, when present, are confined to the corticomedullary junction or renal medulla.
- Also, extrarenal cysts are not common in MCKD.

TREATMENT

- As no specific therapy is available for MCKD, treatment is generally supportive.
- **Maintenance of an adequate fluid volume** is important to replace urinary salt and water losses.

OUTCOME/PROGNOSIS

- **Progression to end-stage renal disease** is the typical pattern for MCKD.
- MCKD1 has a less rapid progression, with a median age of 62 years for end-stage renal disease versus 32 years for MCKD2.

Medullary Sponge Kidney

GENERAL PRINCIPLES

Epidemiology

- MSK is a developmental disorder with cystic dilation of the distal nephron (collecting ducts within the medullary pyramids).
- It is not believed to be a genetically inherited disorder although emerging evidence may suggest an underlying genetic component in some cases.
- Incidence is 1 in 5000 live births with no racial or gender predilection, although many more cases are probably undiagnosed.

Pathophysiology

- The pathogenesis is unknown.
- Only the inner papillary portions of the medulla are affected with cystic dilation, ranging from 1 to 7 mm in size.
- Most cysts communicate directly with the collecting system.
- Abnormalities of distal tubular function are common and account for the typical complications of MSK.
- Defects in urinary concentration may result from impaired vasopressin response (nephrogenic diabetes insipidus).
- Impaired H^+ excretion results in a distal renal tubular acidosis (type I RTA), and the accompanying hypocitraturia and increased calcium filtration can lead to nephrolithiasis.
- Urinary stasis within the cysts predisposes to infection, pyelonephritis, and abscess formation.

DIAGNOSIS

Clinical Presentation

- Patients are typically asymptomatic and the abnormality is frequently picked up on imaging for another cause.
- Complications of the disease, such as nephrolithiasis or recurrent urinary tract infections, can bring these patients to medical attention.
- **Gross hematuria** can occur in up to 20% of patients, either in isolation or in association with a renal stone or infection.
- Renal function is typically normal, and deterioration is not anticipated.

Diagnostic Criteria

- The gold standard for making the diagnosis of MSK is **intravenous excretory pyelography.**
  ○ Dilated collecting ducts appear as linear striations, causing a classic "paintbrush" effect.
  ○ Ectatic areas appear as "bouquets of flowers" or as "bunches of grapes."
- Ultrasonography is generally unable to identify the small cysts.

Differential Diagnosis

- MCKD also involves the deeper portions of the kidney. However, renal dysfunction and a family history are typically absent in MSK.
- MSK can usually be distinguished from ADPKD by the smaller size of the cysts, normal renal function, and absence of a family history.

TREATMENT

- Patients with MSK should be encouraged to **maintain adequate fluid intake** to avoid urinary stasis and reduce stone formation.
- Close vigilance and early eradication of urinary tract infections can reduce infectious complications.
- Persistent hematuria, particularly in patients >50 years of age, should prompt an evaluation for malignancy or other causes.
- **Acid–base balance should be monitored** and **persistent metabolic acidosis treated** in order to protect long-term bone health.

OUTCOME/PROGNOSIS

- As MSK is a developmental disorder and not a progressive one, long-term prognosis is typically excellent.
- Overall patient health is determined by correction of disease complications and not the renal malformations themselves.

Tuberous Sclerosis

GENERAL PRINCIPLES

Epidemiology

- Tuberous sclerosis is an inherited disease complex, involving benign growths in the kidneys (angiomyolipomas), brain, retina, lungs, and soft tissues.

- Two distinct types are defined genetically: TSC1 on chromosome 9 (hamartin) and TSC2 on chromosome 16 (tuberin), with autosomal dominant transmission.
- Incidence is estimated at 1 in 6000 to 10,000 live births, affecting all races and ethnicities.
- The genetic locus for TSC2 is adjacent to the locus for PKD1, and thus approximately 2% of patients with TSC2 will also have PKD1 (with a more severe renal phenotype and earlier progression).

Pathophysiology

- The gene products of TSC1 and TSC2 are tumor suppressors acting on the mammalian target of rapamycin (mTOR) complex.
- Hamartomas, angiomyolipomas, and renal cysts develop from unopposed cell proliferation.

DIAGNOSIS

Clinical Presentation

- Extrarenal manifestations are most characteristic, with **hamartomas** in the brain, retina, soft tissue, and lungs. A history of **epilepsy** is common; developmental delay may be completely absent while some patients exhibit severe disability.
- The kidneys develop angiomyolipomas in 80% of patients by young adulthood, which can lead to **hematuria and pain.**
- Although cyst formation occurs in only 20% to 30% of patients, they can be quite large.
- Symptoms tend to be more severe with mutations in TSC2 as compared to TSC1.

Diagnostic Criteria

- Diagnosis rests on the typical extrarenal manifestations described above.[5]
- **Renal angiomyolipomas** constitute a major criterion for diagnosis, whereas **renal cysts** make up a minor criterion.
- Ultrasonography can define the cystic structures, but angiomyolipomas may be better evaluated with CT scanning or MRI.
- Genetic tests for TSC1 and TSC2 have been available since 2002, although they have a significant false-negative rate.

Differential Diagnosis

- The presence of fat in the renal lesions, as detected on imaging, can help identify them as angiomyolipomas.
- Fat-poor angiomyolipomas may be difficult to distinguish from renal cell carcinoma. Follow-up imaging with CT/MRI every 6 months may prompt a biopsy if the growth rate is more than 5 mm/yr.

TREATMENT

- Early management is primarily centered on the neurologic manifestations.
- In young adults, renal angiomyolipomas become more prevalent, and recent studies have shown efficacy of everolimus, an mTOR inhibitor, in substantially shrinking these lesions.[6] The most common side effects of this medication are stomatitis, nasopharyngitis, and hyperlipidemia; renal function, blood counts, liver enzymes, and lipid levels should be monitored every 3 to 4 months when initiating treatment.

- The risk of a spontaneous life-threatening bleed increases with angiomyolipoma **size >4 cm,** and therefore an intervention with everolimus or arterial embolization should be offered for lesions that exceed this size. For patients on everolimus, interruption of treatment results in the regrowth of the angiomyolipoma to its original size, suggesting that therapy would need to be lifelong.
- **Yearly imaging** with an abdominal MRI is recommended to evaluate for new or growing lesions that may require therapy.

von Hippel–Lindau Syndrome

GENERAL PRINCIPLES

Epidemiology

- The VHL syndrome is an inherited disease complex of cerebellar and retinal hemangioblastomas, adrenal pheochromocytomas (up to 20%), renal/pancreatic cysts and carcinomas (40% incidence).
- Inheritance is autosomal dominant with the genetic abnormality located on chromosome 3.
- The incidence of this disease is 1 in 35,000 live births.

Pathophysiology

- The precise nature of tumor and cyst development has not been fully elucidated.
- Studies have implicated uncontrolled angiogenesis, through abnormal regulation of hypoxia-inducible factors, mTOR overactivity, and microtubular abnormalities during cell division.

DIAGNOSIS

Clinical Presentation

- The VHL syndrome can present with malignancies of the kidney, pancreas, adrenal glands (pheochromocytoma), or brain and retina (hemangioblastoma).
- **Renal cysts** may be large and plentiful, simulating ADPKD with renal dysfunction.
- **Malignant tumors** generally arise separately from the cysts, although renal cysts can show evidence of epithelial dysplasia and progress to solid malignant lesions.
- Not all mutations confer the same risk for developing renal cell carcinoma. Mutations that result in the production of truncated proteins are associated with a higher risk of developing this malignancy, and thus tend to cluster within families.

Diagnostic Criteria

- **CT scans** are preferred over ultrasonography, given their ability to identify smaller lesions.
- However, ultrasonography can be helpful in distinguishing cystic lesions from solid masses.
- **Genetic testing** is available for VHL and can determine the need for cancer screening in at-risk relatives.

Differential Diagnosis

- VHL may be difficult to distinguish from ADPKD when a family history is absent and the cysts are large and numerous. Extrarenal manifestations can be helpful in differentiating between these diseases.
- A high index of suspicion is necessary when evaluating a patient with cysts but without a family history of a cystic syndrome.

TREATMENT

- Screening should begin at age 16 with imaging of the kidneys every 1 to 3 years.
- Once a lesion is identified, imaging with CT scanning every 6 months to 1 year is recommended.
- Suspicious enlarging solid lesions should undergo nephron-sparing surgical removal.

REFERENCES

1. Pei Y, Obaji J, Dupuis A, et al. Unified criteria for ultrasonographic diagnosis of ADPKD. *J Am Soc Nephrol.* 2009;20:205–212.
2. Torres VE, Chapman AB, Devuyst O, et al. Tolvaptan in patients with autosomal dominant polycystic kidney disease. *N Engl J Med.* 2012;367:2407–2418.
3. Torres VE, Chapman AB, Devuyst O, et al. Tolvaptan in later-stage autosomal dominant polycystic kidney disease. *N Engl J Med.* 2017;377:1930–1942.
4. Israel GM, Bosniak MA. An update of the Bosniak renal cyst classification system. *Urology.* 2005;66:484–488.
5. Roach ES, DiMario FJ, Kandt RS, et al. Tuberous Sclerosis Consensus Conference: recommendations for diagnostic evaluation. National Tuberous Sclerosis Association. *J Child Neurol.* 1999;14:401–407.
6. Bissler JJ, Kingswood JC, Radzikowska E, et al. Everolimus for angiomyolipoma associated with tuberous sclerosis complex or sporadic lymphangioleiomyomatosis (EXIST-2): a multicentre, randomised, double-blind, placebo-controlled trial. *Lancet.* 2013;381:817–824.

Renal Diseases in Pregnancy

Deepa Amberker and Will Ross

15

GENERAL PRINCIPLES

- Pregnancy is associated with predictable anatomic changes of the kidney and is characterized by physiologic changes of systemic and renal hemodynamics.
- Hypertension and proteinuria should be considered pathologic, and the presence of these findings must lead to consideration of preeclampsia as well as other conditions.
- Women with mild kidney disease have a slightly higher risk of maternal and fetal complications, but their pregnancies are generally successful.
- More advanced kidney disease is associated with lower fertility rates and worse maternal and fetal outcomes.
- **Normal anatomic renal changes in pregnancy**
  - ○ **Kidney size increases** by 1.0 to 1.5 cm in pregnancy. Kidney volume increases by 30% due to increased renal blood flow and increased interstitial volume.[1]
  - ○ Renal histology and nephron numbers are unchanged.
  - ○ **Dilation of the ureters** (hydroureter) and renal pelvis/calyces (hydronephrosis) occurs due to the smooth muscle relaxing effect of progesterone and relaxin, causing reduced ureteral tone and peristalsis. These are physiologic findings and occur in about 80% of pregnant women, more prominent on the right side.
  - ○ Extrinsic compression of the ureters by the gravid uterus may cause **mechanical obstruction** as the pregnancy progresses, but this is usually of no clinical significance.
  - ○ The dilated collecting system can result in urinary stasis, leading to an **increased risk for ascending infection** of the urinary tract.
- **Normal hemodynamic changes in pregnancy**
  - ○ Systemic hemodynamics:
    - There is **reduction in systemic vascular resistance** in early pregnancy, leading to a drop in mean arterial blood pressure by 10 mm Hg by the second trimester.
    - The reduced systemic vascular resistance leads to increased sympathetic activity, resulting in 15% to 20% **increase in heart rate.**
    - Cardiac output increases by 30% to 50% due to increased heart rate and stroke volume, and reduced afterload.
    - Renin–angiotensin–aldosterone system is activated, leading to **increased sodium and water reabsorption,** resulting in retention of up to 900 mEq of extra sodium during the entire pregnancy and increase of total body water by 6 to 8 L. As a result, **physiologic anemia and edema** are common during normal pregnancy.
  - ○ Renal hemodynamics:
    - Renal vascular resistance decreases during early pregnancy due to incompletely understood mechanisms, leading to a significant **increase in renal blood flow.**
    - Glomerular filtration rate **(GFR) increases** during early pregnancy by 50% because of both increased renal blood flow and increased cardiac output.[2]
    - The increase in GFR results in a decrease in serum creatinine (from 0.8 mg/dL to 0.4 to 0.5 mg/dL), serum blood urea nitrogen (from 13 mg/dL to 8 to 10 mg/dL), and serum uric acid levels (from 4 mg/dL to 2 to 3 mg/dL) (see Table 15-1).

TABLE 15-1 EXPECTED LABORATORY VALUES IN PREGNANCY

	Nonpregnant	Pregnant
Hematocrit (vol/dL)	41	33
Plasma creatinine (mg/dL)	0.7–0.8	0.4–0.5
Plasma osmolality (mOsm/kg)	285	275
Plasma sodium (mmol/L)	140	135
Arterial PCO_2 (mm Hg)	40	30
pH	7.40	7.44
Bicarbonate (mmol/L)	25	22
Uric acid (mg/dL)	4.0	3.0
Plasma protein (g/dL)	7.0	6.0

- Creatinine-based formulas for estimating GFR are less reliable in pregnancy. It is important to remember that **serum creatinine that is considered normal in a nonpregnant female might actually signify significant renal impairment in a pregnant patient.**
- **Changes in water homeostasis**
  - Mild, asymptomatic **hyponatremia** is due to downward resetting of osmotic threshold for antidiuretic hormone (ADH) secretion and thirst (frequently known as the **"reset osmostat"**). This leads to a new steady-state plasma osmolality of 270 to 275 mOsm/kg and fall in serum sodium level by 5 mEq/L. Reset osmostat is thought to be mediated by human chorionic gonadotropin (hCG).
  - During the second half of pregnancy, high levels of placental vasopressinase can lead to increased ADH catabolism. Rarely, **diabetes insipidus** (DI) can ensue but is usually transient.
  - DI in pregnancy can be treated with desmopressin, a vasopressin analog that is resistant to the actions of vasopressinase.
- **Acid–base regulation:** In pregnancy, there is increase in minute ventilation and **mild chronic respiratory alkalosis** (PCO_2 falls to 30 mm Hg, pH increases to 7.44, and serum bicarbonate level decreases to 20 to 22 mEq/L because of compensatory increase in renal bicarbonate excretion). This can occur even in the first trimester, as progesterone directly stimulates central respiratory receptors.
- **Other renal changes**
  - Urinary **protein excretion increases** during pregnancy, **up to 200 mg/24 hrs.** Proteinuria of >300 mg/24 hrs is pathologic.
  - Owing to increased filtered load of glucose and amino acids, as well as less efficient tubular reabsorption, pregnant women may have mild glycosuria and aminoaciduria.

Hypertensive Disorders in Pregnancy

- Absolute blood pressure ≥140/90 mm Hg, taken on two separate occasions 6 hours apart, is considered abnormal.
- **Chronic hypertension** (or pre-existing hypertension): Hypertension diagnosed **prior to 20th week** of gestation, or persisting longer than 12 weeks postpartum.
- **Gestational hypertension:** De novo hypertension occurring **after 20th week** of gestation and resolving within 12 weeks postpartum.

- **Preeclampsia:** New-onset hypertension and proteinuria (>300 mg/24 hrs) occurring after 20th week of gestation. Diagnosis is changed to eclampsia with development of seizures. Preeclampsia may be superimposed on chronic hypertension.

CHRONIC HYPERTENSION IN PREGNANCY

General Principles

- Chronic hypertension occurs in 3% to 5% of all pregnancies and contributes significantly to maternal and fetal morbidity and mortality.
- Pregnancies complicated by hypertension have an increased risk of preeclampsia, intrauterine growth retardation, placental abruption, preterm delivery, and fetal loss.
- Chronic hypertension can be masked in early pregnancy because of the physiologic decrease in blood pressure.
- **Tight blood pressure control does not improve neonatal outcome or prevent superimposed preeclampsia** and **can compromise fetal growth** because of decreased placental perfusion.
- Target blood pressure is ill defined. Most experts recommend a **goal of 140 to 150/ 90 mm Hg.** Kidney Disease: Improving Global Outcomes (KDIGO) recommends that women with CKD without proteinuria should aim for a blood pressure <140/90 mm Hg. KDIGO also recommends this level for patients with an albumin to creatinine ratio >30 mg/mmol.

Treatment

- Pharmacologic treatment is recommended when blood pressure is >150/100 mm Hg to prevent maternal end-organ damage.[3] Please see Table 15-2 for medications.
- Severe hypertension (≥170/110 mm Hg) can be managed using intravenous labetalol, hydralazine, or nicardipine, as these have been extensively used during pregnancy.
- Oral agents that are used to treat elevated blood pressure in pregnancy include methyldopa, labetalol, long-acting nifedipine, and hydralazine.
- Diuretics are generally not recommended during pregnancy because of the risk of volume depletion in the fetus.
- **Angiotensin-converting enzyme (ACE) inhibitors and angiotensin receptor blockers (ARBs) are CONTRAINDICATED** because of extremely high risk of teratogenicity. Other inhibitors of the renin–angiotensin–aldosterone axis also fall into this category.

TABLE 15-2	DRUG OPTIONS FOR HYPERTENSION IN PREGNANCY	
Subacute Antihypertensive Therapy	**Acute Antihypertensive Therapy**	
Methyldopa: 250 mg PO bid or tid; usual dose, 1.0–1.5 g/day; maximum dose, 3 g/day	Labetalol: 20 mg IV; can be repeated at 10–15-min intervals (with escalating doses, i.e., 40 mg, 60 mg, and so forth) to a total cumulative dose of 300 mg	
Nifedipine, long acting: 30 mg/day PO; maximum dose 120 mg/day	Hydralazine: 5–10 mg IV; can be repeated at 15-min intervals to a maximum cumulative dose of 30 mg	
Labetalol: 100 mg PO bid or tid; maximum dose, 1200 mg/day	—	

PREECLAMPSIA

General Principles

- Preeclampsia affects about 5% of all pregnancies and remains the leading cause of maternal and fetal mortality in the world.[4]
- Risk factors for preeclampsia are listed in Table 15-3.
- Initiating events in preeclampsia are poorly understood, but the origin appears to be the placenta and the target is the maternal endothelium.
- In normal pregnancy, cytotrophoblasts invade the uterine spiral arterioles, converting them from small-caliber vessels to large-caliber capacitance vessels capable of carrying larger amount of blood through the placenta.
- In preeclampsia, this process of cytotrophoblast invasion is defective and there is deficient transformation of the spiral arterioles, leading to reduced placental perfusion.
- The diseased placenta secretes an increased amount of antiangiogenic factor (soluble fms-like tyrosine kinase-1), which antagonizes the proangiogenic effects of vascular endothelial growth factor and placental growth factor, resulting in systemic vascular endothelial dysfunction characteristic of preeclampsia.[5]
- Maternal endothelial dysfunction causes increased production of reactive oxygen species, thromboxane, and endothelin-1. Also, there is increased vascular sensitivity to angiotensin II and decreased nitric oxide and prostacyclin bioavailability.
- The end result is potent vasoconstriction and end-organ damage.

Diagnosis

- Symptom onset is usually in the latter part of the third trimester, but can happen anytime after 20th week of gestation, or can be delayed until after delivery.
- Clinical features of preeclampsia are detailed in Table 15-4.
- **Signs and laboratory findings in severe preeclampsia** are:
  - Blood pressure ≥160/110 mm Hg
  - Proteinuria ≥5 g/24 hrs or 3+ protein on urine dipstick results
  - Oliguria <500 mL urine in 24 hours or elevated serum creatinine
  - Hemolysis, elevated liver enzymes, and low platelets (HELLP) syndrome
  - Pulmonary edema, impaired liver function
  - Headaches, visual disturbances, epigastric or right upper quadrant pain
  - Fetal growth restriction

Treatment

- **Definitive treatment is delivery.** Gestational age, severity of preeclampsia, and maternal and fetal condition are all important factors when deciding the appropriate course of action.

TABLE 15-3 RISK FACTORS FOR PREECLAMPSIA

Maternal age ≥40	Multiple gestation
Nulliparity	Diabetes mellitus
Preeclampsia in previous pregnancy	Chronic hypertension
Family history of preeclampsia	Chronic kidney disease
Time between pregnancy >10 yrs	Connective tissue disorder
Obesity	Antiphospholipid syndrome

TABLE 15-4	CLINICAL FINDINGS IN PREECLAMPSIA
Neurologic	Headache, blurred vision, visual scotomata, hyperreflexia, clonus, and seizures. Cerebral edema and intracerebral hemorrhage can be seen
Renal	Proteinuria (>300 mg/day), azotemia (decreased renal blood flow and average GFR decreases by 30–40%), and acute kidney injury—rare and often secondary to acute tubular necrosis. Increased urate reabsorption results in hyperuricemia
Hematologic	Microangiopathic hemolytic anemia, thrombocytopenia, disseminated intravascular coagulation
Hepatic	Elevated liver enzymes (HELLP syndrome)
Cardiovascular	Hypertension, decreased cardiac output
Gastrointestinal	Elevated liver enzymes, epigastric/right upper quadrant pain, subcapsular hemorrhage, liver rupture
Other	Pulmonary edema, peripheral edema—often facial and lower extremity

GFR, glomerular filtration rate; HELLP, hemolysis, elevated liver enzymes, and low platelets.

- **Indications for urgent delivery:** greater than or equal to 37 weeks of gestation, refractory hypertension despite adequate therapy, progressive organ system failure (kidney, liver, hematologic parameters, neurologic dysfunction), eclampsia, HELLP syndrome, fetal compromise, and abruptio placentae.
- Management of hypertension:
  - The **goal of treatment is prevention of cerebrovascular and cardiovascular events.**
  - Treatment **does not change the course of preeclampsia and does not prevent progression to eclampsia.**
  - Aggressive lowering of blood pressure in patients with preeclampsia is NOT recommended, as it can further decrease placental perfusion and compromise fetal growth.
  - The blood pressure level at which treatment should begin is undefined. In general, most experts initiate therapy with blood pressure at ≥150 to 160/100 to 110 mm Hg. **Target blood pressure is usually 140 to 150/90 mm Hg.**
  - Please refer to Chronic Hypertension in Pregnancy for recommendations on antihypertensive therapy.
- **Prevention is key.** Low-dose aspirin has been associated with a significant reduction in preeclampsia and intrauterine growth restriction. The U.S. Preventive Services Task Force now recommends the use of low-dose aspirin (81 mg/day) as preventive medication after 12 weeks of gestation in women who are at high risk for preeclampsia.[6]
- **Mild preeclampsia management:**
  - Supportive therapy until delivery
  - Complete or partial bed rest
  - Frequent fetal monitoring
  - Blood pressure check twice weekly
  - Laboratory tests: hemoglobin and hematocrit, platelet count, creatinine, hepatic enzymes (aspartate aminotransferase, alanine transaminase, lactate dehydrogenase), uric acid, urine dipstick test
- **Severe preeclampsia management** includes:

- ○ Immediate hospitalization
- ○ **Seizure prophylaxis with magnesium sulfate**
- ○ **Corticosteroids between 25 and 34 weeks** to decrease the risk of respiratory distress syndrome in infants
- ○ Acute **management of severe hypertension** with intravenous labetalol, hydralazine, or nicardipine to a target blood pressure of 140 to 150/90 mm Hg
- ○ **Delivery of fetus**

Acute Kidney Injury in Pregnancy

GENERAL PRINCIPLES

- Pregnant patients are susceptible to a variety of causes of acute kidney injury (AKI), including disorders that are pregnancy specific.
- **Prerenal Azotemia:**
  - ○ Hyperemesis gravidarum
  - ○ Other prerenal etiologies
- **Acute Tubular Necrosis:**
  - ○ Hyperemesis gravidarum
  - ○ Hemorrhage
  - ○ Shock/sepsis (e.g., septic abortion, pyelonephritis)
- **Obstructive Uropathy:**
  - ○ Gravid uterus (rare)
  - ○ Large uterine fibroids
  - ○ Stones:
    - These are **usually calcium containing** as urinary calcium excretion increases in pregnancy.
    - They are often located in the distal ureter.
    - Most stones tend to **pass spontaneously.**
    - Ureteral stents can be placed in patients unable to pass the stone; percutaneous nephrostomy may be required to decompress the urinary system.
    - Extracorporeal shock wave lithotripsy is not recommended during pregnancy.
    - Obstructive stones with hydronephrosis/pyonephrosis may require cystoscopic or ureteroscopic stone removal.
    - **Risk of infection is increased.**
- **Acute Pyelonephritis:**
  - ○ Risk factors:
    - **Urinary stasis** due to physiologic hydroureter and hydronephrosis increases risk for upper tract infection.
    - **Anatomic displacement** of ureters by the gravid uterus can also lead to stasis and obstruction, thus increasing risk for pyelonephritis.
    - **Untreated asymptomatic bacteriuria** is a well-known risk factor for urinary tract infections. This is defined by the presence of positive urine culture in an asymptomatic person: $\geq 10^5$ colony-forming units per mL in voided urine on two separate collections or $\geq 10^2$ colony-forming units per mL in a catheterized specimen. It increases risk for adverse fetal outcomes, and routine screen at 12 to 16 weeks is recommended. Treatment is always warranted for asymptomatic bacteriuria.
  - ○ Clinical presentation:
    - Fever, dysuria, flank pain
    - Can lead to sepsis and shock
    - AKI can result from focal microabscesses and sepsis/shock

○ Treatment: Aggressive treatment with intravenous antibiotics and supportive measures

- **Renal Cortical Necrosis:**
  ○ Renal cortical necrosis is secondary to rare catastrophic events resulting in prolonged hypotension and profound renal ischemia, especially to the renal cortex. The **damage is irreversible in most cases,** with survivors often requiring long-term dialysis. The well-described causes for renal cortical necrosis are listed below.
  ○ **Causes:**
    ▪ Septic abortion
    ▪ Amniotic fluid embolism
    ▪ Fetal demise with retained fetus
    ▪ Abruptio placentae
  ○ The precipitating event usually leads to disseminated intravascular coagulation and severe renal ischemia.
  ○ **Clinical presentation** includes:
    ▪ Abrupt onset of oliguria/anuria
    ▪ Flank pain
    ▪ Gross hematuria
    ▪ Hypotension (maybe)
  ○ Diagnosis:
    ▪ Ultrasound or computed tomography scan shows hypoechoic or hypodense areas in the renal cortex.
    ▪ Renal biopsy is not routinely done.
  ○ Treatment:
    ▪ Supportive measures only as there is no effective therapy.
    ▪ A significant percentage of patients will initially require renal replacement therapy.
    ▪ Partial renal recovery can occur, but may take months.
- **Preeclampsia/HELLP Syndrome:** This is a rare cause of AKI, and has been explained in detail under Preeclampsia.
- **Acute Fatty Liver of Pregnancy:**
  ○ This is extremely rare but can be fatal.
  ○ Fatty liver of pregnancy **typically presents in the third trimester.**
  ○ It is extremely important to distinguish from HELLP syndrome and hemolytic uremic syndrome (HUS) (see Table 15-5).
  ○ **Clinical features** include anorexia, jaundice, nausea and vomiting, abdominal pain, and AKI (the mechanism of AKI is unclear and renal pathology is usually unremarkable).
  ○ Etiology: There is extensive microvesicular fatty infiltration of hepatocytes due to defective mitochondrial fatty acid oxidation. The trigger for this is unknown.
  ○ Laboratory data demonstrates elevated transaminases, increased bilirubin/ammonia level, prolonged partial thromboplastin time and prothrombin time, thrombocytopenia (not prominent), and hypoglycemia.
  ○ Treatment:
    ▪ Prompt delivery and supportive care
    ▪ Most patients fully recover, but some may require liver transplantation
- **HUS:**
  ○ HUS usually presents in the near term or in the immediate postpartum period, but can occur at any stage of pregnancy.
  ○ **Clinical features:**
    ▪ Microangiopathic hemolytic anemia
    ▪ Thrombocytopenia
    ▪ AKI: thrombotic microangiopathy is noted on renal pathology
    ▪ Hypertension

TABLE 15-5	DIFFERENTIAL DIAGNOSIS OF AKI IN LATE PREGNANCY		
Features	HUS	HELLP	Acute Fatty Liver of Pregnancy
Time of onset	Usually postpartum	After 20 wks	Third trimester
Hepatic involvement	None	Yes	Yes
Thrombocytopenia	Severe	Moderate	Maybe
Coagulopathy	None	Maybe	Often
Hemolytic anemia	Yes	Yes	No
Hypertension	Maybe	Yes	Maybe
Proteinuria	Maybe	Yes	Maybe
Renal dysfunction	Severe	Mild	Severe
Therapy	Plasmapheresis	Delivery	Delivery

AKI, acute kidney injury; HELLP, hemolysis, elevated liver enzymes, and low platelets; HUS, hemolytic uremic syndrome.

TREATMENT

- Plasma exchange is the primary treatment.
- Pregnancy-associated HUS has a severity at and distribution of complement gene variants similar to those of atypical HUS cases; thus, select cases may be amenable to inhibitors of complement regulatory genes.
- Delivery does not appear to change the course of the disease.

Chronic Kidney Disease and Pregnancy

- **Fertility is diminished in women with chronic kidney disease (CKD),** especially in those with serum creatinine >3.0 mg/dL or who are dialysis dependent. CKD leads to impairment in the hypothalamic–pituitary–gonadal axis, causing decreased fertility.
- If patients with CKD (regardless of underlying etiology) become pregnant, they are at increased risk for adverse maternal and fetal outcomes.
  ○ **Maternal complications** include increased proteinuria, worsening hypertension, increased risk for preeclampsia, and permanently diminished renal function.
  ○ **Fetal complications** include prematurity, intrauterine growth retardation, and an increased risk for fetal loss.
- This risk depends on the severity of baseline renal dysfunction, presence of uncontrolled hypertension, and degree of proteinuria.
- Women with pre-existing mild CKD (creatinine <1.4 mg/dL), normal blood pressure, and no proteinuria generally have good maternal and fetal outcomes.
- Patients with moderate (creatinine 1.4 to 2.5 mg/dL) or severe (creatinine >2.5 mg/dL) CKD have significantly increased risk of developing worsening renal function, proteinuria, hypertension, as well as increased rates of fetal complications.[7]
- In one study, the combined presence of **GFR <40 mL/min/1.73 m^2** (CKD stage 3) and **proteinuria >1 g/day** before conception **predicted faster GFR loss after delivery, shorter time to dialysis, and low birth weight.**[8]

- Necessary discontinuation of certain medications (ACE inhibitor, ARB, or certain immunosuppressants) may lead to renal exacerbation or disease flare.
- Women of reproductive age with CKD should be advised of the potential adverse maternal and fetal effects related to pregnancy.
- **Pregnancy in the dialysis patient:**
  - Conception in dialysis patients is very rare (only 0.3% to 1.5% of all women of childbearing age).
  - Early pregnancy is **difficult to diagnose as β-hCG is not reliable.**
  - **Outcomes** are similar in patients treated with hemodialysis and peritoneal dialysis.[9]
    - **Fetal:** there is a high spontaneous fetal loss rate (50%), high rate of preterm labor (86%), and a risk of fetal growth retardation (30%).
    - **Maternal risks include** severe hypertension (85%) and an increased mortality rate.
  - Management:
    - For patients on hemodialysis, **longer and more frequent dialysis sessions** can improve fetal outcome (>20 hrs/wk).[10] It is important to avoid hypotension, hypocalcemia, and metabolic acidosis.
    - Peritoneal dialysis: Decreased fill volume and frequent exchanges might be beneficial.
    - Anemia:
      - Hemoglobin should be maintained above 10 g/dL.
      - Iron and folic acid supplementation should be administered.
      - Erythropoietin should be prescribed cautiously given the risk of hypertension, but there does not appear to be a risk for teratogenicity.
    - Nutrition: Protein intake should be ~1.8 g/kg/day and supplemented with vitamins.
    - Blood pressure control:
      - Diuretics do not have a significant role in a dialysis patient and should be used with caution in a nondialysis CKD patient.
      - ACE inhibitors and angiotensin II receptor blockers are CONTRAINDICATED in pregnancy.
    - Obstetric care: High-risk obstetric care and serial fetal monitoring during hemodialysis are recommended.

PREGNANCY IN RENAL TRANSPLANT RECIPIENTS AND KIDNEY DONORS

- **After renal transplant**
  - Return of fertility is the rule in female transplant patients of childbearing age, occurring as early as 1 month following renal transplantation.[11]
  - Transplant kidney is an independent risk factor for preeclampsia, even with a good GFR.
  - Patients are advised to **wait for at least 1 year and preferably 2 years following renal transplantation before conception.**
  - Rejection during pregnancy can be treated with corticosteroids and/or antithymocyte globulin.
  - Pregnancy in kidney donors is associated with increased incidence of preeclampsia.
  - Prior to conception:
    - The pregnancy should be planned and the patient should discuss with the treating nephrologist prior to conception.
    - Renal function should be stable with serum creatinine <1.5 mg/dL.
    - Proteinuria should be <500 mg/day.
    - Blood pressure should be controlled with minimal number of medications.

- There should be no recent episodes of rejection or other transplant-related complications.
- **Mycophenolate, sirolimus, cyclophosphamide, rituximab, statins, ACE inhibitor, ARB, and minoxidil should be discontinued prior to pregnancy.**
- It is important to change these medications to others that are considered "safe" in pregnancy ahead of time and to ensure that the serum creatinine and blood pressure are stable, before conception.
- Azathioprine, calcineurin inhibitors, and calcium channel blockers may be continued during pregnancy.
- **After kidney donation**
  ○ Few studies have shown that gestational hypertension and preeclampsia are more likely to be diagnosed in kidney donors compared to healthy individuals with two kidneys.[12]
  ○ KDIGO recommends that potential living donors with childbearing potential should be counseled on risks of gestational hypertension and preeclampsia in the future.

SYSTEMIC LUPUS ERYTHEMATOSUS AND PREGNANCY

- **Best pregnancy outcomes** occur in women with **quiescent lupus for at least 6 months prior to conception.** The PROMISSE study demonstrated that 81% of pregnancies in women with inactive or stable mild and/or moderate disease had positive pregnancy outcomes.[13]
- Systemic lupus erythematosus (SLE) patients with previous kidney disease and low C4 level carry higher risk of lupus nephritis during pregnancy compared to those without past kidney disease and with low C3 level, respectively.
- Pregnancy in women with **active lupus nephritis** is associated with an **increased risk of fetal loss** (up to 75%) and **worsening of both renal and extrarenal manifestations.**
- Women with severe active disease or a high degree of irreversible organ damage, such as symptomatic pulmonary hypertension, heart failure, severe restrictive pulmonary disease, or advanced CKD/lupus nephritis, should avoid pregnancy.
- Maintenance therapy for SLE or lupus nephritis should be continued during pregnancy to prevent flares, although the choice of therapy is frequently limited by teratogenicity.
- When renal function or proteinuria worsens, low complement levels, rising double-stranded DNA antibody levels, and active urine sediment may help differentiate lupus nephritis from preeclampsia.
- There is an **increased risk of thrombosis and fetal loss in the presence of antiphospholipid antibody.**
- The presence of **SSA/SSB antibodies is a risk factor for neonatal heart block.**

OTHER GLOMERULAR DISEASES IN PREGNANCY

- Any active glomerulonephritis will potentially contribute to adverse pregnancy outcomes, and control of the glomerular disease with pregnancy-safe immunosuppression is desirable, whereas all potentially teratogenic medications must be discontinued.[14]
- While kidney biopsy is not contraindicated in pregnancy, it should be considered only when the information obtained is likely to affect the treatment management.
- Urine to protein creatinine ratios can be useful to monitor disease activity.
- Prednisone is considered to be relatively safe in pregnancy, and benefits of continuation usually considerably outweigh any risk. Azathioprine is frequently the drug of choice to maintain disease quiescence during pregnancy.

REFERENCES

1. Bailey RR, Rolleston GL. Kidney length and ureteric dilatation in the puerperium. *J Obstet Gynaecol Br Commonw.* 1971;78:55–61.
2. Baylis C. The determinants of renal hemodynamics in pregnancy. *Am J Kidney Dis.* 1987;9:260–264.
3. Lindheimer MD, Taler SJ, Cunningham FG. Hypertension in pregnancy. *J Am Soc Hypertens.* 2008;2:484–494.
4. Karumanchi SA, Maynard SE, Stillman IE, et al. Preeclampsia: a renal perspective. *Kidney Int.* 2005;67:2101–2113.
5. Gilbert JS, Ryan MJ, LaMarca BB, et al. Pathophysiology of hypertension during preeclampsia: linking placental ischemia with endothelial dysfunction. *Am J Physiol Heart Circ Physiol.* 2008;294:H541–H550.
6. LeFevre ML; U.S. Preventive Services Task Force. Low-dose aspirin use for the prevention of morbidity and mortality from preeclampsia: U.S. Preventive Services Task Force recommendation statement. *Ann Intern Med.* 2014;161:819–826.
7. Zhang JJ, Ma XX, Hao L, et al. A systematic review and meta-analysis of outcomes of pregnancy in CKD and CKD outcomes in pregnancy. *Clin J Am Soc Nephrol.* 2015;10:1964–1978.
8. Imbasciati E, Gregorini G, Cabiddu G, et al. Pregnancy in CKD stages 3 to 5: fetal and maternal outcomes. *Am J Kidney Dis.* 2007;49:753–762.
9. Okundaye I, Abrinko P, Hou S. Registry of pregnancy in dialysis patients. *Am J Kidney Dis.* 1998;31:766–773.
10. Manisco G, Poti M, Maggiulli G, et al. Pregnancy in end-stage renal disease patients on dialysis: how to achieve a successful delivery. *Clin Kidney J.* 2015;8:293–299.
11. McKay DB, Josephson MA. Pregnancy in recipients of solid organs–effects on mother and child. *N Engl J Med.* 2006;354:1281–1293.
12. Shah PB, Samra M, Josephson MA. Preeclampsia risks in kidney donors and recipients. *Curr Hypertens Rep.* 2018;20:59.
13. Buyon JP, Kim MY, Guerra MM, et al. Predictors of pregnancy outcomes in patients with lupus: a cohort study. *Ann Intern Med.* 2015;163:153–163.
14. Blom K, Odutayo A, Bramham K, et al. Pregnancy and glomerular disease: a systematic review of the literature with management guidelines. *Clin J Am Soc Nephrol.* 2017;12:1862–1872.

Nephrolithiasis

16

Seth Goldberg

GENERAL PRINCIPLES

- Kidney stones are crystalline structures in the urinary tract that have achieved sufficient size to cause symptoms or be visible by radiographic imaging techniques.
- Most kidney stones in Western countries are composed of calcium salts and occur in the upper urinary tract. Conversely, in developing countries, most stones are composed of uric acid and occur in the urinary bladder. Dietary factors likely account for this difference, with Western diets high in protein and sodium.
- The immense economic impact of kidney stones includes loss of productivity and emergency department visits, in addition to surgical extraction or fragmentation of stones and the need for preventive treatment.
- Stone formation is associated with increased risk of chronic kidney disease.[1]

Classification

- As specific therapeutic maneuvers depend upon the chemical composition of a patient's kidney stone, extracted or passed stones should be collected and submitted for analysis.
- **Calcium salts:** In Western societies, about 80% of all kidney stones are composed of calcium salts. While a majority of these are of mixed composition (calcium oxalate and calcium phosphate), stones of pure calcium oxalate or calcium phosphate are observed and should prompt a search for an underlying metabolic risk factor.
- **Uric acid stones:** These account for approximately 10% of all stones in the urinary tract, and are notable for their radiolucency and insolubility in acidic urine.
- **Struvite stones:** These are also described as triple phosphate or magnesium-ammonium-phosphate and frequently form a staghorn configuration. They account for approximately 10% of all kidney stones and are associated with an alkaline urine in the setting of urea-splitting bacteria and urinary tract infections (UTIs).
- **Cystine stones:** The hereditary disorder cystinuria (not to be confused with cystinosis) accounts for less than 1% of all stones. Cystinuria is characterized by an amino acid transport defect in the proximal tubule, resulting in a urinary loss of dibasic amino acids.
- **Other:** Rarely, stones can be formed by poorly soluble drugs (e.g., triamterene, indinavir, sulfonamide), xanthine, hypoxanthine, or ammonium urate.

Epidemiology

- Nephrolithiasis is one of the most common diseases in Western countries, with an incidence that is increasing.
- The peak age of onset is the third decade, with increasing prevalence until the age of 70 years. In women, there is a second peak at the age of 55 years.
- Lifetime risk of developing a kidney stone is 12% for men and 6% for women. Historically, men have had a two to three times greater risk than women.[2]
- More recently, an increasing rate of nephrolithiasis has been attributed to larger body mass index. This effect appears to be magnified in women.[3]

Pathophysiology

One can infer from the variety of stones observed that several pathophysiologic mechanisms are responsible for stone formation. Nevertheless, a common pathway leading to stone formation is urinary supersaturation. Crystals form when the amount of solute in the urine exceeds its solubility limits.

Stone Formation

Three steps are necessary to form a stone:

1. Formation of a small initial crystal, or nidus.
2. Retention of a nidus in the urinary tract. If washed away by urine flow, crystal formation would remain a mere physiologic curiosity.
3. Growth of a nidus to a size at which it either becomes symptomatic or visible by imaging.

Solubility

- **Solubility product:** This describes the level of a solution's saturation with solute at which solid-phase material exists in equilibrium with liquid-phase material. The concentration of lithogenic solutes, stone inhibitors, and urine pH may all contribute to the solubility product.
- **Urine pH:** Urinary pH has a variable effect depending on the solutes involved.
  - **Low urine pH** significantly decreases the solubility of uric acid and cystine stones, contributing substantially to the risk of formation. In the case of uric acid stones, a urinary pH below 5.3 is more relevant as a risk factor than the actual amount of uric acid excretion.
  - **High urine pH** significantly decreases the solubility of calcium phosphate and struvite stones, with an increased risk of formation above a urine pH of 6.7 to 7.0. Struvite stones are more commonly associated with the presence of a UTI caused by urea-splitting bacteria.
- **Inhibitors of crystallization:** Several compounds are protective against stone formation.
  - **Citrate,** the primary inhibitor of crystallization of calcium salts, complexes with calcium to form a soluble calcium citrate compound. By doing so, it makes less calcium available to precipitate out as calcium oxalate or calcium phosphate. Hypocitraturia is a common finding among calcium stone formers, particularly when associated with a distal renal tubular acidosis (RTA).
  - **Magnesium** also inhibits crystallization of calcium salts, although its effect is not as significant as that of citrate.

Risk Factors

Risk Factors for Calcium Oxalate Nephrolithiasis

- **Low urinary volume:** As with all stone types, a low urine flow rate increases the risk of stone retention and growth. The commonly accepted threshold is 2 L/day although large randomized controlled trials have not definitively defined the optimum daily urine output.
- **Hypercalciuria:** To understand how hypercalciuria may occur, it is important to consider the normal handling of calcium.
  - Over 99% of the body's calcium is stored in the bone, with the serum concentration tightly regulated by parathyroid hormone (PTH). Dietary fluctuations and gastrointestinal (GI) absorption of calcium will result in the appropriate changes to the PTH level to ensure a steady serum concentration. Thus, **calcium ingestion alone is rarely a cause of hypercalcemia or hypercalciuria.** Instead, **hypercalciuria (>200 to 250 mg/day) is frequently idiopathic** and not associated with concomitant elevations in serum calcium. Recent genetic studies have suggested

TABLE 16-1 DIFFERENTIAL DIAGNOSIS OF HYPERCALCIURIA

Normal serum calcium
Idiopathic hypercalciuria
PTH-dependent elevated serum calcium
Primary hyperparathyroidism: adenoma or hyperplasia
PTH-independent elevated serum calcium
Malignancy: squamous cell carcinoma, breast cancer, bladder cancer, multiple myeloma, lymphoma
Granulomatous disease: sarcoidosis, tuberculosis, berylliosis
Hypervitaminosis D
Hyperthyroidism

PTH, parathyroid hormone.

a role for claudins, which regulate the paracellular reabsorption of calcium within the nephron.[4]

○ Nonetheless, conditions of increased bone turnover (i.e., hyperparathyroidism, metabolic acidosis) can shunt calcium from the skeleton to the urinary tract and should be sought in the evaluation of a patient with calcium-based stones. A number of disease processes can result in hypercalciuria (Table 16-1).

○ Calcium excretion is influenced by dietary sodium intake. Excessive sodium intake leads to extracellular volume expansion and diminished sodium resorption along the nephron. Volume expansion results not only in natriuresis but also in calciuresis. Hence, **dietary salt restriction** can be an effective method of ameliorating hypercalciuria.

○ **Thiazide diuretics** reduce hypercalciuria by increasing calcium resorption at the distal tubule, indirectly through the calcium-selective apical transient receptor potential cation channel subfamily V member 5 (TRPV5) channel. Thiazides, through their diuretic action, also cause a reduction in the extracellular fluid volume, leading to enhanced proximal reabsorption of calcium.

- **Hyperoxaluria** is divided into dietary, enteric, or primary forms (Table 16-2).
  ○ **Dietary hyperoxaluria:** Normal daily urinary excretion of oxalate is <40 mg/day. Excessive dietary intake of oxalate-rich foods can result in a mild form of dietary hyperoxaluria (urinary oxalate excretion of 50 to 60 mg/day). **Oxalate-rich foods** include nuts, sunflower seeds, spinach, rhubarb, chocolate, Swiss chard, lime peel, star fruit, peppers, and tea. Intake of **vitamin C** exceeding 100 mg/day can cause hyperoxaluria due to its conversion to oxalate.
  ○ **Enteric hyperoxaluria:** Fat malabsorption and saponification of calcium in the gut by free fatty acids result in increased free oxalate and its absorption in the colon. The resultant hyperoxaluria is more severe than the dietary form (often exceeding 100 mg/day). Thus, small bowel resection, jejunal bypass surgery, and inflammatory bowel disorders can lead to calcium oxalate nephrolithiasis, and even chronic renal failure due to nephrocalcinosis. In addition to hyperoxaluria, malabsorption has several other consequences that predispose to stone formation, including low urine volumes due to diarrheal loss of water, hypomagnesemia due to magnesium malabsorption, and hypocitraturia due to chronic metabolic acidosis and hypokalemia.
  ○ **Primary hyperoxaluria:** Primary forms of hyperoxaluria result from well-described metabolic defects.[5] These are characterized by **excessive endogenous production of oxalate, resulting in profound hyperoxaluria** (135 to 270 mg/day). Stone

TABLE 16-2 CAUSES OF HYPEROXALURIA

Dietary Hyperoxaluria	Enteric Hyperoxaluria	Primary Hyperoxaluria
Cause: excessive dietary oxalate intake	**Causes:** small bowel malabsorption, Crohn disease, jejunoileal bypass, celiac sprue, short bowel syndrome, chronic pancreatitis, biliary obstruction	**Type I:** deficiency of alanine glyoxylate aminotransferase
Foods rich in oxalate: cocoa, chocolate, black tea, green beans, beets, celery, green onions, spinach, rhubarb, Swiss chard, mustard greens, berries, dried figs, orange and lemon peel, summer squash, nuts, peanut butter	Moderate-to-severe elevation of urinary oxalate excretion; may result in nephrocalcinosis and renal failure	**Type II:** D-glycerate dehydrogenase or glyoxylate reductase deficiency
Mild elevation in urinary oxalate excretion, with increased risk of calcium oxalate nephrolithiasis		Severe hyperoxaluria, resulting in nephrocalcinosis and renal failure

formation often begins in childhood. Deposition of calcium oxalate in the tubulointerstitial compartment of the kidneys (renal oxalosis) often leads to progressive loss of renal function. Deposition of calcium oxalate also occurs in the heart, bone, joints, eyes, and other tissues. Two major defects are worth mentioning:

- **Type I primary hyperoxaluria** is an autosomal-recessive disorder that results from reduced activity of hepatic peroxisomal alanine glyoxylate aminotransferase. This increases the availability of glyoxylate, which is irreversibly converted to oxalic acid. Liver transplantation may ultimately be required to replace the missing enzyme.
- **Type II primary hyperoxaluria** is a much rarer form of the disease, caused by D-glycerate dehydrogenase or glyoxylate reductase deficiency.

- **Hypocitraturia:** This is defined as a **urinary citrate excretion <250 to 500 mg/day.** It is **observed in over 40% of patients with nephrolithiasis.**
  - The presence of hypocitraturia should arouse suspicion of a disorder associated with chronic metabolic acidosis, such as distal RTA or a GI disorder.
  - Hypocitraturia can also be seen in the setting of hypokalemia or with the use of carbonic anhydrase inhibitors such as topiramate.
- **Hyperuricosuria:** This is **seen in up to a quarter of calcium stone formers** defined as a **urinary uric acid excretion >750 mg/day.** Although the stone is not primarily composed of uric acid, this chemical can form the nidus upon which the calcium oxalate builds.
  - The amount of uric acid in the urine is determined by daily production of uric acid and is not necessarily associated with hyperuricemia or gout. High intake of animal proteins or other purine-rich foods or beverages (alcohol) can also lead to hyperuricosuria.
  - **Allopurinol,** a xanthine oxidase inhibitor, significantly reduces the rate of calcium oxalate stone recurrences. The benefits are attributed to a decreased urinary excretion of uric acid.

Risk Factors for Calcium Phosphate Nephrolithiasis
- Calcium phosphate stones have similar risk factors as calcium oxalate stones, including **low urinary volume, hypercalciuria, hypocitraturia, and hyperuricosuria.**

- However, one major distinction is the role of pH in stone formation. Calcium phosphate stones form in relatively **alkaline urine,** with an increased risk at a **urine pH above 6.7.**
- Caution should be taken when treating concomitant hypocitraturia, as the citrate salts can increase the urinary pH. These medications can be both helpful and deleterious, and finding the right balance can be difficult.
- A classic scenario for calcium phosphate nephrolithiasis is a distal RTA, where systemic acidosis results in increased bone resorption (to release buffer) with increased calcium filtration and urinary calcium excretion. Citrate reabsorption in the proximal nephron (to correct the acidosis) leads to hypocitraturia, and a distal urinary acidification defect results in a persistently alkaline urine. An incomplete distal RTA is where the serum bicarbonate is preserved within the normal range. Medullary nephrocalcinosis may occur, with calcification of the renal parenchyma, and subsequent deterioration of renal function.
- Medullary sponge kidney, a developmental defect with dilatation of the distal nephron, can result in urinary stasis and frequent UTIs. A distal RTA may also be present, increasing the risk of calcium phosphate stones.

Risk Factors for Uric Acid Nephrolithiasis

- **Low urinary volume:** As with all other stone types, a low urine volume will predispose to uric acid stone formation.
- **Low urine pH:** Perhaps the most important risk factor for uric acid stones is the **acidity of the urine.** With a pK_a of 5.35, uric acid becomes very insoluble below this pH. Patients with gout, obesity, diabetes, or the metabolic syndrome are at greater risk of forming uric acid stones, presumably secondary to excretion of abnormally acidic urine. Alkalinization of the urine (typically with potassium citrate) remains the cornerstone of therapy, to achieve a urine pH of at least 5.3, and ideally above 6.0.
- **Hyperuricemia and hyperuricosuria:** Uric acid is a product of purine metabolism and is primarily derived from endogenous sources, with dietary purines generally providing comparatively little substrate. However, these risk factors play a smaller role for uric acid stone formation than one might intuitively suspect. As the solubility of uric acid increases substantially as the urine pH rises, **comparatively large amount of uric acid can be excreted in an alkaline urine and still remain in solution.**
  - ○ Dramatically increased uric acid production can, however, lead to stone formation. **Congenital causes** of uric acid overproduction are typically diseases of single-gene defects such as hypoxanthine guanine phosphoribosyltransferase deficiency and other similarly rare diseases.
  - ○ Acquired uric acid overproduction is common in **myeloproliferative disorders,** such as polycythemia vera, or **after chemotherapy** for certain cancers resulting in large-scale cell death (i.e., tumor lysis syndrome).
  - ○ Hyperuricosuria with normal uric acid levels can occur due to **urea-splitting** such as probenecid and high-dose salicylates. Other commonly used medications have uricosuric effects. Several examples include losartan (increases uric acid excretion by approximately 10%), fenofibrate (increases uric acid excretion by 20% to 30%), and atorvastatin.

Risk Factors for Struvite Nephrolithiasis

- **UTI:** Struvite stones form only during a UTI caused by **urea-splitting bacteria,** such as *Proteus* species, *Providencia* species, *Pseudomonas,* and *Enterococcus.* These bacteria cleave ammonia from urea, causing an elevation of **urinary pH >7.0.** Abundant ammonium and magnesium combine with phosphates to give rise to struvite stones. Sometimes, calcium phosphate (apatite) may become incorporated into stones.

- **Urinary stasis:** Factors that lead to urinary retention increase the likelihood of a UTI and struvite stone formation. These include neurogenic bladder, indwelling bladder catheters, ileal conduit, urethral stricture, benign prostatic hyperplasia, bladder and calyceal diverticula, and cystocele.

Risk Factors for Cystine Nephrolithiasis

- Cystinuria is an autosomal-recessive genetic disorder with a prevalence of 1 in 7000 live births.
- Normal urinary cystine excretion is only 30 to 50 mg/day (0.12 to 0.21 mmol/day). Patients with cystinuria often excrete as much as 480 to 3600 mg/day (2 to 15 mmol/day), easily achieving urinary supersaturation.
- Urinary acidification further decreases the solubility of cystine.

Prevention

- The cornerstone of prevention of nephrolithiasis is **maintenance of high urine volumes,** with a goal of at least **2 to 2.5 L/day.**
- High urine volumes lower urine saturation with all salts.
- Patients can be instructed to drink sufficient amounts of fluids **to a point that the urine appears clear.** Patients may take metered quantities of water throughout the day, including in the evenings, to avoid excessive urinary concentration during the night. This is particularly important for those patients who suffer from chronic diarrheal disorders resulting in excessive fluid loss from the GI tract.
- Ingesting a **low-sodium, low-protein, and normal calcium diet** decreases the formation of calcium-based stones. A diet low in animal proteins may also be protective against uric acid and cystine stones by decreasing the acid load and predisposing toward an alkaline urine. Additional therapies to address individual risk factors are listed in Table 16-3.

DIAGNOSIS

Clinical Presentation

- The clinical presentation of nephrolithiasis ranges from incidental diagnosis of otherwise asymptomatic disease to presentation with severe symptoms, such as abdominal

TABLE 16-3	TREATMENT OPTIONS FOR CALCIUM STONE FORMERS

Nonspecific treatment options
Adequate oral liquid intake to maintain urine output of 2 L/day
Restrict sodium intake to <3 g/day
Restrict protein consumption to <12 oz of beef/poultry/fish per day or
  <0.8–1 g/kg/day

Specific risk-factor treatment options
Hypercalciuria: low sodium diet (<3 g/day), thiazide diuretic (i.e., chlorthalidone or
  hydrochlorothiazide 12.5–25 mg/day)
Hyperoxaluria: low oxalate diet, calcium carbonate 500 mg with meals,
  cholestyramine
Hypocitraturia: potassium citrate 10–60 mEq/day in divided doses two to three
  times a day
Hyperuricosuria: low animal-protein/low purine diet, allopurinol 100–300 mg/day

or flank pain (renal colic), macroscopic or microscopic hematuria, UTIs, or even renal failure resulting from bilateral urinary tract obstruction.

- **Asymptomatic disease:** Patients with nephrolithiasis may remain asymptomatic for years. They usually become symptomatic if a calculus or its fragments move along the urinary tract or cause obstruction. However, chronic obstruction may be asymptomatic, eventually resulting in a permanent loss of renal function.
- **Renal colic:** The pain is usually abrupt in onset, colicky in nature, and located in the flank area. It often loops anteriorly and radiates down along the path of the affected ureter; it may migrate inferiorly into the groin and testicles or labia majora. Usually, hematuria, urinary frequency, urgency, nausea, and vomiting accompany the pain.
- **Hematuria:** Trauma to the urinary tract incited by passage of gravel or a stone leads to hematuria. It may be gross or microscopic and can occur even in otherwise asymptomatic patients.
- When interviewing a patient with kidney stones, history of prior stones and dietary history, occupational history, and family history of stones and medicinal use, including supplements such as calcium and vitamin C, should be asked. Clinicians should also **identify various risk factors such as inflammatory bowel diseases, bowel operations, recurrent UTIs, and conditions that predispose toward hypercalcemia.**
- On physical examination, patient with renal colic may have costovertebral tenderness over the affected area.

Differential Diagnosis

In its classic form, the clinical presentation of renal colic is quite suggestive of the diagnosis. However, it is imperative to consider other serious conditions that can masquerade as renal colic in the differential diagnosis: ectopic pregnancy, intestinal obstruction, acute appendicitis, diverticulitis, and many other abdominal catastrophes have been confused with renal colic. The presence of hematuria is suggestive of the diagnosis but not conclusive proof; an imaging study is required to make a positive diagnosis.

Diagnostic Testing

Laboratories

- **Urinalysis:** The presence of hematuria is suggestive of nephrolithiasis, but its presence is insufficient to make the diagnosis.
- **Urine microscopy:** The appearance of specific types of crystals in the urine identifies the type of stone being formed and can guide subsequent therapy. A review of the appearance of various crystals can be found in Chapter 1.
- **Serum chemistries:** A basic chemistry panel should be obtained to assess renal function, as well as any disturbances in electrolyte or mineral balance. Serum levels of calcium, magnesium, phosphate, uric acid, and PTH can be helpful in determining an underlying processes leading to stone formation.

Imaging

- **Plain abdominal radiograph: Approximately 90% of renal stones are radiopaque** and can be seen on plain radiographs of the abdomen. However, the plain radiograph provides no information concerning the presence or absence of urinary obstruction and it may not add significant insight to the differential diagnosis of acute abdominal pain. Thus, plain abdominal films have limited use in the evaluation of acute renal colic.
- **CT scan:** Helical noncontrast CT scans have replaced IV urography as the initial step in evaluation of suspected renal colic. It allows nephrolithiasis to be excluded or confirmed expeditiously and without administration of potentially nephrotoxic radiocontrast material, and may detect other abdominal or pelvic pathology if the symptoms are not related to nephrolithiasis.

- **Renal ultrasound:** Ultrasound is useful to rule out significant hydronephrosis or hydro-ureter. However, the specific site of obstruction may not be clearly delineated and stone sizes tend to be overestimated. Although the sensitivity of ultrasound for stones is low compared to CT scan, it remains very useful for evaluation of patients who cannot receive radiation, such as pregnant women, and is favored as a low-cost alternative for monitoring changes in stone number and size in outpatient clinical follow-up.

TREATMENT

Treatment of Renal Colic

- The treatment of acute renal colic consists of pain management, relief of obstruction, and control of infection, if present.[6,7]
- The larger the stone, the less likely it is to pass spontaneously.
  - If the stone is <5 mm, conservative management is adequate, as 80% to 90% of these stones pass spontaneously. The urine should be strained to retrieve the stone for analysis.
  - Stones 5 to 7 mm only pass spontaneously 50% of the time and if the pain is controlled and the urine is sterile, conservative management can be considered.
  - Stones >7 mm rarely pass spontaneously and urologic consultation is warranted for surgical removal of the obstructing stone. Options commonly include extracorporeal shockwave lithotripsy, percutaneous nephrolithotomy, and ureteroscopic removal, and selection is determined by the size, composition, and anatomic location of the stone, anatomy of the collecting system, health status, and patient preference.
- α-Blockers (e.g., tamsulosin) in addition to supportive therapy may hasten stone passage in those with ureteral stones >5 mm but ≤10 mm but slightly increase the risk of adverse events (e.g., orthostatic hypotension, syncope, palpitations, tachycardia).[8,9]
- Nonobstructing stones within the kidney do not typically cause pain and therefore can be managed more conservatively. Preemptive urologic evacuation can be considered as an elective procedure depending on stone size or number.

Treatment of Calcium-Based Nephrolithiasis

- **Increased urinary flow**
  - All patients should be encouraged to maintain a urine volume of at least 2 to 2.5 L/day.[6,10]
  - Even if urinary levels of calcium, oxalate, phosphate, and uric acid are not ideal, a high urine volume may keep the supersaturation levels low.
- **Dietary measures**
  - Studies have shown that a **low-protein, low-sodium diet** significantly reduces nephrolithiasis recurrence rates in patients with idiopathic hypercalciuria.[6,10]
  - A low-calcium diet may increase the intestinal absorption of oxalate, paradoxically increasing the risk of nephrolithiasis. Therefore, **low-calcium diets are not recommended.**[6,10] Diets containing 700 to 800 mg/day of calcium are adequate for patients with idiopathic hypercalciuria or 1 to 2 dairy servings per day.
- **Thiazide diuretics**
  - Thiazide diuretics have long been the mainstay in treatment of **idiopathic hypercalciuria,** lowering urinary excretion of calcium by at least two mechanisms.[6,10]
    - Thiazides lead to contraction of the extracellular fluid volume. By reducing the extracellular volume, thiazide diuretics increase proximal reabsorption of calcium.
    - Thiazides also increase calcium reabsorption in the distal nephron.
  - The effects of thiazide diuretics can be completely negated by high dietary salt intake. Urinary sodium excretion of ≥200 mEq/day suggests nonadherence to a low-sodium diet.

○ **Hypokalemia and hypocitraturia** may complicate long-term therapy with thiazide diuretics and can be prevented by adding oral potassium citrate. In some cases amiloride may be added in order to enhance the effect of thiazides and to conserve potassium.

- **Citrate supplementation**
  ○ Hypocitraturia is a common finding among patients with calcium-based stones. Specifically, it can occur in patients with GI malabsorption or a distal RTA.
  ○ Citrate supplementation in the form of a potassium salt (**potassium citrate** 10 to 60 mEq/day divided into two or three doses) can be used to correct this abnormality.[6,10] However, care should be taken to avoid overalkalinization of the urine as this could increase the risk of calcium phosphate nephrolithiasis as the pH approaches 6.7 to 7.0.
  ○ Small studies evaluating lemon juice as a source of citrate have not shown consistent benefit in correcting hypocitraturia or reducing stone recurrence. If attempted, patients can mix 4 oz of lemon juice with 2 L of water with sugar added for taste.

- **Oxalate restriction and binding**
  ○ Hyperoxaluria is initially treated with dietary restriction of oxalate-rich foods.
  ○ If this is insufficient to achieve control, particularly in patients with enteric hyperoxaluria from fat malabsorption, administration of intestinal oxalate binders, such as calcium carbonate can be used with meals to form nonabsorbable compounds in the GI tract. If calcium carbonate is ineffective, bile acid sequestrants, such as cholestyramine, may be added.
  ○ Clinical trials evaluating the role of enhancing oxalate excretion by administration of *Oxalobacter formigenes* or reducing synthesis by targeting glycolate oxidase in the management of primary hyperoxaluria are ongoing and may yield alternate treatment options in management of recurrent oxalate stones.

- **Reduction of uric acid excretion**
  ○ For patients with hyperuricosuria, dietary restriction of animal proteins and other purines may reduce the excreted amount of uric acid, making less available in the urine to form a nidus for calcium to build upon.
  ○ If dietary restriction is insufficient, allopurinol, a xanthine oxidase inhibitor that blocks conversion of xanthine to uric acid, can be effective.

Treatment of Uric Acid Nephrolithiasis

- Treatment of uric acid nephrolithiasis is based on attempts to increase the solubility of uric acid and to decrease its excretion. As with other stone types, all patients should maintain a urine volume >2 to 2.5 L/day.[11]
- **Potassium citrate** (10 to 20 mEq PO tid; up to as much as 100 mEq/day) is the preferred alkalinizing agent. A urine pH of at least 6.0 should be targeted.
- **Dietary counseling** about low purine and low protein intake is helpful as this may decrease the acid load that needs to be excreted.
- **Allopurinol** can be employed to reduce uric acid excretion, although urinary volume and urine pH are the more important risk factors to target.

Treatment of Struvite Stones

- **Surgical intervention is usually needed** to remove struvite stones, and their staghorn configuration make them less amenable to the less invasive urologic techniques.[12]
- Once patients are free of stones, they benefit from antibiotic therapy directed against the predominant urinary organism. Most patients with residual stone fragments progress despite treatment with antibiotics. Reducing the bacterial population with antibiotics often slows stone growth but stone resolution with antibiotics alone is unlikely.

Treatment of Cystine Stones

- Preventive medical therapy is directed toward reducing urinary cystine concentration below its solubility limits.
- As with other stone types, patients should attempt to maintain a high urine volume and a low urine sodium. However, the target levels are more stringent, with added benefit observed with urinary volumes >4 L/day and urine sodium levels <70 mEq/day.
- Sulfhydryl drugs (i.e., tiopronin, penicillamine, captopril) cross-link with cysteine and form soluble disulfides. These medications do not lower the total amount of cystine in the urine.
- Urinary alkalinization to a pH 7.0 to 7.5 increases cystine solubility. However, persistently alkaline urine at this level is difficult to attain and could increase the risk of calcium phosphate nephrolithiasis.[13]

MONITORING/FOLLOW-UP

- **Follow-up imaging:** Subsequent imaging studies are recommended at 1 year for evaluation of recurrence. The study may be abdominal radiographs, ultrasound, or helical CT. If there is no evidence of new stones, then imaging studies may be repeated every 5 years. Recurrent nephrolithiasis may mandate more frequent imaging.
- All patients with nephrolithiasis should have a screening evaluation for common problems that can lead to stone formation, although there is no consensus of how extensive evaluation should be after the first episode. Patients with recurrent nephrolithiasis deserve a thorough metabolic evaluation, which should be done once the acute episode has resolved and the patient has returned to his or her daily routine.
- A **24-hour urine** sample should be collected at least 4 weeks after the acute event has resolved and the patient has returned to his or her usual diet and lifestyle.
  - The following **urinary parameters** are routinely determined when performing **stone risk evaluation.** Although the references range may vary among laboratories, commonly accepted targets are listed in parentheses.
    - Volume (>2 L/day)
    - pH (target range depends on stone type)
    - Calcium (<200 mg/day)
    - Oxalate (<40 mg/day)
    - Citrate (>500 mg/day)
    - Uric acid (<750 mg/day)
    - Sodium (<200 mg/day)
    - Phosphate (<1200 mg/day)
  - The 24-hour urine creatinine is also measured to determine the completeness of the sample collection. When in steady-state renal function, the daily creatinine production should equal the excreted load, approximating 20 mg/kg/day for men and 15 mg/kg/day for women. For the day of collection, patients should be instructed to discard the first morning void, save the rest of the urine produced that day and night, then save the first morning void of the following morning to complete the 24 hours.

OUTCOME/PROGNOSIS

Left untreated, kidney stones have high recurrence rate. Patients with a prior episode have a 50% risk of developing a second kidney stone within 7 years. With dietary and lifestyle changes, and with medical management of modifiable risk factors, this recurrence can be reduced.

REFERENCES

1. Rule AD, Bergstralh EJ, Melton LJ, 3rd, et al. Kidney stones and the risk for chronic kidney disease. *Clin J Am Soc Nephrol.* 2009;4:804–811.
2. Curhan GC. Epidemiology of stone disease. *Urol Clin North Am.* 2007;34:287–293.
3. Taylor EN, Stampfer MJ, Curhan GC. Obesity, weight gain, and the risk of kidney stones. *JAMA.* 2005;293:455–462.
4. Thorleifsson G, Holm H, Edvardsson V, et al. Sequence variants in the CLDN14 gene associate with kidney stones and bone mineral density. *Nat Genet.* 2009;41:926–930.
5. Cochat P, Rumsby G. Primary hyperoxaluria. *N Engl J Med.* 2013;369:649–658.
6. Morgan MS, Pearle MS. Medical management of renal stones. *BMJ.* 2016;352:i52.
7. Bultitude M, Rees J. Management of renal colic. *BMJ.* 2012;345:e5499.
8. Campschroer T, Zhu X, Vernooij RW, et al. Alpha-blockers as medical expulsive therapy for ureteral stones. *Cochrane Database Syst Rev.* 2018;4:CD008509.
9. Hollingsworth JM, Canales BK, Rogers MA, et al. Alpha blockers for treatment of ureteric stones: systematic review and meta-analysis. *BMJ.* 2016;355:i6112.
10. Fink HA, Wilt TJ, Eidman KE, et al. Medical management to prevent recurrent nephrolithiasis in adults: a systematic review for an American College of Physicians Clinical Guideline. *Ann Intern Med.* 2013;158:535–543.
11. Heilberg IP. Treatment of patients with uric acid stones. *Urolithiasis.* 2016;44:57–63.
12. Flannigan R, Choy WH, Chew B, et al. Renal struvite stones—pathogenesis, microbiology, and management strategies. *Nat Rev Urol.* 2014;11:333–341.
13. Pereira DJ, Schoolwerth AC, Pais VM. Cystinuria: current concepts and future directions. *Clin Nephrol.* 2015;83:138–146.

Renal Artery Stenosis and Renovascular Hypertension

17

Reem Daloul and Aubrey Morrison

GENERAL PRINCIPLES

- The structural finding of a narrowed renal artery lumen defines renal artery stenosis (RAS).
- **Renal vascular hypertension** (RVHTN) is the increase in blood pressure attributed to reduction in the renal perfusion caused by a stenotic lesion in the renal artery(s).
- In severe cases, reduced renal perfusion can also lead to injury to the renal parenchyma and decrease in kidney function. This is known as **ischemic nephropathy.**
- The presence of a stenotic lesion in the renal artery in patient with HTN does not necessarily reflect a causative relationship. **RAS can be found incidentally in patients without hypertension** and with normal renal function.[1] Moreover, correcting the lesion may or may not improve blood pressure control or renal function.
- **Causes of RAS**
  - **Atherosclerotic renal artery stenosis** (ARAS) is the most common cause of RAS (approximately 80% of cases).
  - **Fibromuscular dysplasia** (FMD) is the second most common cause of RAS (about 20%).
  - **Other causes of** RAS include vasculitis (i.e., polyarteritis nodosa, Takayasu arteritis), aortic or arterial aneurysm (including dissection), embolic disease, trauma, radiation, or mass effect. These are, however, extremely rare.

Epidemiology

- **Atherosclerotic renovascular disease**
  - The prevalence of RAS in the general population is unclear due the asymptomatic nature of the majority of cases. Most data are from autopsy series or patients undergoing angiography for evaluation of other atherosclerotic disease (e.g., cardiac catheterization or lower extremity angiography). In addition, methods and criteria for defining a significant stenosis vary across studies.
  - The prevalence of RAS does not equal the prevalence of RVHTN, because a causal relationship is not always clear. A large autopsy study noted RAS in 4.3% of cases, and if there was a history of type 2 diabetes mellitus, the incidence was as high as 8.3%. A combined history of type 2 diabetes and hypertension was associated with a 10% risk of RAS.[2]
  - Population-based studies using Doppler techniques in persons aged >65 years found RAS in 6.8% (males, 9.1%; females, 5.5%). RAS was unilateral in 88% of cases and bilateral in 12%.[2] Medicare claims from 1999 to 2001 showed an incidence of newly diagnosed ARAS of 3.7 per 1000 patient years. Follow-up of this group for another 2 years showed that cardiovascular events from atherosclerotic heart disease in the incident ARAS patients were higher than in the general population (304 vs. 73 per 1000 patient years).[3]
  - It stands to reason that patients with atherosclerotic disease of other vascular beds would be more likely to have ARAS. For instance, ARAS of >50% can be found incidentally in up to 20% of patients undergoing coronary angiography. **A finding of**

RAS of >75% in this setting is an independent predictor of all-cause mortality.[4] In patients undergoing angiography for atherosclerotic disease in the aorta or legs, RAS of >50% can be seen in up to 50% of the cases.[5,6]

○ **Ischemic nephropathy** is defined as the diminution of renal function due to low blood flow caused by an obstructive lesion in the renal artery. According to the U.S. Renal Data System report from 2000 to 2004, the incidence of ESRD from RAS was 1.8%.[7] Other studies suggest that ischemic nephropathy may be the **cause of ESRD in up to approximately 10% to 15% of cases.** As the elderly population in the United States is steadily increasing, it is also expected that the incidence of RAS and ischemic nephropathy will rise.

● **FMD**
  ○ **FMD is most common in women with onset of hypertension below 30 years of age or in women under the age of 50 years with refractory or suddenly worsening hypertension.** The most common form of FMD is medial fibroplasias, present with the classic string-of-beads appearance on the angiogram. Other arteries may also be affected in this disease.

Pathophysiology

● **Goldblatt model**
  ○ In 1934, Goldblatt experimentally produced hypertension in dogs by clamping their renal arteries, demonstrating that decreasing perfusion to the kidney(s) could cause systemic hypertension.
  ○ The renal blood flow to the kidneys largely exceeds tissue metabolic needs. Hence, for a lesion to cause significant hemodynamic impairment of blood flow through the renal artery, it must occlude the luminal diameter of the artery by 75% to 80%. When this critical level of stenosis is reached, numerous mechanisms are activated in an attempt to restore renal perfusion. Fundamental to this process is the release of renin from the juxtaglomerular apparatus, which then activates the renin–angiotensin–aldosterone system (RAAS).
  ○ Subsequently, systemic arterial pressure increases until renal perfusion is restored or improved. By experimentally blocking the RAAS, medically or by genetic knockout in animal models for the angiotensin II 1A receptor, this rise in systemic arterial pressure can be prevented.[8]
  ○ Mechanisms of continued RVHTN depend on whether the RAS affects one or both kidneys. The terminology that has evolved from experimental animal models illustrates pathophysiologic concepts in human disease.
  ○ The Goldblatt **2-kidney, 1-clip (2K1C) model** represents **unilateral RAS** in a patient with two functioning kidneys. Central to this concept is the fact that the kidney contralateral to the stenosis is normal and experiences increased perfusion pressure. This normal kidney adapts to the increased arterial pressure with local suppression of the RAAS and excretion of excess sodium and water. Because of normalization of volume status, poor perfusion to the stenotic kidney is maintained and persistent activation of the RAAS in this kidney occurs. This model is known as **angiotensin II-dependent RVHTN.**
  ○ The **1-kidney, 1-clip (1C1K) model** means that the entire renal mass is distal to a hemodynamically significant stenosis, whether this is **bilateral RAS in a patient with two functioning kidneys or unilateral RAS in a patient with a single functioning kidney.** In the 1C1K model, the entire renal mass is under-perfused, leading to RAAS activation with sodium retention and volume expansion leading to increased renal perfusion pressure. Once this occurs, the RAAS is then suppressed and hypertension is thought to be more related to persistent volume expansion. This scenario is known as **angiotensin-independent or volume-dependent RVHTN.**[9]

○ The pathophysiology in Goldblatt models is true to the cases of isolated RAS with normal renal parenchyma, such as the case of FMD, or acute renal artery occlusion due to an aneurysm rupture. The pathophysiology underlying HTN in ARAS is more complicated.

• **ARAS**
  ○ The pathophysiology underlying hypertension in ARAS is multifactorial and does not result solely from the reduction in renal perfusion as seen in Goldblatt models. This is evident by the failure of angioplasty procedures to cure hypertension in many patients with ARAS.
  ○ The atherosclerotic milieu that results in the development of atherosclerotic plaques in the variable vascular beds, is part of a systemic inflammatory environment that does not only affect vascular beds but also several tissues and organs. In the kidneys, it results in renal parenchymal damage by means of endothelial injury, increased generation of reactive oxygen species and oxidative stress. This damage to the renal parenchyma is the primary culprit for hypertension and reduced renal function.[10]
  ○ ARAS may superimpose hypoxic injury upon the pre-existing atherosclerotic tissue injury in cases of severe luminal stenosis.

DIAGNOSIS

Clinical Presentation

• There are no clinical characteristics that absolutely differentiate RVHTN from other causes of hypertension. RVHTN shares many of the features seen with other etiologies of secondary hypertension such as **acute onset of moderate-to-severe hypertension early or late** in life, and hypertension **refractory to standard therapy** (Table 17-1).
• Some of the features that should raise suspicion of ARAS per se are as follows
  ○ Unexplained malignant or accelerated hypertension with or without renal failure in patients with previously well-controlled blood pressure should raise suspicion for

TABLE 17-1	CLINICAL CHARACTERISTICS SUGGESTIVE OF RENOVASCULAR HYPERTENSION
Abrupt onset of HTN <30 females (FMD)	
Abrupt onset of HTN >50 yrs of age (ASRVD)	
No family history for HTN	
Worsening of previously controlled HTN	
HTN refractory to multiple medications	
Recurrent flash pulmonary edema	
Unexplained heart failure	
Evidence of end-organ damage from malignant HTN	
Abdominal bruit	
Hypokalemia and metabolic alkalosis with HTN	
Increase in serum creatinine after initiation of ACE inhibitor or ARB	
Renal asymmetry of >1.5 cm	

ACE, angiotensin-converting enzyme; ARB, angiotensin receptor blocker; ASRVD, atherosclerotic renovascular disease; FMD, fibromuscular dysplasia; HTN, hypertension.

acute severe renal ischemia such in the cases of renal artery plaque rupture or aneurysm dissection.

○ Increase in antihypertensive requirements in patient with previously stable blood pressure control that is not explained by medication or dietary noncompliance or worsening renal function could signify progression of underlying ARAS.

○ Rapid deterioration of renal function (>30% reduction in estimated glomerular filtration rate [eGFR] over ≤3 months) in patients with previously stable or slowly progressive renal disease and background of atherosclerotic milieu.

○ Episodes of **recurrent flash pulmonary edema** with accelerated hypertension should raise the suspicion of RVHTN and are more commonly found in patients with bilateral disease. This is related to the pathophysiology of the 1C1K model (see Pathophysiology) and the resultant tendency toward volume overload and to left ventricular hypertrophy with diastolic dysfunction.

○ A **significant and persistent rise (>30%) in serum creatinine after initiation of an angiotensin-converting enzyme (ACE) inhibitor or angiotensin II receptor blocker (ARB)** suggests the presence of bilateral RAS or RAS in a patient with a single functioning kidney.

• Other characteristics associated with RVHTN include smoking, elevated cholesterol, increased body mass index, and progressive unexplained renal failure.

• Reports suggest that RVHTN may rarely be associated with nephrotic range proteinuria.

• Patients may have polydipsia with hyponatremia secondary to the dipsogenic properties of angiotensin II and **may have hypokalemia** related to increased aldosterone activity.

Diagnostic Testing

• Before embarking on an extensive diagnostic evaluation for renal artery disease, the clinician should consider whether further intervention would occur if disease were found. Renal artery disease is a relatively common unsuspected finding in certain high-risk groups, as discussed above.

• Most experts **advocate looking for RAS only if the patient would be a candidate for revascularization therapy.** Factors such as comorbid conditions, age, and risk of intervention should be considered in the decision process (Table 17-2).

• Given that functional tests measuring renin activity in the blood lack statistical power for diagnosis, **radiographic imaging of the renal vasculature** has become the primary approach to RAS diagnosis. The test chosen depends on institutional expertise but less-invasive tests are generally preferred initially.

• Functional testing, such as the **captopril radionuclide renogram,** is most helpful in patients with **unilateral disease** and **normal renal function.**

Laboratories
• Although increased renin production, measured as **plasma renin activity** (PRA), is fundamental to the initial rise in blood pressure, the chronic elevation of blood pressure

TABLE 17-2	CHARACTERISTICS OF PATIENTS NOT LIKELY TO BENEFIT FROM REVASCULARIZATION
Pre-existing longstanding hypertension (>3 yrs) well controlled with medical management	
Pre-existing chronic kidney disease that is stable or slowly progressive over time	
Kidney size <8 cm	
Physiologically insignificant stenosis on noninvasive imaging (stenosis <70%)	

in RVHTN is thought to be from other mechanisms, as noted in the pathophysiology section in this chapter. Renin levels can fall within a few weeks, despite persistently elevated blood pressure. Renin levels are also **highly dependent on other factors** such as sodium intake, posture, age, race, gender, and medications.

- Consequently, **the usefulness of PRA alone in the evaluation of RVHTN is extremely limited** and this test has been largely abandoned in clinical practice.

Imaging

- **Renal ultrasound with Doppler**
  - Ultrasound is an excellent initial assessment tool as it is widely available, relatively inexpensive, extends little, if any, risk to the patient, and provides both structural and functional assessments of the kidneys.
  - Ultrasound allows for assessment of kidney size, asymmetry, as well as other structural abnormalities such as cysts or obstruction. Small kidneys suggest chronic damage, with low likelihood of improvement in renal function after revascularization.
  - Measurement of blood flow velocities in the renal arteries using Doppler technique can evaluate the presence of RAS and roughly estimate the severity of the lesion. Higher velocities indicate a narrowed luminal diameter.
  - **Peak systolic velocities** (PSVs) have been reported to carry the highest sensitivity (85%) and specificity (92%) for the diagnosis of RAS >50%.[11] Cutoffs correlating with hemodynamically significant stenosis of ≥70% have varied among studies anywhere between 180 to 320 cm/s. Recently, studies using blood oxygen level dependent MRI (BOLD-MRI), which enables direct evaluation of tissue oxygenation, reported that a PSV of >384 cm/s correlates with cortical and medullary ischemia.[12] To this date, the optimal PSV to correlate with hemodynamically significant stenosis is yet to be determined. Elevated PSV should be interpreted in the light of the overall clinical picture and the level of clinical suspicion.
  - **Renal to Aortic ratio (RAR)** is a ratio of the PSV in the renal artery to the aorta. It is used to eliminate the effect of cardiac output on measurement of PSV. A RAR of >3.5 has been reported to correlate with hemodynamically significant stenosis with an AUC of 0.94 ± 0.043 (CI; 0.83–0.99).[13]
  - **Resistive index** (RI) can be measured by Doppler ultrasonography and is defined as the PSV minus the end diastolic velocity (EDV) divided by the PSV. RI represents a measure of the overall resistance to renal arterial blood flow in the microcirculation, beyond the main RAS. Elevated RI may indicate intrinsic parenchymal or small vessels disease. RI has been proposed as a measure to predict response to angiography in the setting with ARAS. Preangioplasty RI >0.8 was reported to confer worse renal outcome compared to patients with RI <0.8.[14] However, this finding was not reproducible in other clinical trials. Hence, the use of RI as a predictive parameter in the management of ARAS is not recommended.
  - **Disadvantages** of renal Doppler ultrasonography are that it is highly dependent on patient body habitus, operator skill, interpreter expertise, and the type of equipment. For these reasons, the sensitivity and specificity vary in the literature but can be as high as 98% when proficiency is great. Technology and expertise with Doppler ultrasound is growing and it is now **often utilized as an initial test for RAS.**
- **Spiral computed tomography (CT) scan and CT angiography**
  - CT angiography (CTA) with 3D reconstruction is a highly sensitive and specific tool for the diagnosis of RAS. However, it is expensive and requires administration of iodinated contrast, which places the patient at risk for contrast-induced nephropathy.
  - Additionally, CTA does not provide any functional information regarding the hemodynamic effect of the lesion. The use of CTA maybe best applied prior to planned angiography to accurately characterize the vascular anatomy or in patients with very high clinical suspicion for ARAS when the question is whether or not ARAS exists.

○ Dynamic contrast-enhanced CT is a new technique currently limited to research use. This technique uses kinetic modeling of the injected contrast to estimate single kidney perfusion, volume, and eGFR. Studies to validate this technique for clinical use are still needed.

- **Magnetic resonance angiography (MRA)**
  ○ MRA is being increasingly used as the initial test for the diagnosis of RAS. It is a highly sensitive and specific noninvasive test that is less operator dependent compared with Doppler ultrasound.
  ○ MRA utilizes gadolinium in lieu of iodinated contrast. Gadolinium has been associated with nephrogenic systemic fibrosis in patients with advanced chronic kidney disease (CKD) and should not be used in patients with eGFR <30 mL/min/1.73 m^2.
  ○ Similar to CTA, MRA provides only structural information. It tends to slightly overestimate the severity of a stenotic lesion when compared with angiography because of issues related to maximum spatial resolution.
  ○ Limitations include lack of functional data, slow acquisition compared to CTA, patient intolerance in case of claustrophobia, advanced CKD, and implanted ferromagnetic material such as pacemakers, cochlear implants, intracranial aneurysm clips, or other metallic implants.
  ○ New MRA techniques such as 4D flow MRI, dynamic contrast-enhanced MRI, and BOLD-MRI are currently under investigation. These techniques can provide noninvasive functional data such as velocity, flow, single kidney eGFR, and tissue oxygenation.

- **Renal angiography**
  ○ Renal angiography is considered **the gold standard for the diagnosis of RAS** and a key inclusion criterion in clinical trials. Stenosis is usually categorized into mild (<50%), moderate (50% to 70%), and severe (>70%).
  ○ Angiography as a diagnostic test carries multiple limitations. It is an invasive procedure that carries risk for catheter-induced injury (atheroemboli and arterial dissection) and contrast-induced nephropathy. Digital imaging procedures and use of carbon dioxide as the contrast medium can minimize the later complication.
  ○ Angiography is also operator dependent and vulnerable to interobserver variability and performer bias. It tends to overestimate the severity of the stenosis. In the CORAL trial roll-in period for example, the stenosis was decreased by core laboratory from an average of 72.5% to 67.3%.[15]
  ○ The assessment of luminal stenosis does not adequately identify hemodynamic significance. Translesional pressure gradient measured during angiography can help identify functionally significant lesions. Different pressure measurements have been studied and reported including:
    ■ A ratio between the pressure distal (Pd) and proximal to the stenosis (aortic pressure, Pa) of >0.9[16]
    ■ Resting mean pressure gradient of >10 mm Hg
    ■ Hyperemic systolic gradient >20 mm Hg[17]
  ○ Angiography is now usually performed only at the time of percutaneous intervention after another less-invasive test has made the diagnosis of RAS very likely. If noninvasive testing is inconclusive despite high degree of clinical suspicion, angiography could be considered.

- **Captopril radionuclide renogram**
  ○ Radionuclide imaging of the kidneys can be helpful in evaluating the individual contribution of each kidney to overall GFR.
  ○ In the kidney distal to a stenosis, GFR is maintained by the efferent arteriolar constrictive effects of angiotensin II. When angiotensin II is blocked by captopril, efferent arteriolar dilatation occurs and GFR in the stenotic kidney often decreases, usually with a corresponding increase in GFR in the nonstenotic kidney.

○ When a radioactive isotope such as Tc-99m diethylenetriamine-penta-acetic acid (DTPA) is given in this setting to measure GFR, the **stenotic kidney will exhibit decreased uptake with a delayed peak time and a slower washout time** compared with the precaptopril baseline and the nonstenotic kidney.

○ ACE inhibitors or ARBs must be held prior to this test but other antihypertensive agents can be continued and loop diuretics may even enhance the sensitivity.

○ A **positive captopril renogram indicates the presence of a physiologically significant stenosis** and has been proposed as a predictor for good blood pressure response after percutaneous transluminal renal angioplasty (PTRA).

○ Captopril renography cannot distinguish unilateral from bilateral disease. It can only detect difference between the two kidneys which can simply represent a worse stenosis on one side. Additionally, the sensitivity and specificity of the test decrease with reduction in renal function.

○ The test is **now rarely used in clinical practice** due to its limitations and lower performance characteristics compared to other noninvasive studies such as CTA and MRA.

TREATMENT

• Recent prospective studies using Doppler ultrasound show that **progression of ARAS may not occur as frequently and rapidly as was once thought.**

• Progression can occur in as many as 30% of higher-risk patients at 3 years, or as little as 4% in lower-risk patients followed up to 8 years.[18]

• **Progression of disease is related to the initial degree of stenosis.** Progression to complete occlusion may develop in up to 3% to 7% of patients. Risk factors for progression are still poorly understood, but appear to be similar to risk factors for general atherosclerotic disease.

• Complicating matters further, **progression of a stenotic lesion may not translate clinically into worsening hypertension or renal function.** In a group of patients with high-grade RAS (>70%) followed up for just over 3 years, only 8% eventually required revascularization for refractory hypertension. In the entire group, antihypertensive medication requirement increased but blood pressure remained relatively unchanged and creatinine rose from 1.4 to 2 mg/dL. This increase in serum creatinine was more pronounced in patients with bilateral RAS. Mortality in this group was 30% and was primarily due to other cardiovascular-related disease.[19]

• It is possible that the long-term neuroendocrine defects caused by ARAS could contribute to worsening cardiovascular disease. Therefore, end points of therapy should not only be targeted at blood pressure control and preservation of renal function but should also include reduction in cardiovascular events overall.

• Based on the available body of evidence, **in patients with stable renal function and adequate control of blood pressure, the presence of anatomic evidence for RAS does not mandate intervention.** These patients are best managed with optimal medical therapy.

• Patients with clinical presentations highly suspicious for functional RAS lesion (Tables 17-1 and 17-3) should be considered for intravascular intervention if the presence of hemodynamically significant lesion is confirmed with a noninvasive study such as renal US with Doppler. The benefit of intravascular intervention should be weighed against the procedural risks in each patient individually.

• The decision to perform revascularization with **PTRA or surgery for FMD** is less controversial than for atherosclerotic disease and **is usually recommended.** Intervention results in a cure or improvement of hypertension in 70% to 90% of patients.[20]

TABLE 17-3	CHARACTERISTICS OF PATIENTS LIKELY TO BENEFIT FROM REVASCULARIZATION

Recent onset of resistant, accelerated, or malignant hypertension in patient with previously stable blood pressure control

Recent onset of unexplained acute or subacute deterioration in renal function in patient with previously normal or stable chronic kidney disease

Significant rise in creatinine following administration of ACE inhibitors or ARBs

Recurrent flash pulmonary edema in the context of patient compliance

Recent increase in blood pressure medication requirements in patient with previously stable blood pressure control

ACE, angiotensin converting enzyme; ARB, angiotensin receptor blocker.

Medications

- **Aggressive medical therapy** targeted at reducing atherosclerotic disease is recommended in all patients with ARAS. This includes **smoking cessation, control of dyslipidemia, glycemic control, aspirin, and blood pressure control** according to Joint National Committee (JNC) 8 goals.
- ACE inhibitors and ARBs are the preferred first-line agents, as they have proven benefit in RAS and cardiovascular disease. It is rare for patients to experience a clinically significant drop in their GFR after initiation of these agents but **close monitoring of serum creatinine** and **optimization of volume status** after initiation of these drugs is recommended.[21]
- If GFR does decline, it is usually in a patient with bilateral disease or RAS in a single functioning kidney. In such situations, revascularization should be considered.
- Refractory hypertension is generally defined as **inadequate control of blood pressure despite maximally tolerated dose of three antihypertensive medications including a diuretic.** Refractory hypertension should be confirmed by 24 hours ambulatory blood pressure monitoring. Twenty-four-hour urinary sodium is also recommended to ensure patient compliance with low salt diet. Once confirmed, refractory hypertension should raise suspicion of ARAS.

Other Nonpharmacologic Therapies

- PTRA is the preferred revascularization procedure in most institutions. **Owing to high rates of restenosis with balloon angioplasty alone, especially with ostial lesions, stent deployment has been increasingly used.** This has improved technical success and is now the most widely used procedure for revascularization of RAS.
- Before the era of interventional radiology, surgery was the definitive treatment for RAS. Now, it is reserved for situations in which revascularization is necessary but cannot be achieved by the percutaneous route.
- Response to intravascular intervention is related to the underlying etiology of RAS. On the one hand, PTRA in the case of FMD has been shown to provide cure or at least moderate improvement in blood pressure control. On the other hand, in the case of ARAS, multiple large randomized clinical trials have failed to show improvement in blood pressure control, renal function, cardiovascular or renal events when compared to optimal medical management. Two of such landmark trials are the ASTRAL and CORAL trials.[22,23]
- It is important to be cognizant of the specific patient population studied across the contemporary clinical trials. Due to relatively similar inclusion and exclusion criteria, all

recent studies excluded patients with malignant or accelerated hypertension, advanced renal failure, history of unstable heart failure (such as recent admission for pulmonary edema or heart failure exacerbation), or recent acute coronary syndrome. The resulting studied cohorts consisted predominately of patients with normal to moderate renal dysfunction and hypertension. It is worth noting that patients with these exclusion criteria are the population more likely to have clinically significant ARAS.[24,25]

- Another limitation that is important to watch for in all previous and future coming clinical trials is the diagnostic method/technique used to diagnose clinically significant ARAS. As discussed previously, the mere presence of a stenotic lesion whether above or below 70% does not automatically translate into a functional lesion. A functional test such as PSV, RAR or one of the new MRA or CTA techniques along with a clinical suspicion score should be taken into account.

- **Risks of PTRA**
  - ○ **Restenosis** is estimated to occur in 15% to 20% of cases. **Contrast nephropathy** complicates the procedure up to 13% of the time but is usually self-limited. Conversely, acute and progressive **deterioration in renal function** has been reported to have an incidence of up to 20% in some series.
  - ○ **Atheroembolic disease** is thought to be responsible for a majority of these cases. Studies using distal filter devices after stent placement showed that atheroembolic debris can be recovered with less frequent deterioration of postprocedural renal function.
  - ○ Other complications are **renal artery dissection, renal artery thrombosis, and segmental renal infarction.** Periprocedural death or cardiovascular events each occur with a reported incidence of up to 3%. In the ASTRAL trial, 23 patients out of 403 patients in the revascularization arm experienced serious complications, including 2 deaths and 3 amputations.[22] In the CORAL trial, the most common complication was arterial dissection that occurred in 2.2% of the patients. There was no procedure-related death.[23]

REFERENCES

1. Lorenz EC, Vrtiska TJ, Lieske JC, et al. Prevalence of renal artery and kidney abnormalities by computed tomography among healthy adults. *Clin J Am Soc Nephrol.* 2010;5:431–438.
2. Hansen KJ, Edwards MS, Craven TE, et al. Prevalence of renovascular disease in the elderly: a population-based study. *J Vasc Surg.* 2002;36:443–451.
3. Kalra PA, Guo H, Kausz AT, et al. Atherosclerotic renovascular disease in United States patients aged 67 years or older: risk factors, revascularization, and prognosis. *Kidney Int.* 2005;68:293–301.
4. Conlon PJ, Little MA, Pieper K, et al. Severity of renal vascular disease predicts mortality in patients undergoing coronary angiography. *Kidney Int.* 2001;60:1490–1497.
5. Olin JW, Melia M, Young JR, et al. Prevalence of atherosclerotic renal artery stenosis in patients with atherosclerosis elsewhere. *Am J Med.* 1990;88:46N–51N.
6. Zanoli L, Rastelli S, Marcantoni C, et al. Non-hemodynamically significant renal artery stenosis predicts cardiovascular events in persons with ischemic heart disease. *Am J Nephrol.* 2014;40:468–477.
7. United States Renal Data System. National Institutes of Health, *National Institute of Diabetes and Digestive and Kidney Diseases.* Bethesda, MD. Available at https://www.usrds.org/adr.aspx. Accessed January 16, 2019.
8. Balk E, Raman G, Chung M, et al. Effectiveness of management strategies for renal artery stenosis: a systematic review. *Ann Intern Med.* 2006;145:901–912.
9. Safian RD, Textor SC. Renal-artery stenosis. *N Engl J Med.* 2001;344:431–442.
10. Lerman LO, Textor SC, Grande JP. Mechanisms of tissue injury in renal artery stenosis: ischemia and beyond. *Prog Cardiovasc Dis.* 2009;52:196–203.
11. Williams GJ, Macaskill P, Chan SF, et al. Comparative accuracy of renal duplex sonographic parameters in the diagnosis of renal artery stenosis: paired and unpaired analysis. *AJR Am J Roentgenol.* 2007;188:798–811.

12. Gloviczki ML, Glockner JF, Crane JS, et al. Blood oxygen level-dependent magnetic resonance imaging identifies cortical hypoxia in severe renovascular disease. *Hypertension.* 2011;58: 1006–1072.

13. Drieghe B, Madaric J, Sarno G, et al. Assessment of renal artery stenosis: side-by-side comparison of angiography and duplex ultrasound with pressure gradient measurements. *Eur Heart J.* 2008;29:517–524.

14. Radermacher J, Chavan A, Bleck J, et al. Use of Doppler ultrasonography to predict the outcome of therapy for renal-artery stenosis. *N Engl J Med.* 2001;344:410–417.

15. Murphy TP, Cooper CJ, Cutlip DE, et al. Roll-in experience from the Cardiovascular Outcomes with Renal Atherosclerotic Lesions (CORAL) study. *J Vasc Interv Radiol.* 2014;25:511–520.

16. De Bruyne B, Manoharan G, Pijls NH, et al. Assessment of renal artery stenosis severity by pressure gradient measurements. *J Am Coll Cardiol.* 2006;48:1851–1855.

17. Mangiacapra F, Trana C, Sarno G, et al. Translesional pressure gradients to predict blood pressure response after renal artery stenting in patients with renovascular hypertension. *Circ Cardiovasc Interv.* 2010;3:537–542.

18. Pearce JD, Craven BL, Craven TE, et al. Progression of atherosclerotic renovascular disease: a prospective population-based study. *J Vasc Surg.* 2006;44:955–962.

19. Plouin PF, Chatellier G, Darné B, et al. Blood pressure outcome of angioplasty in atherosclerotic renal artery stenosis: a randomized trial. Essai Multicentrique Medicaments vs Angioplastie (EMMA) Study Group. *Hypertension.* 1998;31:823–829.

20. Slovut DP, Olin JW. Fibromuscular dysplasia. *N Engl J Med.* 2004;350:1862–1871.

21. Textor SC. Stable patients with atherosclerotic renal artery stenosis should be treated first with medical management. *Am J Kidney Dis.* 2003;42:858–863.

22. Wheatley K, Ives N, Gray R, et al. Revascularization versus medical therapy for renal-artery stenosis. *N Engl J Med.* 2009;361:1953–1962.

23. Cooper CJ, Murphy TP, Cutlip DE, et al. Stenting and medical therapy for atherosclerotic renal-artery stenosis. *N Engl J Med.* 2014;370:13–22.

24. Daloul R, Morrison AR. Approach to atherosclerotic renovascular disease: 2016. *Clin Kidney J.* 2016;9:713–721.

25. Sag AA, Sos TA, Benli C, et al. Atherosclerotic renal artery stenosis in the post-CORAL era part 2: new directions in Transcatheter Nephron Salvage following flawed revascularization trials. *J Am Soc Hypertens.* 2016;10:368–377.

Secondary Causes of Hypertension

Randy Laine and Patricia F. Kao

18

Introduction

- This chapter will cover nonrenovascular etiologies of secondary hypertension (sHTN), focusing specifically on hormonal and monogenic causes.
- The work-up for secondary causes can be expensive and time consuming. Thus, the cost-effective diagnosis and management of sHTN requires a thorough knowledge of the clinical signs and symptoms, risk factors, and diagnostic tools available.
- sHTN is defined as high blood pressure (BP) from an identifiable cause, unlike primary, or essential hypertension, which has no clear identifiable etiology.
- A secondary cause can be identified in about 15% of prevalent patients with hypertension (HTN).[1]
- In hypertensive adults <age 40 the prevalence of sHTN is approximately 30%.
- The prevalence rates of specific forms of sHTN are highly variable and remain unclear, likely due to heterogeneity in diagnostic criteria and sampling bias.
- **Renal parenchymal disease** has been reported as the most common cause of sHTN. It is unclear whether HTN is the cause or the result for the chronic kidney disease (CKD) in most patients.
  - All patients who present with HTN should be screened for renal disease.
  - In the large longitudinal Chronic Renal Insufficiency Cohort (CRIC) the prevalence of HTN increased with decreasing glomerular filtration rate (GFR): 67% in patients with an estimated GFR (eGFR) >60 mL/min/1.73 m^2, 92% in those with eGFR <30 mL/min/1.73 m^2.[2]
  - The various forms of renal parenchymal diseases that are classically associated with HTN are discussed in other chapters extensively, and will not be discussed further here. These are typically a high renin type of HTN and may cause a secondary hyperaldosteronism.
- **Renal artery stenosis** has been reported as the second most common cause of sHTN. (See Chapter 17.)
- Various **medications,** as outlined in Table 18-1, are associated with secondary or resistant hypertension and patients should be asked about use of these medications during evaluation.[3]
- This chapter will focus primarily on **endocrine/hormonal causes** of sHTN: primary and familial hyperaldosteronism, Cushing syndrome, and rare conditions, such as pheochromocytoma, syndrome of apparent mineralocorticoid excess (SAME), Liddle syndrome, glucocorticoid-remediable aldosteronism (GRA), pseudohypoaldosteronism type II (Gordon syndrome), and activation mutation of mineralocorticoid receptor (MR, sometimes referred to as Geller syndrome).
- **Obstructive sleep apnea** (OSA) and **thyroid disease** are two common and important medical conditions that are often overlooked as causes of sHTN. Since etiology of hypertension associated with these conditions does not have a direct correlation with renal pathophysiology, they are outside of the scope of this chapter, and will not be discussed. Patients who have risk factors for OSA and have uncontrolled HTN should be referred for a sleep study.
- A comprehensive list of causes of secondary and resistant HTN is shown in Table 18-1.

TABLE 18-1	COMMON ETIOLOGIES OF SECONDARY OR RESISTANT HYPERTENSION
Renal disorders	• Renal disease of any etiology • Glomerular disease • Polycystic kidney disease • Renal artery stenosis (fibromuscular dysplasia or atherosclerotic disease)
Systemic disorders	• Obstructive sleep apnea • Hypo- or hyperthyroidism • Coarctation of the aorta • Pheochromocytoma
Medications	• Oral contraceptives • Attention deficit disorder medications (e.g., amphetamine, methylphenidate, etc.) • NSAIDs • Corticosteroids • Nasal decongestants (sympathomimetic agents such as phenylephrine and pseudoephedrine) • Erythropoietin-stimulating agents (i.e., erythropoietin, darbepoetin) • Tyrosine kinase inhibitors • Calcineurin inhibitors • Herbal products (e.g., ephedra, ginseng) • Caffeine (excessive use) • Weight loss agents (e.g., phentermine) • Illicit drugs (e.g., cocaine, methamphetamine) • Anabolic steroids
Disorders associated with renin–aldosterone–angiotensin system	• Primary hyperaldosteronism • Adrenal adenoma (aldosteronoma or Conn syndrome) • Idiopathic aldosteronism • Unilateral or bilateral adrenal hyperplasia • Adrenal carcinoma • Glucocorticoid-remediable aldosteronism • Syndrome of apparent mineralocorticoid excess • Renin-secreting tumor • Congenital adrenal hyperplasia • Liddle syndrome • Gordon syndrome • Activating mutation of mineralocorticoid receptor gene

Primary Aldosteronism

GENERAL PRINCIPLES

- Primary aldosteronism (PA, also known as Conn syndrome) occurs when aldosterone secretion is independent of the normal regulatory pathway of the renin–angiotensin–aldosterone system. Specifically, the feedback signals that normally suppress aldosterone, such as volume expansion an increased sodium intake are ineffective in PA.

- **Aldosterone secretion is autonomous.** Renin levels are low due to negative feedback exerted by the excess aldosterone.
- PA is one of the few potentially curable forms of sHTN, so it is important to detect and initiate treatment in a timely manner.
- Prevalence is unclear but it has been estimated that PA is present in about 5% to 10% of patients with HTN.
- Aldosterone is a mineralocorticoid that is produced by the zona glomerulosa, the outer region of the adrenal gland.
- The primary action of aldosterone is on the principal cell of the cortical collecting tubule (CCT). When it binds the MR, this results in increased activity of basolateral Na-K-ATPase, the epithelial sodium channel (ENaC), and the renal outer medullary potassium channel (ROM-K). The net effect is increased reabsorption of sodium and increased secretion of potassium in the renal CCT.
- There are several pathophysiologic etiologies of PA. In PA, aldosterone secretion is independent of renin.
- **The most common cause of PA is hyperactivity of one or both adrenal glands.**
  - ○ **Unilateral** disease is typically the result of an **aldosterone-producing adenoma** (APA, also referred to as an adrenal adenoma, adrenocortical adenoma, or aldo-steronoma). These benign tumors are generally <2 cm in diameter. They are more common in women than men.
  - ○ **Bilateral** disease is typically characterized by bilateral micro- or macronodular **adrenal hyperplasia.** This is also sometimes referred to as idiopathic aldosteronism. This is more common in men than women, and presents later in life.
  - ○ There are conflicting reports in the literature as to whether adrenal adenomas or bilateral adrenal hyperplasia is more common, but these are the two most common causes of PA.
- Less common causes of PA include unilateral adrenal hyperplasia, malignant adrenal carcinoma, familial hyperaldosteronism, and ectopic aldosterone-producing tumor, each of which account for only 1% to 2% of cases of PA.
  - ○ **Familial hyperaldosteronism type I** (FH-I) is a rare, genetic, autosomal dominant form of PA and is also referred to as **glucocorticoid-remediable aldosteronism** (GRA).[4] In this disease, a chimeric gene encoding 11-beta hydroxylase and aldosterone synthase results in a hybrid form of aldosterone synthase that is adrenocortico-tropic hormone (ACTH)-sensitive. Normally, ACTH is only a minor regulator of aldosterone secretion in an acute and transient fashion. However, in GRA, secretion of aldosterone is regulated completely by ACTH rather than by the renin–angiotensin system. This results in oversecretion of aldosterone.
  - ○ Other forms of hyperaldosteronism such as FH-II (familial occurrence of aldosterone adenomas), FH-III (mutations of the potassium channel) and the newly characterized FH IV (mutations of genes that code for calcium channel) are exceedingly rare.[5,6]

DIAGNOSIS

Clinical Presentation

- The classic presentation of PA is **moderate or severe hypertension, hypokalemia, and metabolic alkalosis.**
- However, **patients may be asymptomatic, some patients are normotensive, and most patients are not overtly hypokalemic.**[7,8]
- Patients rarely present with malignant hypertension.
- Serum sodium levels are normal or on the high end of the normal range.
- OSA prevalence is increased in patients with PA.[9]

TABLE 18-2	HIGH-RISK PATIENTS WHO SHOULD BE SCREENED FOR PRIMARY ALDOSTERONISM

- Sustained elevated BP (SBP ≥150 mm Hg and/or DBP ≥100 mm Hg)
- Hypertension (BP >140/90 mm Hg) resistant to three conventional antihypertensive drugs, including a diuretic
- Controlled BP (BP <140/90 mm Hg) with ≥4 antihypertensive drugs
- HTN and spontaneous or diuretic-induced hypokalemia
- HTN and adrenal incidentaloma identified on imaging
- HTN and OSA
- HTN and a family history of early-onset HTN or cerebrovascular accident (<40 yrs old)
- Case detection for all hypertensive first-degree relatives of patients with PA

BP, blood pressure; DBP, diastolic blood pressure; HTN, hypertension; OSA, obstructive sleep apnea; SBP, systolic blood pressure.
Adapted from Young WF, Calhoun DA, Lenders JWM, et al. Screening for endocrine hypertension: an Endocrine Society Scientific Statement. *Endocr Rev.* 2017;38:103–122.

- Most patients with PA present in their third to sixth decades of life.
- In children with hypertension, with or without a family history of HTN, GRA should be suspected. Patients may be asymptomatic or they may present with failure to thrive, weakness, and hypokalemia in infancy.

Diagnostic Testing

- Evaluation for PA involves initial screening tests, followed by confirmatory testing in some cases, and then localization using radiologic techniques and imaging.
- Table 18-2 shows which high-risk patients should be screened for PA, as recommended by the Endocrine Society clinical practice guideline.[10]
- Other guidelines have also recommended screening for PA in any patient with untreated HTN with low normal serum potassium levels of unknown cause.

Laboratories

- In PA, **the plasma renin level is low,** due to the effect of negative feedback from excess aldosterone. However, random plasma renin and aldosterone levels are not sensitive for detection of PA.
- The **aldosterone to renin ratio** (ARR) is the most readily available and commonly used screening test for PA. **ARR >30 is highly suggestive of PA,** with some studies reporting 1-hour upright ARR ≥35.90 as having 100% sensitivity and 92.3% specificity.[11] In order to maximize the sensitivity of the ratio, the ARR **should be repeated more than once** and should be checked under the following conditions:
  - Hypokalemia must be corrected
  - Encourage the patient to follow a liberal sodium diet, which suppresses aldosterone in normal circumstances
  - Secretion of aldosterone is positional and follows a circadian rhythm (peaks during sleep), so plasma levels of aldosterone and renin should be checked in the morning in seated patients who have been in the upright position (i.e., sitting, standing, or walking) for 2 to 4 hours
  - Diuretics should be withdrawn for at least 4 weeks
  - Antihypertensive medications that block the renin–angiotensin system, dihydropyridine calcium channel blockers, β-blockers, and clonidine should be held for 2 weeks

TABLE 18-3	FACTORS THAT AFFECT THE RELIABILITY OF THE ALDOSTERONE TO RENIN RATIO (ARR)

False-Negative ARR	False-Positive ARR
Dietary salt restriction	β-Adrenergic blockers
Uncorrected hypokalemia	α-Methyldopa
Concomitant malignant or renovascular hypertension	Clonidine
Pregnancy	Nonsteroidal anti-inflammatories
Potassium sparing diuretics	CKD
Dihydropyridine calcium channel blockers	Age >65 yrs old
Angiotensin-converting enzyme inhibitors (ACE-I)	Luteal phase of menstruation
Angiotensin receptor antagonists (ARB)	Familial hyperkalemic hypertension (pseudohypoaldosteronism type II, Gordon syndrome)
Selective serotonin reuptake inhibitors (SSRI)	

prior to testing if possible. If antihypertensive medications are required during this period, use nondihydropyridine calcium channel blockers (e.g., verapamil), hydralazine, and prazosin or doxazosin, where possible

○ In cases where antihypertensive medications cannot be altered or held prior to testing, refer to Table 18-3 for the potential effects of interfering medications on the ARR.

○ Note that **screening for PA using an ARR is not recommended in all patients with hypertension,** since the prevalence of this disease remains relatively low compared to essential hypertension and this testing is not cost effective in low clinical suspicion. In addition, it is important to screen with the ARR only in high-risk patients, as the withdrawal of hypertensive agents in preparation of collecting the ARR may lead to adverse outcomes in patients with severe hypertension.

• If a patient has a positive blood or urine screening test for PA, **confirmatory testing** may be performed using one of four methods or the patient **may proceed directly to lateralization** methods discussed in Imaging (this will also depend on the medical center and the availability of specific lateralization techniques). There is no established gold standard for confirmatory testing and some authors suggest that confirmatory testing does not add additional diagnostic value and that all patients should proceed to imaging and lateralization.

• The selection of one of the somewhat controversial confirmatory testing methods depends on time, cost, patient compliance, the presence of severe HTN, coronary artery disease, or advanced CKD.

○ **Oral sodium loading test:** Dietary sodium intake is increased to about 6 g/day and hypokalemia is corrected for 4 days. A 24-hour urine is collected from the morning of day 3 to the morning of day 4. **Urinary Na excretion >200 mEq per day** indicates the patient is adequately salt loaded. Under normal circumstances, the urinary aldosterone excretion should be <10 mcg/day if the patient is adequately salt loaded. **Urinary aldosterone >12 mcg/24 hrs** is highly suggestive of PA. As with all 24-hour urine collections, a concomitant 24-hour urine creatinine and creatinine clearance should be collected to validate the sample as a 24-hour urine collection.

○ **Saline infusion test:** The patient is in the recumbent position for at least 1 hour before and during a 2-L normal saline infusion over 4 hours in the morning. Plasma renin, aldosterone, cortisol, and potassium are drawn at time zero and after 4 hours with BP and heart rate monitored throughout. Postinfusion plasma aldosterone levels

<5 ng/dL make the diagnosis of PA unlikely and levels >10 ng/dL are highly suggestive of PA.

○ **Fludrocortisone suppression test:** Patient receives fludrocortisone 0.1 mg orally every 6 hours for 4 days, with potassium supplementation and a high salt diet. On day 4, plasma aldosterone concentration and plasma renin activity are measured in the seated position at 10:00 AM, and serum cortisol concentration at 7:00 AM and 10:00 AM. If plasma renin activity is <1 ng/mL/hr and plasma cortisol concentration at 10:00 AM is lower than the value obtained 7:00 AM, an upright plasma aldosterone concentration of >6 ng/dL confirms the diagnosis of PA.

○ **Captopril challenge test:** Captopril 25 to 50 mg is given orally to a patient who has been upright for 1 hour. Plasma aldosterone concentration, plasma renin activity, and serum cortisol concentration are measured at time zero and 1 to 2 hours after captopril. If plasma aldosterone concentration is not suppressed by 30% with captopril, this confirms a diagnosis of PA.

○ The latter 2 tests (fludrocortisone suppression test and captopril challenge test) are rarely used nowadays in establishing diagnosis of PA.

• Additional testing for **GRA** (FH-I) is recommended in patients with a positive screening test for PA who:
  ○ Lack a demonstrable tumor on imaging
  ○ Are young/pediatric
  ○ Have a family history of cerebral hemorrhage or HTN before age 30 years
  ○ Have a known family history of GRA

• **GRA** testing includes a dexamethasone suppression test, genetic testing for the chimeric gene, and 24-hour urinary 18-hydroxycortisol and 18-oxocortisol levels.

Imaging

• **All patients diagnosed with PA should have a high-resolution CT scan of MRI of the adrenal glands** to classify the subtype of PA, evaluating for nodules, adenomas, carcinomas and lateralizing the disease.

• The management of PA depends on **lateralization** of the source of the excessive aldosterone secretion, therefore it is critical to distinguish between unilateral and bilateral disease.

• Imaging alone is inadequate in determining laterality, as an adenoma noted on CT may be inactive and the real disease might be caused by the hyperplasia in the contralateral adrenal gland. In one study, approximately 15% of patients would have undergone unnecessary adrenalectomy, solely based on CT scan finding.[12]

• **Adrenal vein sampling** (AVS) is now considered the gold standard for lateralization.[13,14] However, AVS requires highly skilled radiologists, and there are complications associated with cannulation of the adrenal vein.

• Some authors recommend that the following patients do not require AVS:
  ○ Age <40 with clear unilateral adrenal adenoma and normal contralateral gland on high-resolution CT or MRI
  ○ Nonsurgical candidates with high operative risk
  ○ Patients with suspected adrenocortical carcinoma
  ○ Patients with an established diagnosis of familial hyperaldosteronism

TREATMENT

Natural History

• Aldosterone excess leads to increased cardiovascular and renal morbidity and mortality. This is due to both the effects of hypertension, and in part from the direct effects of aldosterone-associated inflammation, remodeling, and fibrosis in cardiovascular and renal tissues that lead to end-organ damage.

- Cardiovascular morbidity and mortality are higher in patients with PA versus those with essential hypertension when matched for BP level. This **increased CV morbidity in PA is reversed after treatment of PA,** which makes early detection and initiation of treatment particularly important.

Indications for Intervention

- **Adrenalectomy in patients with unilateral adrenal adenomas or unilateral adrenal hyperplasia** is curative of HTN in 30% to 60% of patients, and results in normalization of hypokalemia in all patients.[15]
- Available surgical approaches include lateral transperitoneal laparoscopy, posterior retroperitoneoscopy, or robotic-assisted surgery.

Medical Management

- Medical management is recommended in bilateral adrenal adenomas or bilateral idiopathic hyperaldosteronism, or in patients who are poor surgical candidates.
- **MR antagonists,** such as spironolactone and eplerenone, are the first-line agents.
- Spironolactone dosages from 75 to 225 mg/day have been shown to be more efficacious than eplerenone at 100 to 300 mg/day for hypertension control.[16] Eplerenone may be a reasonable alternative in patients with significant gynecomastia and dysmenorrhea on spironolactone.
- Hypertension control may take several months on an MR antagonist. Approximately 50% of patients with PA require a second agent, such as a low-dose thiazide diuretic. Other adjunctive antihypertensive medications that may be required include ENaC inhibitors (e.g., amiloride and triamterene), calcium channel blockers, ACE inhibitors and ARBs.
- For **GRA** patients, medical treatment includes glucocorticoids (dexamethasone 0.125 to 0.25 mg, or prednisolone 2.5 to 5 mg daily, titrated to normotension), MR antagonist, ENaC antagonists, additional antihypertensive medications (e.g., β-blockers, ACE-I, ARB, dihydropyridine calcium channel blockers).

Disorders That Resemble Mineralocorticoid Excess

GENERAL PRINCIPLES

- When the clinical suspicion for PA is high but the ARR is not consistent with PA, evaluation for other endocrine disorders that resemble mineralocorticoid excess is indicated.[4]
- Endocrine disorders and syndromes that fall into this category are rare and include
  ○ SAME
  ○ Licorice ingestion
  ○ Liddle Syndrome
  ○ Congenital adrenal hyperplasia (11-beta hydroxylase deficiency and 17-hydroxylase deficiency)
  ○ Deoxycorticosterone-producing tumors
  ○ Mutation in MR gene (Geller syndrome)[4,17]
  ○ Mutations in WNK (with no lysine kinase) kinase gene (pseudohypoaldosteronism type II or Gordon syndrome)[17]
- Table 18-4 summarizes the plasma renin activity and aldosterone levels for each of these disorders.
- **SAME** is due to impaired activity of the enzyme **11-beta hydroxysteroid dehydrogenase,** which converts cortisol to cortisone in the kidney. Cortisone does not bind the MR. However, cortisol has the same binding affinity for the MR as aldosterone and,

TABLE 18-4	SUMMARY OF PLASMA RENIN AND ALDOSTERONE LEVELS IN VARIOUS ETIOLOGIES OF SECONDARY HYPERTENSION		
Condition		Plasma Renin Activity	Plasma Aldosterone
Renal parenchymal disease		↑	↑
Renovascular disease		↑	↑
Primary aldosteronism		↓	↑
Renin secreting tumor (Conn syndrome)		↑	↑
Syndrome of mineralocorticoid excess (SAME)		↓	↓
Liddle syndrome		↓	↓
Congenital adrenal hyperplasia		↓	↓
Deoxycorticosterone-producing tumor		↓	↓
Pseudohypoaldosteronism type 2 (Gordon Syndrome)		↓	↓
Autosomal dominant pseudohypoaldosteronism type 1 (Geller syndrome, usually occurs in pregnancy)		↓	↓

therefore, cortisol when present in high levels can serve as a potent mineralocorticoid, mimicking aldosterone excess. 11-beta hydroxysteroid dehydrogenase can be genetically deficient (autosomal recessive) or its activity blocked by **glycyrrhizic acid** found in **black licorice.** There have also been reports that 11-beta hydroxysteroid dehydrogenase activity may be blocked in some cases of preeclampsia.[18]

- **Liddle syndrome** is an autosomal dominant mutation of the amiloride-sensitive ENaC. Enhanced activity of this channel results in increased distal sodium reabsorption in the CCT, leading to potassium wasting, hypokalemia; and hypertension.
- **Congenital adrenal hyperplasia** is a group of autosomal recessive disorders in which there is a lack of inhibitory feedback by cortisol on the hypothalamus and pituitary gland, and excess ACTH secretion. Two of these disorders, **11-beta hydroxylase deficiency and 17-hydroxylase deficiency,** result in hypersecretion of the mineralocorticoid **deoxycorticosterone** (DOC) that can bind the MR.
- **Deoxycorticosterone-producing tumors** are adrenal tumors that cosecrete androgens and estrogens, in addition to DOC.
- **Gordon syndrome** is also known as **familial hyperkalemic hypertension** (FHH), or **pseudohypoaldosteronism-II** (PHA-II). Several forms have been described, including loss of function mutations in the WNK kinase family (specifically WNK1 and WNK4). This results in uninhibited activity of the Na-Cl cotransporter (NCC) in the distal tubule. A so-called chloride-shunt develops, decreasing distal delivery of chloride and lowering the anion load in the CCT lumen. Lumen negativity in this portion of the nephron normally drives potassium and hydrogen ion secretion in the CCT down the electrical gradient across the apical membrane into the lumen. Since the CCT lumen is less negative in Gordon syndrome, renal tubular potassium and hydrogen ion secretion are impaired and patients develop **hyperkalemia** and a non–anion gap **metabolic acidosis. Salt-sensitive hypertension** is thought to be a result of uninhibited sodium reabsorption through the NCC.

DIAGNOSIS

- **SAME:** A 24-hour urine collection will demonstrate an abnormally high ratio of cortisol and cortisone or >10-fold the normal value. Congenital forms present in childhood, and acquired forms are most commonly suspected in patients with a history of excessive black licorice ingestion.
- **Liddle syndrome:** A clinical diagnosis can be established with reasonable certainty if empiric amiloride or triamterene results in marked improvement in hypertension. A lack of response to MR antagonists and dexamethasone as well as a normal 24-hour urine cortisone/cortisol ratio help to support a diagnosis of Liddle syndrome. Genetic testing is available for confirmatory testing.
- **Congenital adrenal hyperplasia:** An initial screening test is for blood levels of DOC, 11-deoxycortisol, androstenedione, testosterone, and dehydroepiandrosterone sulfate (DHEA-S), all of which should be increased above the upper limit of normal. Confirmatory testing includes germline mutation testing.
- **Deoxycorticosterone-producing tumors:** A diagnosis is established by high levels of plasma DOC or urinary tetrahydrodeoxycorticosterone, and a large adrenal tumor on CT scan.
- **Gordon syndrome:** A sensitivity to thiazide diuretics in a patient with hyperkalemia, non–anion gap metabolic acidosis, and salt-sensitive hypertension is suggestive of Gordon syndrome. Genetic testing is necessary for definitive diagnosis.

TREATMENT

- Medical treatment in all of these disorders that mimic mineralocorticoid excess is aimed at the site of the abnormal activity or enzyme deficiency, with either a mineralocorticoid MR antagonist or an ENaC antagonist.
- However, in Geller syndrome, the mutation of MR may lead to a paradoxical increase in BP with spironolactone and other agents may need to be used.
- In the case of Gordon syndrome, salt restriction and thiazide diuretics are recommended.

Reninoma

- **Renin-secreting tumors** (reninomas) are rare juxtaglomerular (JG) cell tumors that are seen in the pediatric population.[19]
- The autonomous renin production from these tumors leads to excess aldosterone production and elevated BP.
- A diagnosis of reninoma is established by high-resolution CT scan and renal vein sampling with lateralization for renin. Reninomas are often missed on ultrasonography.
- Nephron-sparing surgical removal of the JG tumor is curative and restores normal BP in majority of the patients.

Pheochromocytoma

GENERAL PRINCIPLES

- Pheochromocytomas and paragangliomas (collectively referred to as PPGLs) are neuroendocrine tumors of the chromaffin system that produce catecholamines.

- 80% to 85% arise from the adrenal medulla; 15% to 25% arise from the paravertebral ganglia of the sympathetic chain.[20]
- About 10% of pheochromocytomas are **malignant.** The most frequent metastases are to lung, bone, lymph nodes, brain or liver through hematogenous spread.
- Pheochromocytomas are very rare with an incidence of 1 to 10 per million/yr and a prevalence of 1 in 10,000.[21]
- The prevalence is higher in those who have an incidental adrenal mass, about 500 in 10,000.[20]
- Only about 0.1% to 0.5% of patients with hypertension are found to have a pheochromocytoma.[20]
- Equal incidence in both genders; patients typically presents in their 30s to 60s.[20,22]
- At least a quarter to one-third of pheochromocytomas are **inherited.** Pheochromocytomas are present in numerous familial syndromes, including in 50% of **multiple endocrine neoplasia type 2 (MEN2),** in 10% to 30% of **von Hippel–Lindau,** and in 1% of neurofibromatosis type 1 (NF1) patients. These 3 syndromes are all autosomal dominant.[22]
- Other rare conditions include the Carney triad (i.e., gastrointestinal stromal tumor, pulmonary chondroma, and extra-adrenal paragangliomas) and mutations of the succinate dehydrogenase subunits.
- PPGLs can be biochemically categorized as **adrenergic or noradrenergic** tumors.
  ○ The adrenergic type are located in the adrenal medulla and usually produce epinephrine, metanephrine (major metabolite of epinephrine), and varying amounts of norepinephrine.
  ○ The noradrenergic type are located either in the adrenal medulla or at extra-adrenal sites and produce norepinephrine and normetanephrine.
- PPGLs produce metanephrines constantly, whereas catecholamines are produced in surges and are, therefore, harder to detect.
- Paragangliomas located in the neck and skull base are usually hormonally inactive; some produce dopamine.

DIAGNOSIS

Clinical Presentation

- **Clinical presentation is highly variable,** ranging from no symptoms (5% to 10% of adrenal incidentalomas are pheochromocytomas) to life-threatening manifestations.[22]
- More than 50% of patients with pheochromocytomas present with secondary or paroxysmal HTN.
- Clinical manifestations range from **headaches, sweating, dizziness, palpitations, and weakness** to hypercalcemia, orthostatic hypotension, and dilated cardiomyopathy.
- The classic triad suggestive of pheochromocytoma includes a pounding headache, profuse sweating, and palpitations/tachycardia. The symptoms may last from a few minutes to an hour and may occur a few times per day to a few times per month. Patients are asymptomatic between episodes.
- The associated medical emergencies are myocardial infarctions, cardiomyopathy, stroke, and pulmonary edema.
- Patients may develop sustained or resistant HTN, hypertensive crisis, enhanced BP variability, and paradoxical BP responses to drugs, surgery, anesthesia, or some foods (e.g., with tyramine).
- Suggestive clinical symptoms should trigger a high index of suspicion, especially if coupled with a family history.
- One should suspect inherited pheochromocytoma and screen all first-degree relatives if:
  ○ the presentation is before 45 years of age or

○ there are multifocal tumors (including bilateral pheochromocytoma), extra-adrenal sites, and/or a malignant tumor.

Diagnostic Testing

Laboratories

• Biochemical laboratory testing should generally precede imaging procedures for localization.
• The primary laboratory tests are **plasma-free metanephrines** or **24-hour urinary fractionated metanephrines**—both tests have equally very high sensitivity.
• The Endocrine Society of America considers the urine and plasma test equal in diagnostic power but some experts warn that the specificity of the plasma test may be lower (<90%) and may decrease with age, especially after 60s (leading to a higher risk of false positives if there is low clinical suspicion).[20]
• Testing with liquid chromatography with tandem mass spectrometry has higher specificity.[23]
• **False negatives** are seen in:
  ○ very small tumors; hereditary pheochromocytomas tend to be smaller than acquired ones
  ○ incorrect sample collection
  ○ asymptomatic patients screened because of family history
• **False positives** seen in:
  ○ association with certain medications (Table 18-5)
  ○ incorrect sample collection (e.g., stress, patient recently stood up)
  ○ stress states/comorbidities (e.g., severe illness, hospitalization/intensive care unit admission, OSA, heart failure, myocardial infarction, stroke)
• **Normal plasma-free metanephrines and/or 24-hour urinary fractionated metanephrines levels in symptomatic patient essentially exclude pheochromocytoma,** but there could be false negative as mentioned above and labs should be repeated during symptomatic episodes (presuming the patient has such episodes).
• **If normal levels are found in asymptomatic patients, then they should be retested later** as a negative result does not exclude the disease; these patients are usually screened because of a family history of pheochromocytoma.

TABLE 18-5	MEDICATIONS ASSOCIATED WITH FALSE-POSITIVE SERUM OR URINE METANEPHRINE TESTING

Monoamine oxidase inhibitors (MAO-I, especially with tyrosine rich diet)

Amphetamines

Tricyclic antidepressants (TCA)

Metoclopramide

Sympathomimetic amines

Catecholamine reuptake inhibitors (e.g., cocaine and derivatives)

Anesthetics (e.g., lidocaine, halothane gas)

Antihypertensive drugs (e.g., α- or β-blockers, especially clonidine and propranolol)

Withdrawal from levodopa or sedative drugs (e.g., alcohol, benzodiazepines, opioids)

Levodopa

- **When plasma-free metanephrine levels are >3 times the upper normal or urine 24-hour fractionated metanephrines levels are >2 times the upper limit of normal, proceed to imaging studies to localize tumor.**
- For elevated levels that do not meet the above criteria, retest after eliminating possible causes of false positives and/or repeat during a spell (presuming the patient has such episodes). Other laboratory tests may also be considered to aid in confirming the diagnosis.
  - 24-hour fractionated metanephrine urine test if initial test was a free metanephrine plasma test
  - Plasma chromogranin A
  - Plasma and urinary catecholamines
  - Urinary vanillylmandelic acid
  - Clonidine suppression test to distinguish elevated catecholamines from a pheochromocytoma as opposed to sympathetic activation[24]
  - Dopamine and its metabolite 3-methoxytyramine (some rare tumors selectively secrete dopamine)

Imaging

- **CT abdomen/pelvis with and without contrast and MRI with contrast** are equivalent and usually locate the lesion.
- The large majority of neuroendocrine tumors occur in the abdomen/pelvis most of these are in the adrenal glands.
- If an adrenal mass >10 cm or a paraganglioma is found also obtain ^{123}I-metaiodobenzylguanidine (MIBG) scan due to the increased risk of metastases.
- If both CT and MRI are negative but high clinical suspicion, consider ^{123}I-MIBG scan, whole-body MRI, ^{18}F-fluoro-dihydroxyphenylalanine (^{18}F-FDOPA)-positron emission tomography (PET), ^{18}F-fludeoxyglucose (FDG)-PET, or pentetreotide scan. Radioactive tracers are especially useful in genetic syndromes and extra-adrenal tumors.

TREATMENT

- Treatment eliminates paroxysms and pheochromocytoma-associated HTN.
- Unilateral or bilateral pheochromocytoma
  - Complete tumor removal is usually curative but high risk and needs adequate preoperative preparation with α- and β-blockade.
  - Partial adrenalectomy (if bilateral pheochromocytoma) can preserve some native adrenal function.
- Metastatic disease is hard to treat and surgery is not usually curative. A combination of ^{131}I-nuclear treatment, chemotherapy, and medical management is often used. Palliation is achieved in about half of patients and the 5-year survival ranges from 30% to 60%.[25]
- Medical management for hypertensive crises
  - **Nitroprusside:** 0.5 to 5 mcg/kg/min infusion titrated with BP, but <3 mcg/kg/min for prolonged infusion
  - **Phentolamine:** 1-mg test dose, then 5 mg boluses or infusion; lasts 10 to 15 minutes
  - **Nicardipine:** 5 mg/hr infusion, titrated to BP

REFERENCES

1. Young W, Calhoun DA, Lenders JWM, et al. Screening for endocrine hypertension: an Endocrine Society Scientific Statement. *Endocr Rev.* 2017;38:103–122.
2. Muntner P, Anderson A, Charleston J, et al. Hypertension awareness, treatment, and control in adults with CKD: results from the Chronic Renal Insufficiency Cohort (CRIC) Study. *Am J Kidney Dis.* 2010;55:441–451.

3. Calhoun DA, Jones D, Textor S, et al. Resistant hypertension: diagnosis, evaluation, and treatment: a scientific statement from the American Heart Association Professional Education Committee of the Council for High Blood Pressure Research. *Circulation.* 2008;117:e510–e526.

4. Lifton RP, Gharavi AG, Geller DS. Molecular mechanisms of human hypertension. *Cell.* 2001;104:545–556.

5. Monticone S, Tetti M, Burrello J, et al. Familial hyperaldosteronism type III. *J Hum Hypertens.* 2017;31:776–781.

6. Perez-Rivas LG, Williams TA, Reincke M. Inherited forms of primary hyperaldosteronism: new genes, new phenotypes and proposition of a new classification. *Exp Clin Endocrinol Diabetes.* 2019;127:93–99.

7. Mulatero P, Stowasser M, Loh KC, et al. Increased diagnosis of primary aldosteronism, including surgically correctable forms, in centers from five continents. *J Clin Endocrinol Metab.* 2004;89:1045–1050.

8. Rossi GP, Bernini G, Caliumi C, et al. A prospective study of the prevalence of primary aldosteronism in 1,125 hypertensive patients. *J Am Coll Cardiol.* 2006;48:2293–2300.

9. Di Murro A, Petramala L, Cotesta D, et al. Renin-angiotensin-aldosterone system in patients with sleep apnoea: prevalence of primary aldosteronism. *J Renin Angiotensin Aldosterone Syst.* 2010;11:165–172.

10. Funder JW, Carey RM, Mantero F, et al. The management of primary aldosteronism: case detection, diagnosis, and treatment: an Endocrine Society clinical practice guideline. *J Clin Endocrinol Metab.* 2016;101:1889–1916.

11. Yin G, Zhang S, Yan L, et al. One-hour upright posture is an ideal position for serum aldosterone concentration and plasma renin activity measuring on primary aldosteronism screening. *Exp Clin Endocrinol Diabetes.* 2012;120:388–394.

12. Kempers MJ, Lenders JW, van Outheusden L, et al. Systematic review: diagnostic procedures to differentiate unilateral from bilateral adrenal abnormality in primary aldosteronism. *Ann Intern Med.* 2009;151:329–337.

13. Rossi GP, Sacchetto A, Chiesura-Corona M, et al. Identification of the etiology of primary aldosteronism with adrenal vein sampling in patients with equivocal computed tomography and magnetic resonance findings: results in 104 consecutive cases. *J Clin Endocrinol Metab.* 2001;86:1083–1090.

14. Kline G, Holmes DT. Adrenal venous sampling for primary aldosteronism: laboratory medicine best practice. *J Clin Pathol.* 2017;70:911–916.

15. Zhou Y, Zhang M, Ke S, et al. Hypertension outcomes of adrenalectomy in patients with primary aldosteronism: a systematic review and meta-analysis. *BMC Endocr Disord.* 2017;17:61.

16. Parthasarathy HK, Menard J, White WB, et al. A double-blind, randomized study comparing the antihypertensive effect of eplerenone and spironolactone in patients with hypertension and evidence of primary aldosteronism. *J Hypertens.* 2011;29:980–990.

17. Melcescu E, Phillips J, Moll G, et al. 11Beta-hydroxylase deficiency and other syndromes of mineralocorticoid excess as a rare cause of endocrine hypertension. *Horm Metab Res.* 2012;44:867–878.

18. Kosicka K, Siemiatkowska A, Glówka FK. 11β-hydroxysteroid dehydrogenase 2 in preeclampsia. *Int J Endocrinol.* 2016;2016:5279462.

19. Trnka P, Orellana L, Walsh M, et al. Reninoma: an uncommon cause of renin-mediated hypertension. *Front Pediatr.* 2014;2:89.

20. Lenders JW, Duh QY, Eisenhofer G, et al. Pheochromocytoma and paraganglioma: an Endocrine Society clinical practice guideline. *J Clin Endocrinol Metab.* 2014;99:1915–1942.

21. Beard CM, Sheps SG, Kurland LT, et al. Occurrence of pheochromocytoma in Rochester, Minnesota, 1950 through 1979. *Mayo Clin Proc.* 1983;58:802–804.

22. Kiernan CM, Solórzano CC. Pheochromocytoma and paraganglioma: diagnosis, genetics, and treatment. *Surg Oncol Clin N Am.* 2016;25:119–138.

23. Taylor RL, Singh RJ. Validation of liquid chromatography-tandem mass spectrometry method for analysis of urinary conjugated metanephrine and normetanephrine for screening of pheochromocytoma. *Clin Chem.* 2002;48:533–539.

24. Eisenhofer G, Goldstein DS, Walther MM, et al. Biochemical diagnosis of pheochromocytoma: how to distinguish true- from false-positive test results. *J Clin Endocrinol Metab.* 2003;88:2656–2666.

25. Goffredo P, Sosa JA, Roman SA. Malignant pheochromocytoma and paraganglioma: a population level analysis of long-term survival over two decades. *J Surg Oncol.* 2013;107:659–664.

Onconephrology

Monica Chang-Panesso
and Benjamin D. Humphreys

19

Introduction

- The advent of numerous targeted chemotherapy agents and improvements in hemato-poietic stem cell transplants over the past two decades have significantly improved the survival of patients with malignancies.
- Renal involvement in the setting of malignancies is broadly divided into: (1) renal manifestations of the primary malignancy and (2) renal manifestations from chemotherapy agents and other treatments.
- Renal involvement may result in acute kidney injury (AKI), chronic kidney disease (CKD), hypertension, proteinuria, and/or electrolyte disturbances.
- The American Society of Nephrology has a detailed online resource on onconephrology topics covered in this chapter.[1]

Acute Kidney Injury

- AKI and CKD in patients with malignancy are more common than in the general population, especially elderly patients.
- Some malignancies have a much higher risk of AKI. Multiple myeloma, liver, and renal cell carcinoma have the highest risk.[2]
- **Prerenal causes**
  - Volume depletion related to nausea, vomiting, or diarrhea as a consequence of chemotherapy.
  - Medications that might increase the risk of prerenal azotemia include nonsteroidal anti-inflammatory drugs, diuretics, angiotensin-converting enzyme (ACE) inhibitors or angiotensin receptor blockers (ARBs).
  - Hypercalcemia, a frequent cancer complication, causes AKI by direct renal vasoconstriction and natriuresis-induced volume depletion.
- **Intrinsic causes**
  - Cast nephropathy is the most common presentation of AKI related to multiple myeloma.
  - Tumor lysis syndrome (TLS) is an oncologic emergency. It can occur spontaneously but much more often seen after induction chemotherapy or other targeted therapies, particularly in the setting of bulky disease.
  - Lymphomatous infiltration of the kidney is less common but should not be overlooked. It is characterized by enlarged kidneys, AKI, and subclinical proteinuria and is almost always diagnosed by renal biopsy.
- **Postrenal causes:** Obstructive uropathy is most common in prostate, bladder, and kidney cancers or from extrinsic compression of the urinary tract from either primary or metastatic abdominal or pelvic malignancies.
- **AKI after hematopoietic cell transplantation** (HCT)
  - Early after HCT (within the first 30 days) AKI is commonly caused by sepsis, hypotension, and nephrotoxins. It may also be rarely caused by TLS and hepatic sinusoidal obstruction syndrome, though frequency of the latter is decreasing.

○ AKI later after HCT (>3 to 4 months) is usually due to **thrombotic microangiopathy (TMA)** or **calcineurin inhibitor toxicity.**
- The management of AKI in this setting is similar to those without malignancy and is discussed elsewhere.

Tumor Lysis Syndrome

General Principles

- TLS occurs when malignant cells rapidly release cytosolic contents into the extracellular space. TLS is an oncologic emergency.[3]
- Cellular release of adenosine triphosphate also causes hyperphosphatemia, which is also nephrotoxic through precipitation in tubules (phosphate nephropathy).
- Nucleic acid breakdown can lead to severe hyperuricemia.
- Uric acid is poorly soluble in an acidic milieu and crystallizes at high concentrations.
- Hyperuricemia leads to urate crystal formation within the nephron as well as the vasa recta, causing AKI.
- Cellular release of potassium can cause rapid-onset hyperkalemia, which is life threatening and may require hemodialysis.

Diagnosis

- TLS is defined as a collection of metabolic complications that occur in the setting of a rapidly proliferating neoplasm and large tumor burden.
- It is characterized by hyperuricemia, hyperphosphatemia, hypocalcemia, hyperkalemia, elevated uric acid, and lactate dehydrogenase (LDH).
- TLS occurs most frequently in hematologic malignancies such as lymphoma (especially Burkitt lymphoma), acute lymphocytic leukemia, and acute myeloid leukemia.
- It most commonly develops in the setting cytotoxic chemotherapy or radiotherapy, but can also occur spontaneously in rapidly growing cancers.

Treatment

- Patients at high risk require frequent monitoring of electrolytes and aggressive intravenous fluid administration (at least 3 L/day) if no contraindications to volume expansion.
- **Allopurinol** (xanthine oxidase inhibitor) can be used prophylactically to prevent acute hyperuricemia during treatment in high-risk patients.
- **Febuxostat** is another xanthine oxidase inhibitor and might have a role in TLS treatment given hepatic rather renal excretion; however, no clinical trials evidence supports its efficacy in this setting to date.
- **Rasburicase** is recombinant urate oxidase that enzymatically degrades uric acid and rapidly reduces elevated uric acid levels. Rasburicase should be avoided in patients with glucose-6-phosphate dehydrogenase deficiency. It is also occasionally used prophylactically in high-risk patients.[4,5]
- **Urine alkalinization** can improve uric acid solubility; however, this will also increase intratubular calcium phosphate deposition therefore normal saline is preferred over sodium-bicarbonate–containing solutions.

Chemotherapy Toxicities and the Kidney

ANTIANGIOGENIC THERAPIES

General Principles

- Antiangiogenic therapies typically target the vascular endothelial growth factor (VEGF) pathway.[6]

- Examples include bevacizumab, sunitinib, sorafenib, axitinib, and pazopanib.
- The VEGF pathway is important for maintenance of glomerular function in the kidney as well as maintenance of endothelial cell health in the systemic vasculature.
- Blocking the pathway therefore has kidney and vascular toxicities, including **proteinuria, kidney dysfunction, and hypertension.**

Diagnosis

- New or exacerbated hypertension is relatively common after patients start antiangiogenic therapies, usually within the first few months of starting therapy. In some cases, blood pressure rise can occur much later.
- Urinalysis should be performed at baseline and quarterly on patients receiving antiangiogenic therapies in order to detect new proteinuria. A positive result should be followed up with a spot urine protein to creatinine ratio.
- Kidney function should also be routinely monitored on this class of targeted therapy.
- The kidney lesion induced by antiangiogenic therapy is **TMA,** which is typically diagnosed by renal biopsy. In most cases this is not required because the clinical picture is sufficient to make a diagnosis.

Treatment

- The vast majority of patients developing new or exacerbated hypertension on antiangiogenic therapies can be treated medically. First-line agents include **ACE inhibitors, ARBs, and calcium channel blockers,** with second-line agents including diuretics. β-Blockers are less effective and should not be used for first-line therapy, though combined α and β blockade such as labetalol is effective.
- Patients that develop proteinuria should be monitored closely but do not necessarily need to be taken off therapy. Proteinuria is typically subnephrotic. An ACE inhibitor or ARB should be started as long as tolerated and proteinuria monitored by urine protein to creatinine ratio at each visit. If proteinuria rises to nephrotic levels or is accompanied by a fall in estimated glomerular filtration rate (eGFR), referral to a nephrologist and/or dose reduction or drug holiday should be considered.
- Some patients develop AKI on antiangiogenic therapy, which reflects a TMA. In this situation, referral to a nephrologist is suggested. Some patients can continue on a lower dose but others may develop CKD if continued on therapy.

PLATINUM COMPOUNDS

General Principles

- Cisplatin (cis-diamminedichloroplatinum II) is both the most frequent platinum-based chemotherapy used and the most nephrotoxic.[7]
- Cisplatin becomes activated within cells, reacting with DNA to cause intra-strand cross-linking leading to cytotoxicity.
- Cisplatin is concentrated in the renal cortex in proximal tubule via organic cation transporter 2 and this partly explains its predilection for nephrotoxicity.[8]
- Renal dysfunction occurs in up to one-third of patients and is characterized by a stuttering rise in serum creatinine 1 to 2 weeks after starting therapy.
- Carboplatin is another platinum-based agent with a safer nephrotoxic profile but can induce renal toxicity at high doses (>800 mg/m^2).
- Oxaliplatin has the least risk of nephrotoxicity.

Diagnosis

- Nephrotoxicity is characterized by **delayed but often progressive azotemia.** The urine sediment is bland and there is minimal proteinuria.

- **Electrolyte disturbances** are common including partial or full **Fanconi syndrome,** characterized by hypomagnesemia, hyponatremia, and **nephrogenic diabetes insipidus.** Glycosuria and hypomagnesemia are clues to the diagnosis.
- Long-term cisplatin exposure may lead to interstitial fibrosis and CKD.
- Hypomagnesemia is a frequent complication, can be severe, and may persist for years even after discontinuation.

Treatment

- Efforts to prevent cisplatin-induced AKI center on **hydration during treatment,** with the goal to induce high urine flow.
- Forced diuresis with saline plus furosemide or saline plus mannitol is also used in many centers, based on older studies; however, the effectiveness of mannitol is still an open question and prehydration with normal saline is current standard of care.

IMMUNE CHECKPOINT INHIBITORS

General Principles

- Immune checkpoint inhibitor (ICIs) antibodies such as ipilimumab (anticytotoxic T-lymphocyte–associated protein 4, CTLA-4), nivolumab, and pembrolizumab (anti-programmed death 1, PD-1) are increasingly used to treat nonsmall cell lung cancer, melanoma, and renal cell cancer; renal toxicity is a known complication of these therapies.
- The overall incidence of renal toxicity has been estimated to range between 13% and 29%, with a higher incidence reported in patients receiving combination therapy with ipilimumab and nivolumab.[9]
- The injury from ICIs **resembles acute interstitial nephritis** (AIN). CTLA-4 blockade leads to an uncontrolled activation of T cells (Tregs), which then migrate and infiltrate the kidney. PD-1 inhibition leads to increase proliferation of T cells and cytotoxicity to the kidney.

Diagnosis

- **Elevated creatinine and pyuria** are the major clues. Hematuria, eosinophilia, and hypertension have also been reported.
- With CTLA-4 inhibitors, renal injury presents in about 2 to 3 months, whereas PD-1 inhibitors have a later onset occurring in about 3 to 10 months.[9,10]
- AKI has also been reported in renal transplant patients receiving these ICIs.
- **Renal biopsy** should be considered to confirm the diagnosis in the appropriate clinical setting and if risk is low.
- Ipilimumab has been associated with AIN and podocytopathies such as lupus-like nephritis, minimal change disease, and TMA. PD-1 inhibitors also induce an AIN-like picture.

Treatment

- Rule out all other potential causes of AKI.
- If AIN is present on renal biopsy, **discontinuation of the ICIs** is recommended along with a course of **corticosteroids.** In some cases, continuation of therapy along with low to moderate steroid doses may also be effective, though this is based on clinical experience and no trial data exist.
- There is no recommended dosing for the corticosteroid treatment but case reports had used prednisone 1 mg/kg tapered over 1 to 2 months.

Paraprotein Disease and the Kidney

CAST NEPHROPATHY

General Principles

- Cast nephropathy, or myeloma kidney, is an **inflammatory tubulointerstitial renal lesion** that is characterized by the presence of multiple **intraluminal proteinaceous casts** mainly in the distal portion of the nephrons.
- The glomeruli are usually normal in appearance.
- The casts are precipitates of **monoclonal free light chain (FLC)** and Tamm–Horsfall glycoprotein and they cause tubular toxicity as well as intratubular obstruction.
- Persistence of casts produces giant cell inflammation and tubular atrophy.

Diagnosis

- Cast nephropathy often presents with an **acute and rapid rise in creatinine**; however, a renal biopsy may be required to make the diagnosis when patients are not known to have myeloma.
- Below are the clinical tests often used in the screening for cast nephropathy and other paraproteinemias.
  - ○ **Serum protein electrophoresis** (SPEP) is the most commonly used test for M proteins. It is used in both diagnosis and to monitor disease response since it is a quantitative test. However, it is not sensitive enough as a single screening tool and the M-band does not distinguish the isotype (immunofixation is required).
  - ○ **Urine protein electrophoresis** (UPEP) is also used for diagnosis and monitoring of response in multiple myeloma. It has the lowest sensitivity of all tests, because M proteins are not always found in the urine of patients with monoclonal gammopathy. New renal impairment, a urinary M spike, and low albumin are highly suggestive of a tubulointerstitial process such as cast nephropathy.
  - ○ **Serum and urine immunofixation electrophoresis** (IFE) is a useful qualitative (not quantitative) adjunct in the diagnosis of paraproteinemias. It increases the detection rate of patients with multiple myeloma and immunoglobulin light chain (AL) amyloidosis. It also allows for identification of the type of monoclonal protein.
  - ○ **Serum FLC** used along with SPEP and serum IFE increases the sensitivity in the detection of multiple myeloma and other paraproteinemias. It is a quantitative test and thus is used to monitor disease. Its speed of normalization has been considered an important predictor of renal recovery in cast nephropathy.[11] It has some limitations such as not being able to differentiate between polyclonal or monoclonal FLCs. Renal insufficiency can increase the ratio of FLCs since they are cleared by the kidney. This rise is not symmetric since κ FLCs are cleared more rapidly than λ FLCs. A FLC ratio of between 0.37 and 3.1 has been suggested as a reference range during renal impairment.[12]

Treatment

- The mainstay of therapy remains includes steroids and chemotherapy to reduce the circulating levels of the monoclonal FLC.
- A role for plasmapheresis to rapidly lower FLC is debated, with many centers avoiding it due to lack of clinical trial data supporting its use.[13,14]
- Increasingly, therapies that include the proteasome inhibitor bortezomib are used especially in the setting of kidney damage and reduced renal function.
- A clinical feature of cast nephropathy is that recovery of renal function correlates with the degree of FLC proteinuria. With successful treatment, normalization of renal function occurs in 31% to 58% of patients.[11] Even severe renal failure from cast nephropathy is a

potentially reversible process, particularly with effective reduction in serum monoclonal FLC levels.

- Because tubulointerstitial atrophy and fibrosis may develop rapidly in cast nephropathy, the speed with which reduction of the serum monoclonal FLC is achieved appears to be another critical element in predicting recovery.[11]
- Recovery of renal function is also associated with improved patient survival.

AMYLOIDOSIS

General Principles

- Amyloid proteins represent a family of insoluble fibrillar molecules derived from more than 20 different naturally occurring precursor proteins.
- Amyloid formation under physiologic conditions reflects a sequence-specific process.
- Amyloid precursor proteins have amino acid sequences that promote misfolding, permitting aggregation into fibrillar amyloid.
- In AL-type amyloid, only a small portion of all FLC forms amyloid and the **tendency to polymerize to produce amyloid resides specifically within the variable domain.** While κ FLC may cause amyloidosis, λ FLC more frequently forms amyloid.

Diagnosis

- Tests such as serum and urine IFE, quantitative serum FLCs, and SPEP are useful screening tools; however, diagnosis requires tissue biopsy and microscopic examination by immunofluorescence.
- A critical element in the determination of the type of amyloidosis includes careful **immunofluorescence microscopy.**
- Confirmation of the type of amyloidosis is critical and may require genotyping to evaluate for a familial amyloidosis or extraction of the amyloid from the injured tissue and analysis of the composition of the amyloid using tandem mass spectrometry.

Treatment

- First ensure that the patient has AL-type amyloidosis (vs. secondary amyloidosis).
- Next, stage the extent of disease process with bone marrow biopsy, echocardiography, and assessment of renal function.
- In general, patients with **AL-type amyloidosis are treated similarly to patients with multiple myeloma,** which centers in chemotherapy designed to reduce tumor burden and decrease the circulating offending FLC.
- While plasma exchange or hemodialysis using dialyzers that have high–molecular-weight cutoff may remove FLC, there are no data to support their use in AL-type amyloidosis.

MONOCLONAL IMMUNOGLOBULIN DEPOSITION DISEASE

General Principles

- Monoclonal immunoglobulin deposition disease (MIDD) refers to a group of diseases that are characterized by deposition of monoclonal immunoglobulin fragments as electron-dense granular deposits in basement membranes in the glomerulus and along the tubular basement membrane.[15]
- When the protein involved is a monoclonal FLC, the term **light chain deposition disease** (LCDD) is used. The term **light and heavy chain deposition disease** (LHCDD) is applied when both monoclonal heavy chains and light chains are identified in the biopsy. **Heavy chain deposition disease** (HCDD) is used in the very rare situation when only monoclonal heavy chains are present in the biopsy.

- As in AL-type amyloidosis, MIDD is the result of changes in the glomerulus induced by the FLC. The pathogenesis, however, is different from AL-type amyloidosis. It has been proposed that it is characterized by glomerulosclerosis with accumulation of extracellular matrix proteins in the mesangium.
- κ is the predominant FLC isotype involved in LCDD and LHCDD.

Diagnosis

- Glomerular diseases related to monoclonal immunoglobulin deposition may be classified according to their ultrastructural pattern (Table 19-1).
- Although MIDD is a systemic disease process, renal manifestations, including proteinuria, hematuria, and renal failure, dominate the clinical picture.
- Kidney failure can occur rapidly in some patients, giving the clinical impression of a rapidly progressive glomerulonephritis.
- Often the diagnosis is entertained only after analyzing kidney tissue and subsequent search identifies a hematologic abnormality. An associated lymphoplasmacytic malignancy is identified in about 50% of patients with LCDD and LHCDD and perhaps only 25% in HCDD.[15]
- Detection of the monoclonal protein in the circulation may be challenging in MIDD. In one study, SPEP, serum IFE, and UPEP, and urine IFE were positive only in 86% of

TABLE 19-1	CLASSIFICATION OF PARAPROTEIN-ASSOCIATED GLOMERULAR DISEASES		
Ultrastructural Pattern	Disease	Monoclonal Protein	Ultrastructural Appearance
Organized deposits	AL-type amyloidosis	Free light chains	Fibrils
	AH-type amyloidosis	Monoclonal heavy chain	Fibrils
	Cryoglobulinemia, types I and III	Ig or Ig fragment	Microtubules
	Immunotactoid glomerulopathy	Ig or Ig fragment	Microtubules
	Fibrillary glomerulonephritis	Free light chains alone or Ig light chain and heavy chain	Fibrils
Electron-dense granular deposits	MIDD (includes LCDD, LHCDD, and HCDD)	Free light chains alone or Ig light chain and heavy chain	Amorphous
	Proliferative glomerulonephritis with monoclonal Ig deposition	Monoclonal Ig or only free light chains	Amorphous
	HCDD	Ig heavy chain	Amorphous

AL, amyloid light chain; AH, heavy chain amyloid; Ig, immunoglobulin; MIDD, monoclonal immunoglobulin deposition disease; LCDD, light chain deposition disease; LHCDD, light and heavy chain deposition disease; HCDD, heavy chain deposition disease.

TABLE 19-2 COMMON ELECTROLYTE ABNORMALITIES ASSOCIATED WITH MALIGNANCY AND CHEMOTHERAPY

Electrolyte Abnormality	Associated Malignancy or Medications	Mechanism of Electrolyte Abnormality	Treatment
Hyponatremia	1. Primary or metastatic brain tumors 2. Small cell lung cancer 3. Other pulmonary tumors	SIADH	See Chapter 3, Disorders of Water and Sodium Balance
Hypercalcemia	1. Lung, breast, renal cell, squamous cell carcinoma	PTHrP-mediated hypercalcemia	IV fluids IV furosemide once volume replete
	2. Lymphoma, leukemia 3. Multiple myeloma	Local bone destruction	IV bisphosphonates Denosumab
Hypomagnesemia	1. Cisplatin	Renal magnesium wasting and reduced gastrointestinal absorption[8]	Oral or IV magnesium repletion Consider alternate chemotherapy regimen if available
	2. Epidermal growth factor receptor inhibitors (e.g., cetuximab, panitumumab)	EGFR activation is required for TRPM6 activity; TRPM6 mediates magnesium reabsorption in the loop of Henle and distal convoluted tubule[17]	
Hypophosphatemia	1. Tyrosine kinase inhibitors (e.g., imatinib)	Mechanism unclear; may be mediated through FGF-23, however this is speculative[18,19]	Oral and IV supplementation Replete vitamin D If related to chemotherapy, consider alternatives if hypophosphatemia is severe
	2. Mesenchymal tumors	Release of FGF-23 by tumor cells leads to down regulation of sodium-phosphorus transporter and cause phosphaturia[20]	Treatment of underlying malignancy

SIADH, syndrome of inappropriate anti-diuretic hormone; PTHrP, parathyroid hormone–related peptide; EGFR, epidermal growth factor receptor; TRPM6, transient receptor potential cation channel, subfamily M, member 6; FGF-23, fibroblast growth factor 23.

patients, although the commercially available nephelometric assay that quantifies serum κ and λ FLC was abnormal in every patient including those with HCDD.[15]

• Recurrence of MIDD in kidney allografts is common.

Treatment

• Treatment begins with an assessment of the size and aggressiveness of the plasma cell clone producing the nephrotoxic paraprotein.

• When MIDD coexists with multiple myeloma, patients are treated with chemotherapy that targets the myeloma. Some patients have been treated with high-dose chemotherapy with autologous stem cell transplantation.

• Those patients with a proliferative glomerulonephritis, but no clinical evidence of a plasma cell dyscrasia other than kidney deposition of an intact monoclonal IgG are most difficult to treat, as there is paucity of evidence to guide therapy, but it has been suggested that they may respond to novel agents.[16]

ELECTROLYTE ABNORMALITIES IN MALIGNANCY

• Various electrolyte abnormalities are observed in setting of malignancy, either secondary to the underlying malignancy or secondary to the treatment regimen.

• Table 19-2 outlines the most common electrolyte abnormalities and underlying mechanisms.[8,17–20]

REFERENCES

1. Perazella M. Online curricula: onco-nephrology. Available at https://www.asn-online.org/education/distancelearning/curricula/onco/. Accessed January 2, 2019.
2. Christiansen CF, Johansen MB, Langeberg WJ, et al. Incidence of acute kidney injury in cancer patients: a Danish population-based cohort study. *Eur J Intern Med.* 2011;22:399–406.
3. Wilson FP, Berns JS. Tumor lysis syndrome: new challenges and recent advances. *Adv Chronic Kidney Dis.* 2014;21:18–26.
4. Cortes J, Moore JO, Maziarz RT, et al. Control of plasma uric acid in adults at risk for tumor Lysis syndrome: efficacy and safety of rasburicase alone and rasburicase followed by allopurinol compared with allopurinol alone—results of a multicenter phase III study. *J Clin Oncol.* 2010;28:4207–4213.
5. Lopez-Olivo MA, Pratt G, Palla SL, et al. Rasburicase in tumor lysis syndrome of the adult: a systematic review and meta-analysis. *Am J Kidney Dis.* 2013;62:481–492.
6. Cosmai L, Gallieni M, Liguigli W, et al. Renal toxicity of anticancer agents targeting vascular endothelial growth factor (VEGF) and its receptors (VEGFRs). *J Nephrol.* 2017;30:171–180.
7. Manohar S, Leung N. Cisplatin nephrotoxicity: a review of the literature. *J Nephrol.* 2018;31:15–25.
8. Oronsky B, Caroen S, Oronsky A, et al. Electrolyte disorders with platinum-based chemotherapy: mechanisms, manifestations and management. *Cancer Chemother Pharmacol.* 2017;80:895–907.
9. Wanchoo R, Karam S, Uppal NN, et al. Adverse renal effects of immune checkpoint inhibitors: a narrative review. *Am J Nephrol.* 2017;45:160–169.
10. Izzedine H, Mateus C, Boutros C, et al. Renal effects of immune checkpoint inhibitors. *Nephrol Dial Transplant.* 2017;32:936–942.
11. Hutchison CA, Cockwell P, Stringer S, et al. Early reduction of serum-free light chains associates with renal recovery in myeloma kidney. *J Am Soc Nephrol.* 2011;22:1129–1136.
12. Hutchison CA, Harding S, Hewins P, et al. Quantitative assessment of serum and urinary polyclonal free light chains in patients with chronic kidney disease. *Clin J Am Soc Nephrol.* 2008;3:1684–1690.
13. Clark WF, Stewart AK, Rock GA, et al. Plasma exchange when myeloma presents as acute renal failure: a randomized, controlled trial. *Ann Intern Med.* 2005;143:777–784.

14. Bridoux F, Carron PL, Pegourie B, et al. Effect of high-cutoff hemodialysis vs conventional hemodialysis on hemodialysis independence among patients with myeloma cast nephropathy: a randomized clinical trial. *JAMA*. 2017;318:2099–2110.

15. Nasr SH, Valeri AM, Cornell LD, et al. Renal monoclonal immunoglobulin deposition disease: a report of 64 patients from a single institution. *Clin J Am Soc Nephrol*. 2012;7:231–239.

16. Nasr SH, Satoskar A, Markowitz GS, et al. Proliferative glomerulonephritis with monoclonal IgG deposits. *J Am Soc Nephrol*. 2009;20:2055–2064.

17. Jian DM, Dennis K, Steinmetz A, et al. Management of epidermal growth factor receptor inhibitor-induced hypomagnesemia: a systematic review. *Clin Colorectal Cancer*. 2016;15:e117–e123.

18. Alemán JO, Farooki A, Girotra M. Effects of tyrosine kinase inhibition on bone metabolism: untargeted consequences of targeted therapies. *Endocr Relat Cancer*. 2014;21:R247–R259.

19. Bellini E, Pia A, Brizzi MP, et al. Sorafenib may induce hypophosphatemia through a fibroblast growth factor-23 (FGF23)-independent mechanism. *Ann Oncol*. 2011;22:988–990.

20. Hautmann AH, Hautmann MG, Kölbl O, et al. Tumor-induced osteomalacia: an up-to-date review. *Curr Rheumatol Rep*. 2015;17:512.

Hemodialysis

20

Frank O'Brien

GENERAL PRINCIPLES

- The loss of kidney function in end-stage renal disease (ESRD) results in uremia and an impairment in regulation of fluids and electrolytes. Without intervention, ESRD is inevitably fatal.
- Therapeutic options include hemodialysis (HD), peritoneal dialysis, transplantation, and supportive/palliative care. HD is the most commonly utilized form of renal replacement therapy in the United States.
- Of the 678,000 patients with ESRD in the United States, over 430,000 are currently on HD.[1]
  - Like the general ESRD population, the prevalent HD population is predominately white (56% white, 37% black, and 5% Asian), with a slightly higher proportion of males (57%).
  - Diabetes is the most common cause of ESRD, followed by hypertension, glomerulonephritis, and congenital and cystic kidney diseases.
  - The largest age group of HD patients is between 45 and 64 years. This is similar to the general ESRD population and younger patients are more likely to be on peritoneal dialysis or to receive a kidney transplant.
- Despite advances in care, the mortality rate in HD patients is startling.
  - **Cardiovascular disease is the leading cause of death** among patients on HD, followed by sepsis.
  - The average lifespan after commencing dialysis is approximately 8 years in those aged 40 to 44 years, dropping to 4.5 years in those aged 60 to 64 years.[2]
  - The probability of death in the first 5 years after starting HD is 63%.[3]
  - Among diabetics on HD, this probability rises to 71%.
  - Dialysis patients over the age of 65 have a mortality rate seven times higher than the general Medicare population. Dialysis patients between the ages of 20 and 64 have a mortality rate eight times higher.

WHO REQUIRES DIALYSIS?

- Given the poor outcomes for patients on HD, **every effort should be undertaken to preserve renal function.**
  - Early nephrology referrals, patient education, and serious consideration of transplant options may be helpful in attenuating the progression to ESRD.
  - Even with aggressive early medical care, dialysis may become necessary to relieve uremic symptoms, electrolyte imbalances, or fluid accumulation due to declining renal function.
- The majority of patients who require maintenance HD have pre-existing chronic kidney disease (CKD) with a gradual but progressive loss of renal function over time.
  - Patients usually develop **uremic symptoms** and require dialysis initiation, when their estimated glomerular filtration rate **(eGFR) falls below 10 mL/min/1.73 m^2. This varies considerably between patients.**

○ Patients with **significant comorbidities,** particularly heart failure, may require dialysis initiation at an earlier stage for volume management.

○ Timing of the initiation of maintenance dialysis requires incorporation of both patient's uremic symptom burden and eGFR. Studies have shown no difference in outcomes in patients commenced on HD with an average eGFR of 9 mL/min versus 7 mL/min.[4]

○ **Uremic symptoms** develop presumably to the accumulation of toxic metabolites that are no longer adequately cleared by the failing kidney.

  ▪ This may manifest in a variety of ways, including nausea, vomiting, poor energy levels, decreased appetite, lethargy, pruritus, impaired cognition, and a metallic aftertaste.

  ▪ Motor neuropathies may be elicited on physical examination, while asterixis, tremor, and myoclonus suggest uremic encephalopathy.

  ▪ Uremic pericarditis manifests as a pericardial friction rub or pericardial effusion, and is a clear indication for urgent initiation of dialysis.

● **Acute kidney injury** (AKI) may also require dialytic support, particularly in those who develop pulmonary edema, hyperkalemia, or metabolic acidosis and other indications.

● **Acute indications** for the initiation of dialysis can be remembered with the **mnemonic AEIOU.**

  ○ **Acidosis:** life-threatening metabolic acidosis with a pH <7.2, not responsive to conservative treatments.

  ○ **Electrolyte abnormalities:** life-threatening hyperkalemia, not responsive to conservative treatment or with associated electrocardiogram (ECG) changes and symptomatic hypercalcemia.

  ○ **Intoxications:** There are a limited number of intoxications for which HD is indicated. It should be considered in patients with deteriorating medical status, those whose measured levels of a substance are indicative of poor outcomes, or those with metabolic derangements (e.g., metabolic acidosis caused by intoxication). Substances that are effectively cleared with dialysis have the following characteristics:

  ▪ Low molecular weight (<500 Da).

  ▪ High water solubility.

  ▪ Low degree of protein binding.

  ▪ Small volumes of distribution (<1 L/kg).

  ▪ High dialysis clearance relative to endogenous clearance.

  ▪ The following substances can be cleared with dialysis: methanol, ethylene glycol, lithium, theophylline, dabigatran, and salicylates.

  ○ **Overload:** fluid overload or pulmonary edema not responsive to aggressive diuresis.

  ○ **Uremia:** mental status changes attributable to uremia, uremic pericarditis, or neuropathy, bleeding diatheses, or vomiting associated with uremia.

DIALYSIS MODALITIES FOR PATIENTS WITH ESRD

● Choosing the appropriate HD modality is an important decision that should be made with the consideration of both patient preference and a practical assessment of patient resources and capabilities. The primary variables that differentiate the various modalities are location, independence, duration, and cumulative dialysis dose.

● **Intermittent in-center HD** is the most common form of HD.

  ○ This form of HD typically involves treatments two to three times per week, with each session averaging between 3 and 4 hours.

  ○ Patients receive HD at a dialysis center, where trained staff are able to set up and supervise each treatment. For patients new to HD, this is often the modality of choice to acclimate patients to a supervised and controlled HD session.

- **Short daily HD** exposes patients to more frequent treatments (usually six times per week), although with a shorter duration of each session.
  - The cumulative weekly dose of dialysis is similar to that obtained on intermittent HD. However, dividing the treatments into frequent, shorter treatments may prevent intradialytic complications, particularly hypotension and cramping.
  - This modality is predominately performed at home, although some in-center locations are able to accommodate the daily treatments.
  - This modality is associated with increased frequency of vascular complications.
- **Nocturnal HD** is different, in that it offers a larger cumulative dose of dialysis each week.
  - Patients who undergo nocturnal HD at home typically have longer treatment time periods, averaging 6 to 8 hours, performed six nights per week.
  - This modality does have the added convenience of allowing the patient greater freedom during the day.
  - Like short daily HD, nocturnal HD is predominately done at home, although in-center locations are available. In-center nocturnal HD typically offers 8-hour treatments, three nights per week.
- The decision to dialyze patients with acute renal failure is often performed based on acute indications, and the selection of modalities is often done in consideration of the patient's hemodynamic status. Other options for renal replacement are discussed in Chapter 22.

DIALYSIS ACCESS

- For HD to be effective, there must first be an effective system of blood delivery from the patient to the machine, and vice versa. This is referred to as a dialysis access.
- There are **three types of dialysis access:** arteriovenous fistulas (AVFs), arteriovenous grafts (AVGs), and dialysis catheters.
  - Fistulas and grafts are vascular conduits that can support a high flow of blood. They are cannulated at each dialysis treatment with two needles—one through which arterial blood is pumped through the dialyzer and the other through which blood is returned into the venous system.
  - Catheters are placed in a central venous position, typically in the internal jugular location, with flow through separate luminal ports to simulate arterial output and venous return. Specific characteristics of each type of access are described below.
- **The AVF is the most desirable form of vascular access.** It is created by the surgical manipulation of the patient's native vasculature.
  - Construction is performed under regional anesthesia by an experienced vascular surgeon and can consist of either a side-to-side anastomosis between an artery and vein or a side-of-artery to end-of-vein anastomosis.
  - The goal is to provide an access site that can withstand repeated cannulation with large bore needles and can sustain the high blood flow necessary for dialysis. Flow through an AVF averages between 600 and 800 mL/min.
  - Complications with thrombosis, infection, and vascular steal are lower in comparison to the AVG.
  - Placement of an AVF requires careful planning, as they can take 3 to 4 months to mature. Furthermore, the construction of an adequate AVF may be impossible if the patient lacks healthy vasculature. In particular, elderly patients or patients with peripheral vascular disease may not have vessels that are amenable to the creation of a fistula.
- The **AVG** can be placed in patients for whom an AVF cannot be created.
  - In lieu of the patient's native vasculature, a synthetic graft (frequently created from polytetrafluoroethylene) is placed for the arteriovenous connection.

- ○ Long-term patency rates are less impressive than those obtained with AVF. However, the AVG does have a few advantages, including a large surface area for cannulation and can be used earlier than an AVF, with a shorter maturation time of 2 to 3 weeks.
- ○ Flow rates through an AVG are typically 1000 to 1500 mL/min, with thrombosis occurring at flows less than 600 to 800 mL/min.
- ○ The average graft survival rate is approximately 2 years.
- **A catheter is the least desirable form of vascular access for HD.**
- ○ Cuffed tunneled dialysis catheters are typically placed in the right internal jugular vein, with a tunneled exit site just below the ipsilateral clavicle.
- ○ These can be placed in patients requiring HD who do not yet have a site for a permanent vascular access. However, given variable success with flows, difficulties with recirculation, catheter dysfunction, and significant risk of infection, the catheter should not be used except as an access of last resort.

BASIC MECHANISM OF HD

- The goal of HD is to replace the basic functions of the failing kidney including clearance uremic substances, adjustment of serum electrolytes, and offloading accumulated fluid.
- The dialysis machine maintains two compartments throughout treatment, a blood compartment and a dialysate compartment. These are separated by a semipermeable dialyzer. Each HD treatment is composed of two parts that operate independently: diffusion and ultrafiltration.
  - ○ **Diffusion** uses the difference in solute concentration between blood and dialysate to drive the movement of small solutes.
    - To maximize the gradient between blood and dialysate compartments, the blood and dialysate flow in a countercurrent fashion.
    - Although any solute smaller than the membrane pore is capable of moving between compartments, diffusion favors the movement of smaller solutes, as they possess a higher particle velocity and a greater likelihood of contact with the membrane surface.
    - The lower concentration of potassium and higher concentration of bicarbonate in dialysate fluid are responsible for removal of potassium and correction of metabolic acidosis in the blood.
  - ○ **Ultrafiltration uses a hydrostatic pressure gradient to move fluid from the blood to the dialysate compartment.**
    - Ultrafiltration is used to remove fluid from the patient.
    - When fluid moves from blood to dialysate, the flow of fluid "drags" solutes across the dialysis membrane. This is also known as convection.
    - Both small and larger solutes are cleared to the same degree with convection.
    - The extent of ultrafiltration or fluid removal can be controlled by the dialysis machine.

DIALYSIS PRESCRIPTION

The dialysis prescription should be tailored to the specific goals of attaining adequate clearance of toxins, maintaining electrolyte balance, and removing excess fluid gains (Table 20-1).

Attaining Dialysis Adequacy: Time, Flow, and Choice of Dialyzer

- For chronic HD, the adequacy of dialysis dose is assessed using two metrics, urea reduction ratio (URR) and the Kt/V_{urea}.

TABLE 20-1	GUIDELINES FOR MAINTENANCE HEMODIALYSIS PRESCRIPTION		
Goal	Variable	Typical Prescription	Comments
Dialysis adequacy (Kt/V_{urea} > 1.2 or URR >65%)	Time	3–4 hrs	Can be adjusted in 15-min increments
	Frequency	3 times/week	Consider adding weekly treatments for large volumes of distribution
	Dialyzer	Variable by institution	High-efficiency dialyzers have larger surface areas
	Blood flow	350–450 mL/min	AV grafts and fistulas: 400–500 mL/min Catheters: 350–400 mL/min
	Dialysate flow	500–800 mL/min	Little benefit for dialysate flow rates >800 mL/min
Electrolyte balance	Dialysate [K]	2–3 mEq/L	1 mEq/L can be used for severe hyperkalemia but requires monitoring of serum [K] at 30- to 60-min intervals
	Dialysate [Na]	140–145 mEq/L	Should be no more than 15–20 mEq/L higher than serum [Na] in patients with chronic hyponatremia
	Dialysate [Ca]	2.5 mEq/L	Consider higher Ca content in hypocalcemia
	Dialysate [HCO_3]	35–38 mEq/L	Can be lowered to 28 mEq/L for alkalotic patients
Volume regulation	Ultrafiltration	Based on EDW; typically 2–3 L	UF >4 L during a single treatment may lead to uncomfortable fluid shifts and hypotension

AV, arteriovenous; Ca, calcium; EDW, estimated dry weight; HCO_3, bicarbonate; K, potassium; Kt/V_{urea}, volume of cleared plasma (Kt) to the volume of urea distribution (V_{urea}); Na, sodium; UF, ultrafiltration; URR, urea reduction rate.

- The **URR** reflects the reduction of urea levels during dialysis and is calculated using blood urea nitrogen (BUN) levels from pre- and postdialysis treatments:

$$URR = (BUN_{pre} - BUN_{post})/BUN_{pre}$$

  ○ The **Kt/V$_{urea}$** value is the dialyzer clearance (K) multiplied by dialysis time (t) divided by the volume of distribution of urea (V). Kt/V$_{urea}$ is closely related to the URR.
    ▪ The guidelines instituted by the National Kidney Foundation's Kidney Disease Outcomes Quality Initiative (KDOQI) set the minimal Kt/V$_{urea}$ for a patient dialyzed thrice weekly at 1.2 for each dialysis treatment, with a target goal of 1.4.[5]
    ▪ A Kt/V$_{urea}$ of 1.3 roughly correlates to a URR of 70%. KDOQI guidelines recommend the attainment of a minimal URR of 65% and a target URR of 70%.
- The parameters of the dialysis prescription that can be modified to achieve an adequate Kt/V$_{urea}$ or URR are increased treatment time and increased dialytic clearance.
- A typical dialysis treatment time (t) is between 3 and 4 hours in length and is administered thrice weekly. Time on dialysis can be increased if Kt/V$_{urea}$ or URR reflect inadequate dialysis.
- Increases in dialytic clearance can be achieved in three main ways, as noted below.
  ○ Increasing blood flow rate
    ▪ Blood flow rate is largely dependent on the access used. Most grafts and fistulas can support blood flow between 400 and 500 mL/min. Catheters are less predictable, and, on average, support flows of 350 to 400 mL/min.
    ▪ Patients with decreasing dialysis adequacy and poor blood flows from their access should be evaluated for vascular stenosis or thrombosis.
    ▪ Correction of flow-limiting complications or changing the type of access from a catheter to an AVG/AVF permits higher blood flows.
  ○ Increasing dialysate flow rate
    ▪ Dialysate flow rate is generally between 500 and 800 mL/min.
    ▪ Titrating the dialysate flow rate is an option, particularly in those with a prescribed dialysate flow under 800 mL/min but increasing the rate beyond 800 mL/min will not significantly improve urea clearance.
  ○ Use of a larger dialyzer
    ▪ Dialyzer size refers to the amount of exposed surface area between blood and dialysate.
    ▪ A larger surface area increases solute transport from blood to dialysate.
    ▪ The availability of various dialyzers is institution dependent, though most dialysis facilities are stocked with large surface area dialyzers.

Attaining Electrolyte Balance: The Dialysate Composition

- The choice of dialysate is the key variable for the balance of serum electrolytes and the correction of conditions such as hyperkalemia.
- Potassium, sodium, calcium, and bicarbonate levels are the primary components that can be controlled in the choice of a dialysate solution.
- **Potassium concentration** in the dialysate can vary widely depending on the patient's pre-HD potassium concentration.
  ○ For a patient with a potassium of ≥5.5 mEq/L, a dialysate potassium concentration of 2 or 3 mEq/L is appropriate.
  ○ In those with a tendency to develop arrhythmias, the 3 mEq/L bath is preferred to avoid precipitating hypokalemia.
  ○ A dialysate potassium concentration of 4 mEq/L is appropriate for patients with hypokalemia or persistent serum potassium <3.5 mEq/L.
  ○ In those with a potassium of >6.5 to 7.0 mEq/L or ECG changes concerning for hyperkalemia, a 1 mEq/L potassium bath may be required for a rapid correction. However, this can cause a rapid fall in potassium levels, and serum potassium levels should be monitored every 30 to 60 minutes.

- It is important to also acknowledge that there is a rebound in potassium levels 1 to 2 hours after dialysis. Further supplementation of potassium based on laboratory results drawn immediately after a dialysis treatment is unwise.
- A dialysate **sodium concentration** of 140 to 145 mEq/L is appropriate in most circumstances but can be adjusted in patients with pre-existing dysnatremias to prevent overcorrection.
  - Low serum sodium levels in dialysis patients are often indicative of excessive free water intake in the context of limited, or absent, capacity for renal water handling.
  - The majority of these patients can be managed through the enforcement of a fluid restriction.
  - Initiating dialysis on patients with chronic hyponatremia requires caution. When dialyzing patients with a chronic serum sodium of <130 mEq/L, the dialysate sodium concentration should be no more than 15 to 20 mEq/L above the serum levels.
  - Patients with hypernatremia should also be corrected slowly. Dialysate sodium should be between 3 and 5 mEq/L lower than serum levels.
- Most dialysate preparations are available with 2.5, 3, or 3.5 mEq/L **calcium concentrations.**
  - A 2.5 mEq/L calcium concentration is equivalent to an ionized calcium concentration of 5 mg/dL.
  - In chronic HD patients, there are concerns about positive calcium balance contributing to vascular calcification and cardiovascular morbidity and mortality. Because of this, a 2.5 mEq/L Ca bath is generally recommended.[6]
  - In patients with persistent hypocalcemia, as in patients who have had a parathyroidectomy, this may need to be increased to maintain serum calcium levels in a safe range.
  - A higher calcium bath of 3 or 3.5 mEq/L is also used in patients who undergo HD acutely or have a significant concurrent acidosis, as the correction of acidosis on dialysis further lowers the plasma calcium concentrations.
- Most chronic dialysis centers use dialysate solutions containing **bicarbonate levels** of 35 to 38 mEq/L. This is usually sufficient to correct the metabolic acidosis associated with chronic renal failure.
  - There are patients who are susceptible to alkalosis, particularly those who are receiving total parenteral nutrition (TPN), have vomiting or nasogastric suction, have poor protein intake, or have respiratory alkalosis.
  - To avoid detrimental effects of alkalemia, including arrhythmias, headaches, soft tissue calcifications, a lower bicarbonate bath of 20 to 28 mEq/L can be used.

Attaining Appropriate Volume Status: Prescribing Ultrafiltration

- The goal of volume removal in dialysis patients is to attain the patient's estimated dry weight (EDW).
  - **The dry weight (DW) refers to a weight in which the patient is clinically euvolemic** and does not demonstrate symptomatic volume contraction (particularly cramping).
  - Ultrafiltration to the EDW allows physicians to remove fluid weight that is gained in between dialysis treatments.
  - Patients should restrict fluid intake to limit intradialytic weight gains to <4 kg, as excessive fluid gains may exceed the capacity to ultrafiltrate during a single treatment.
  - Attempts to remove >4 to 5 L of fluid during a standard 3- to 4-hour treatment may cause uncomfortable fluid shifts and intradialytic hypotension.
- It is also important to acknowledge that a patient's **DW is not a fixed number.**
  - As a result of improved or worsened nutritional status, a patient's DW may increase or decrease. This is a result of true weight that is gained and not merely fluid retention.

○ Patients with limited intradialytic fluid gains and no edema, who note hypotension, lightheadedness, or severe cramping, should be considered for an increase in their DW.

○ Patients who are attaining their usual DW but develop worsening edema or shortness of breath should be challenged with fluid removal to a lower DW.

Anticoagulation

- Heparinization during HD minimizes clotting of the dialysis circuit during the treatment.
- Clotting is particularly problematic among patients with a high hemoglobin and hematocrit, a high rate of ultrafiltration, and a low blood flow on dialysis.
- In the United States, unfractionated heparin is most commonly used to prevent this, although low–molecular-weight heparins can also be used.
- Heparin may be given as a bolus of 1000 to 2000 units, followed by a constant infusion of 1000 to 1200 units per hour.
- It may be necessary to hold heparin in hospitalized HD patients who are undergoing surgery or other interventions.

COMPLICATIONS

Access Complications

Poor Flow

- **Stenosis** of an AVG or AVF can affect both arterial and venous flow. It should be suspected in patients with a decreased rate of blood flow on dialysis, declining dialysis adequacy, or elevated venous pressures on dialysis.
- Prolonged bleeding time periods from the access after needle removal may also indicate vascular congestion as a result of a venous outflow obstruction.
- Patients with a suspected stenosis should have an evaluation of their access with an **angiogram.**
- A **percutaneous transluminal angioplasty or surgical revision** is warranted in lesions that are >50% of the luminal diameter, with associated clinical findings.
- If angioplasty is required more than two times within a 3-month period, the patient should be referred back to vascular surgery for a possible revision.
- Stents are sometimes placed for surgically inaccessible lesions, limited access, or patients with surgical contraindications.

Thrombosis

- Thrombosis can be detected by the absence of a bruit or thrill, and should be addressed promptly to salvage the access.
- Evaluation with an angiogram is necessary to evaluate the cause of the thrombosis.
- Thrombectomies can be performed to treat AVG thrombosis, though they have limited success in AVF. Thrombosis of a fistula may require referral to the access surgeon for reevaluation. If extensive surgical revision or new fistula placement is necessary, the patient may require a tunneled catheter for access until the new access is ready.
- Poor flow from a catheter can result from malpositioning, thrombus formation, and central venous stenosis.
- Early malfunction, preventing successful use shortly after catheter placement, may require positional adjustments or an exchange over a guide wire.
- Thrombosis and stenosis should be suspected in previously functional catheters that are now unable to sustain flows >300 mL/min.
- Intraluminal thrombosis is a common complication that can be treated by instilling the catheter with a thrombolytic drug, such as alteplase.

- A dwell time of 30 minutes is usually sufficient to restore flow, although a repeated trial for 30 to 60 minutes is warranted if suspected catheter thrombosis does not respond to the initial treatment.
- Persistent tunneled catheter failure should be managed with exchange of a new catheter over a guidewire or placement of a new catheter.
- The placement of stiff, non-silicone catheters—particularly in the subclavian position increases the risk of central stenosis. Although this may remain clinically silent during catheter use, it can cause dysfunction in subsequent arteriovenous accesses. For this reason, subclavian catheters should be avoided for HD.

Recirculation
- Recirculation describes a phenomenon by which blood returning to the patient through the venous needle is taken back up by the arterial needle and recirculated through the dialysis circuit.
- Recirculation reduces the efficiency and adequacy of dialysis and can occur from different mechanisms.
- Stenosis at the venous end of an access can impair flow and allow the blood to be pulled back through the extracorporeal circuit.
- Recirculation can also occur if the site of venous return is in close proximity to the arterial outflow.
- Correction of stenosis, proper needle placement, and repositioning of dialysis catheters are useful in decreasing the likelihood of access recirculation.

Infection
- Infections represent the second most common cause of mortality in ESRD patients and are an important part of management in dialysis patients.
- **Exit-site infections** are identified by wound cultures at the site of an erythematous or tender catheter.
  - Infected sites should be cleaned thoroughly and topical antibiotics should be applied.
  - In the presence of an exudate or discharge, wound cultures should be sent and intravenous (IV) antibiotics initiated.
  - If there is discharge from the actual tunnel site, the catheter should be removed.
- **Catheter-related bacteremia** is identified by constitutional symptoms along with growth from blood cultures and signs of catheter infection (e.g., purulence, erythema, or tenderness).
  - Initial antibiotic coverage should include gram-positive organisms, particularly *Staphylococci*, as well as gram-negative organisms.
  - Dual coverage with vancomycin and either ceftazidime or gentamicin is recommended as empiric therapy.
  - Blood culture growth, speciation, and antibiotic sensitivities should guide continued therapy.
  - **Removing an infected catheter is more successful than attempts to salvage catheters with antibiotics alone.** However, as dialysis patients require regular access for treatment sessions, some find it impractical to remove all catheters.
    - In a stable patient who demonstrates prompt clinical improvement and has no indications of a tunnel infection, immediate removal of the catheter may not be necessary and the patient should be started on a 2- to 3-week course of antibiotics.
    - Patients who demonstrate a poor clinical response after 36 hours of antibiotic therapy or any deterioration of clinical status should have the catheter promptly removed.
    - If dialysis is necessary prior to clinical improvement, a temporary dialysis catheter may be placed for individual treatment sessions.
    - **Catheters should also be removed as soon as possible for all catheter-related infections due to *Staphylococcus aureus*.**[7]

- **Any staphylococcus-related catheter infection should prompt examination for signs of septic emboli.**
  ○ Infections of grafts or fistulas are less common.
    - Areas of fluctuance should be evaluated with ultrasound for evidence of an abscess.
    - Extensive graft infections may require partial or complete graft excisions.
    - Infections of AVFs are rare and require a course of 6 weeks of antibiotics. There should be a cautious examination for septic emboli or metastatic infections, particularly endocarditis and osteomyelitis. Occasionally, fistula resection is required.

Hemodynamic Complications

- Limb ischemia as a result of a **steal syndrome** is an important complication of vascular access.
- This occurs when an AVF or graft "steals" the blood supply of the arm distal to the AVF.
- Patients with mild symptoms, such as coldness or paresthesia, can be followed conservatively.
- **Pain and poor wound healing require surgical evaluation and motor/sensory loss is considered a surgical emergency.**
- The high flows through vascular access may also be problematic for patients with cardiovascular disease. High output cardiac failure may be exacerbated due to the placement of an AVG and may require ligation to restore hemodynamic stability.

Aneurysms and Pseudoaneurysms

- Aneurysms and pseudoaneurysms can develop in fistulas and grafts, stimulated by the trauma of repetitive cannulation. Generally, these can be managed with observation and by avoiding cannulation at the site of aneurysmal dilation.
- In patients who demonstrate rapid growth of the aneurysm, poor eschar formation, or spontaneous bleeding, surgical evaluation should be made urgently. Rupture of an aneurysm or pseudoaneurysm can result in prompt exsanguination and imminent death.

Complications of Urea Clearance

- **Dialysis disequilibrium syndrome** occurs in response to an acute reduction of uremic solutes in patients with CKD.[8,9]
- This is typically seen after the initiation of dialysis, when aggressive treatment prescriptions result in a rapid reduction of uremic solutes. Cells that have accommodated to the uremic milieu may not be able to rapidly respond to the dramatic osmolal change, resulting in symptoms of dialysis disequilibrium.
- The syndrome may manifest with headache, nausea, restlessness, confusion, or, in the most serious cases, seizure and coma. In rare circumstance, the condition can be fatal.
- This syndrome can be prevented by using a lower dialysis dose for the first treatment, thus preventing a dramatic shift in uremic solute concentration.

Dialyzer Reactions

- **Type A reactions**
  ○ Type A reactions, characterized by severe dyspnea, pruritus, abdominal cramping, and angioedema, occur in the first 30 minutes of treatment.
  ○ They have previously been attributed to ethylene oxide used in device sterilization, contaminated dialysate, latex allergy, and bradykinins, particularly in patients taking angiotensin-converting enzyme inhibitors in conjunction with exposure to the AN69 dialysis membrane.[9,10]
  ○ Treatment of suspected type A reactions includes cessation of dialysis, diphenhydramine (25 mg IV for pruritus), oxygen as needed, and 200 mL normal saline if hypotensive. Blood should not be returned.

- ○ To prevent subsequent reactions, an alternate sterilizing agent may be tried, and dializers should be thoroughly rinsed before use.
- **Type B reactions**
  - ○ These are characterized by mild back pain and chest pain and occur in the first hour of dialysis.
  - ○ One may attempt to treat through symptoms with supplemental oxygen and antihistamine therapy as needed. Symptoms should diminish during the remainder of therapy.
  - ○ As the etiology of type B reactions is uncertain, methods for prevention are also uncertain, although trial of an alternate membrane may help.

REFERENCES

1. United States Renal Data System. *2016 USRDS Annual Data Report: Epidemiology of Kidney Disease in the United States.* National Institutes of Health, National Institute of Diabetes and Digestive and Kidney Diseases: Bethesda, MD, 2016. Available at https://www.usrds.org/2016/view/default.aspx (Last Accessed December 20, 2019).
2. Collins AJ, Foley RN, Herzog C, et al. Excerpts from the US renal data system 2009 annual data report. *Am J Kidney Dis.* 2010;55:S1–420, A6–7.
3. Bradbury BD, Fissell RB, Albert JM, et al. Predictors of early mortality among incident US hemodialysis patients in the Dialysis Outcomes and Practice Patterns Study (DOPPS). *Clin J Am Soc Nephrol.* 2007;2:89–99.
4. Cooper BA, Branley P, Bulfone L, et al. A randomized, controlled trial of early versus late initiation of dialysis. *N Engl J Med.* 2010;363:609–619.
5. National Kidney F. KDOQI clinical practice guideline for hemodialysis adequacy: 2015 update. *Am J Kidney Dis.* 2015;66:884–930.
6. Ok E, Asci G, Bayraktaroglu S, et al. Reduction of dialysate calcium level reduces progression of coronary artery calcification and improves low bone turnover in patients on hemodialysis. *J Am Soc Nephrol.* 2016;27:2475–2486.
7. Miller LM, Clark E, Dipchand C, et al. Hemodialysis tunneled catheter-related infections. *Can J Kidney Health Dis.* 2016;3:2054358116669129.
8. Patel N, Dalal P, Panesar M. Dialysis disequilibrium syndrome: a narrative review. *Semin Dial.* 2008;21:493–498.
9. Saha M, Allon M. Diagnosis, treatment, and prevention of hemodialysis emergencies. *Clin J Am Soc Nephrol.* 2017;12:357–369.
10. Butani L, Calogiuri G. Hypersensitivity reactions in patients receiving hemodialysis. *Ann Allergy Asthma Immunol.* 2017;118:680–684.

21

Peritoneal Dialysis and Home Hemodialysis

Lisa Koester and Brent Miller

Peritoneal Dialysis

GENERAL PRINCIPLES

- Peritoneal dialysis (PD) is a form of renal replacement therapy that utilizes the patient's peritoneal membrane and capillaries as a semipermeable membrane between the blood and an infused dialysis solution in the peritoneal space.
- Equilibration of solutes across the peritoneal membrane has long been known. The development of sterile, physiologic solutions and reliable peritoneal access allowed for the use of PD first in the acute setting and then in the chronic setting in the 1970s.[1]
- With technical advancements over the ensuing decades, PD has become a viable option for patients with end-stage renal disease; however, less than 15% of dialysis patients in the United States utilize PD as opposed to hemodialysis (HD).
- Unlike HD, PD is a continuous dialysis treatment usually performed all day, 7 days weekly.
- As compared to HD, actual treatment costs of PD are similar; however, the overall cost of care is higher for HD when vascular access complications and medication usage are factored. Essentially, the supply costs of PD counterbalance the fixed overhead and labor costs of center-based HD.
- Patients on PD require fewer hospitalizations and shorter durations of stay.
- Although neither dialysis modality offers a survival advantage over the other, greater satisfaction and flexibility are qualities often promoted by patients on PD as compared to those on HD.

PHYSIOLOGY

- **Diffusion**
  - Most solute (except sodium and calcium) removal in PD occurs by diffusion via the peritoneal capillaries with a small component of convection.
  - Substances retained in renal failure (e.g., urea, creatinine, potassium, and phosphorus) are present in higher concentrations in the blood and thus diffuse down the gradient into the dialysis solution.
  - Dextrose, which is present in high concentrations (up to 3860 mg/dL) in the dialysis solution, diffuses inwardly over time during a PD exchange.
  - The alkaline equivalent, usually lactate, also diffuses inwardly, correcting the metabolic acidosis present in renal failure. PD fluid may contain both D- and L-lactate, though patients rarely have issues converting them to bicarbonate or symptoms due to mild elevations of either.
- **Ultrafiltration**
  - A plasma ultrafiltrate removes water and solute from the body.
  - As opposed to HD, where hydrostatic pressure across the dialysis membrane drives ultrafiltration, osmotic pressure, typically from dextrose, drives ultrafiltration.

○ The hyperosmolar gradient is produced most commonly by the high dextrose concentration in the dialysis solution, although colloidal oncotic pressure from icodextrin and osmotic pressure from amino acids are also utilized.
- **Absorption**
  ○ Absorption of peritoneal fluid via the lymphatics of the abdominal wall can account for over 1 L/day of fluid absorbed.
  ○ This counteracts the removal via diffusion and osmosis through the peritoneal capillaries, making dialysis less efficient.
  ○ Increased abdominal pressure via position (sitting > standing > supine) or large volumes promotes absorption of peritoneal fluid.

PATIENT SELECTION

- Patients need to be highly motivated and capable of performing regular treatments within their home environment, without direct supervision of a trained medical specialist.
- Patients who prefer PD over HD tend to be more independent, as the flexible schedule is more conducive to employment and travel as compared to the rigid schedule of in-center HD.
- Some **relative and absolute contraindications for PD** include the following:
  ○ The presence of uncorrectable mechanical defects (irreparable abdominal hernia).
  ○ Recent intra-abdominal surgery (including aortic vascular graft).
  ○ Frequent diverticulitis and/or other intra-abdominal infections and pathology.
  ○ Abdominal wall cellulitis.
  ○ A history of repeated abdominal operations with adhesion formation.
  ○ Patients who are physically unable to perform their own exchanges and who lack a suitable caregiver at home.

APPARATUS

Catheter and Setup
- Most centers use a two-cuff, silastic intraperitoneal catheter. Many different shapes are available and no shape has proven more efficacious than another.
- Laparoscopic placement of the catheter is generally preferred to ensure proper positioning and allow repair of subclinical hernias, defects, adhesions, and redundant omentum. Percutaneous placement under ultrasound and fluoroscopy has also been effective. Open surgical placement of PD catheters is no longer routinely performed.
- The intra-abdominal portion contains many side-port perforations to maximize fluid flow.
- Although catheters can be used immediately after surgical placement, a preferred healing period of 10 to 28 days prior to initiation of dialysis allows healing of the exit-site and reduces the incidence of early subcutaneous leaks or infection.
- The deep cuff is placed in the abdominal wall musculature and after healing secures the catheter in its position.
- The subcutaneous superficial cuff allows for granulation tissue to form, creating an additional barrier to infection; however, externalization of this cuff may occur.
- The exit-site may be placed anywhere and must be visible to the patient for hygiene and not where the catheter is subject to irritation (e.g., belt line).
- Tunneled presternal catheters are associated with reduced infectious complications in obese patients.
- The Y-set is the standard setup in manual PD (Fig. 21-1).

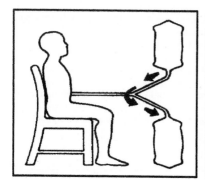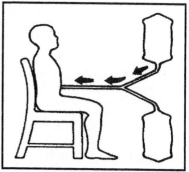

FIGURE 21-1. The Y-set for peritoneal dialysis (PD), with demonstration of the "flush-before-fill" technique.

- Infection risk is reduced as there is only one connection point (at the stem emerging from the patient) where sterile technique may accidentally be broken.
- The flush-before-fill technique is where the patient first flushes air out of the tubing by allowing a small amount of dialysis solution to pass into the drain bag; the drain bag is then clamped and the rest of the dialysis solution is infused into the peritoneal cavity via gravity (10 to 15 minutes).
- Between exchanges, the bags are disconnected and the stem is capped.
- When the specified dwell time is complete, a new transfer set is attached and the peritoneal cavity is drained via gravity (20 to 25 minutes) before a new infusion is started, again with the flush-before-fill technique.
- It is generally recommended that the catheter should not be submerged in water, although many physicians allow swimming in salt water.

Dialysis Solution

- Standard PD solutions contain sodium, chloride, lactate, magnesium, calcium, and varying concentrations of dextrose (Table 21-1).
- Most commercial solutions contain a sodium concentration of 132 mEq/L to allow a net sodium diffusion; this protects against hypernatremia that might otherwise occur, particularly with the more hypertonic solutions.

TABLE 21-1	STANDARD PERITONEAL DIALYSIS SOLUTION COMPONENTS
Sodium	132 mEq/L
Potassium	0 mEq/L
Chloride	Variable (95–105 mEq/L)
Calcium	2.5 mEq/L (1.25 mMol/L) or 3.5 mEq/L (1.75 mMol/L)
Phosphorus	0 mEq/L
Magnesium	1.5 mEq/L or 0.5–0.75 mEq/L
Lactate	35 mEq/L or 40 mEq/L
Dextrose	Variable (1.5%, 2.5%, 4.25%)

TABLE 21-2 PERITONEAL DIALYSIS SOLUTIONS

Dextrose	Glucose (g/dL)	Osmolarity (mOsm/L)	Color Code
1.5% (1.5 g/dL)	1.36	346	Yellow
2.5% (2.5 g/dL)	2.27	396	Green
4.25% (4.25 g/dL)	3.86	485	Red
Icodextrin (non-dextrose solution)		282	Purple

- Potassium is not present in standard solutions and hypokalemia is usually corrected with oral supplementation.
- Phosphorus is also absent but PD is not able to remove the daily dietary load and most patients require both dietary restriction and oral phosphorus binders.
- In the present era of wide-spread calcium-containing phosphorus binders, a PD solution with a lower calcium concentration (2.5 mEq/L) is preferred to prevent placing a patient in positive calcium balance.
- Lactate has been the primary alkaline equivalent used in PD because of technical difficulty with bicarbonate in the manufacturing process; the resultant acidic pH of 5.5 can cause inflow pain and may be damaging to the mesothelium.
- Newer dual-chamber bags with bicarbonate are available, allowing for mixing at the time of use, although they are not yet available in the United States.
- The hypertonic dextrose concentration can be 1.5%, 2.5%, or 4.25%, with the higher concentrations providing a stronger osmotic force leading to more ultrafiltration.
- Most commercially available solutions have color-coded tabs with which patients may be more familiar rather than the actual percentage of dextrose (Table 21-2).
- A drawback of dextrose-containing solutions is that 60% to 80% can diffuse inwardly during a dwell, thereby dissipating the osmotic gradient, limiting the achieved ultrafiltration and giving the patient a glucose load.
- Newer solutions with long-chain glucose polymers (icodextrin) allow for a more sustained colloid oncotic effect, roughly equivalent to the ultrafiltration of a 2.5% dextrose solution over 12- to 18-hour period. The metabolic products of icodextrin can lead to falsely elevated glucose measurements on some diabetic test strips and blood sugar results in patients on icodextrin must be interpreted cautiously.
- Amino acids can also be used as an osmotic agent, particularly in malnourished patients, although frequent or long-term use may lead to a metabolic acidosis and elevations in the serum urea concentration; ultrafiltration capacity is limited, roughly equivalent to a 1.5% dextrose solution.

Peritoneal Membrane

- The membrane separating the blood in the capillaries from the solution in the peritoneal cavity consists of many layers.
  - Unstirred layer in the blood
  - Capillary endothelium
  - Capillary basement membrane
  - Interstitium
  - Peritoneal basement membrane
  - Peritoneal mesothelium
  - Unstirred layer in the peritoneal solution
- Most resistance to solute movement occurs at the capillary endothelium (via filtration pores) and interstitium (which may be of variable thickness).

TABLE 21-3 PERITONEAL MEMBRANE TYPES

Membrane Type	D/P Creatinine Ratio	Characteristics
High	>0.81	Transports solutes quickly, poor ultrafiltration and problems with protein loss
High average	0.65–0.81	Transports solutes well, with adequate ultrafiltration
Low average	0.50–0.64	Transports solutes somewhat slowly, with good ultrafiltration
Low	<0.50	Transports solutes slowly, with excellent ultrafiltration

D/P, dialysate-to-plasma.

- The total surface area in adults is about 2 m², consisting of both the parietal and visceral layers although most exchange is through the parietal peritoneum. Not all capillaries are readily available to participate in solute exchange as some may be too far from the cavity under baseline conditions.
- Larger dwell volumes can stretch the membrane, recruiting more capillaries to participate in solute exchange. Peritonitis increases the vascularity of the membrane thus increasing peritoneal transport. Patients will often ultrafiltrate less during an episode of peritonitis.
- The "three-pore model" describes large pores (>25 nm) through which proteins and other macromolecules pass, small pores (4 to 6 nm) for electrolytes and solutes like urea and creatinine, and ultra-small pores (0.3 to 0.5 nm), aquaporins, allowing only solute-free water to pass, acting like a sieve.
- The peritoneal cavity can typically accommodate 2 to 3 L of fluid without discomfort or respiratory compromise.
- Not all membranes are alike, and there is considerable amount of patient-to-patient variability in the character of the peritoneal membrane. Patients' peritoneal membrane transport characteristics also change with time and events, usually increasing over time.
- Four classes of membrane transport characteristics are defined based on the rate of creatinine diffusion and glucose absorption (Table 21-3).
  ○ A **peritoneal equilibration test** (PET) allows one to determine the type of membrane a patient possesses and then tailor the PD prescription to maximize efficiency.[2]
    ▪ A 2-L infusion of 2.5% dextrose solution is allowed to dwell for 4 hours.
    ▪ The dialysate-to-plasma (D/P) ratio of creatinine is calculated.
    ▪ The ratio of dialysate glucose at 4 hours to 0 hours is also calculated.
  ○ Higher D/P values correlate with better solute diffusion and clearance; however, the osmotic gradient is also more rapidly lost, limiting ultrafiltration. Lower D/P values correlate with slower solute diffusion and clearance but a maintained osmotic gradient with better ultrafiltration.
- The Canada-USA (CANUSA) Study Group found a greater risk of technique failure or death in patients with high transport membranes undergoing long, manual exchanges; the underlying mechanism for this increased risk is thought to involve poor ultrafiltration (with resultant hypertension and left ventricular hypertrophy) and increased protein losses.[3] Most patients with high transport characteristics are placed on short, automated exchanges with no long dwells to counteract this physiology.

MODALITIES AND PRESCRIPTION

Manual Exchanges

- **Continuous ambulatory peritoneal dialysis** (CAPD) involves patient-operated manual exchanges performed throughout the day.
- Fluid volumes of 2 to 3 L are typical, with dwell times each ranging from 6 to 8 hours.
- Most patients are first educated and trained in CAPD prior to learning other modalities, as this can be used as a backup or emergency modality in the event of a power outage or machine malfunction.
- Patients admitted to the hospital overnight can resort to CAPD if nurse staffing or machine availability is limited.
- A sample prescription would be 2 L of 2.5% dextrose solution with four exchanges of approximately 6 hours each (or can be unevenly spaced at more convenient times of the day such as awakening, noon, dinner, and bedtime, with the longest dwell overnight).
- Patients with significant residual renal function can be started on 2 or 3 exchanges instead.

Automated Cycler Exchanges

- In **continuous cycling peritoneal dialysis** (CCPD), also known as **automated PD,** the patient undergoes automated exchanges overnight, with three or more relatively short cycles.
- The final exchange remains in the peritoneal cavity on awakening, and the patient disconnects from the machine and is free to go about doing daily activities.
- The "continuous" label in the name of this modality refers to the retained daytime dwell that allows for solute transfer to occur around the clock.
- An extra manual exchange is sometimes added during the day if clearance or ultrafiltration targets are not reached. In general, anuric patients have day dwells.
- A sample prescription would have four dwells of 2 hours each, with 2.5 L of 2.5% dextrose solution, and a final fill (daytime dwell) of 2 L of icodextrin prior to disconnecting.

Prescriptions

- In choosing a PD modality, the patient's membrane type should be known, as determined from the results of the PET.
- Those with **high transport membranes** dissipate their osmotic gradients more rapidly, and **short repeated dwells** may be required to achieve adequate ultrafiltration (bringing in fresh hypertonic solution); these patients fare better on CCPD.
- Those with **low transport membranes** have difficulty with solute diffusion and would benefit from the **long, evenly spaced dwells of CAPD.**
- Patients with either high-average or low-average membranes can usually achieve adequate solute removal and ultrafiltration with either modality; thus, selection can generally depend on patient preference.

ADEQUACY OF PD

Clearance Targets

- The 2006 Kidney Disease Outcomes Quality Initiative (KDOQI) guidelines, as do multiple other medical society guidelines, recommend a **weekly clearance of urea (Kt/V_{urea}) of at least 1.7,** reflecting combined contribution from PD and residual renal function in patients producing >100 mL of urine per day.[4] The Centers for Medicare and Medicaid Services (CMS) also deduct payment to dialysis centers if a percentage of PD patients do not reach Kt/V_{urea} of 1.7. However, no rigorous trial has established an "adequate" target for PD clearance and clinical parameters are paramount.

- Clearance adequacy should be **measured within the first month** after initiating therapy, then **at 4-month intervals,** unless there has been a change in the prescription or in the clinical status of the patient.
- The clearance is calculated from the 24-hour Kt/V_{urea} shown below, where V_D is the total volume of dialysate used (in L), D_{urea} is the dialysate urea concentration, P_{urea} is the plasma urea concentration, and V_{urea} is the estimated volume (in L) of distribution of urea (total body water or from Watson or Hume formulae).
  - **24-hour** $Kt/V_{urea} = (V_D)(D_{urea})/(P_{urea})(V_{urea})$
  - The 24-hour Kt/V_{urea} is then multiplied by 7 for the weekly clearance.
  - Residual renal function is calculated with the same equation, substituting urine values for V_D and D_{urea}, then multiplied by 7 and added to the dialysate clearance.
  - Note the similarity of this equation to the generic creatinine clearance (UV/P) equation.
- Protection of residual renal function is important in the PD population, with avoidance of nephrotoxic medications and radiographic contrast as prudent. Similar to HD, the adequacy of PD in Mexico (ADEMEX) study showed a statistically significant association between loss of residual renal function and death.[5]
- Improved clearance can be achieved by increasing the amount of dialysis solution used over the 24-hour period. For example, this can be achieved by adding an extra exchange or by using larger dwell volumes. Computer prescription modeling programs are available to optimize the PD prescription.
- However, there are diminishing returns to adding more exchanges, as more time is lost draining and filling the peritoneal cavity or when larger volumes increase the intra-abdominal pressure such that the balance is tilted toward more fluid reabsorption by the lymphatics.

Ultrafiltration Targets

- Ultrafiltration targets are less clearly defined than clearance, although a minimum of 750 mL of net fluid removal per day has been associated with better outcomes in anuric patients.[6]
- To enhance ultrafiltration, a higher dextrose concentration can be used (4.25% solution). Shorter dwell times (particularly in patients with high transport characteristics) can also aid in increasing ultrafiltration; however, since water moves during the first part of the PD exchange, short exchanges may leave sodium behind and cause thirst and hypertension. This phenomenon is termed sodium sieving.
- In volume-overloaded patients, restricting sodium and water may help, as may administering diuretics in patients with residual urine production.
- **Ultrafiltration failure** is a term used to describe a condition of fluid overload in association with net ultrafiltration of <400 mL after a 4-hour dwell of 2 L of 4.25% dextrose. This can be the result of rapid loss of the osmotic gradient (high transporters), decreased peritoneal membrane water permeability (peritonitis, fibrosis, adhesions), or from increased reabsorption by the lymphatics. True ultrafiltration failure is a rare event in PD.
- Failure of adequate ultrafiltration may necessitate a switch to HD.

COMPLICATIONS

Infectious Complications

Peritonitis
- Table 21-4 describes some of the common signs and symptoms found of peritonitis in PD patients.

TABLE 21-4	COMMON SIGNS AND SYMPTOMS IN PERITONEAL DIALYSIS PATIENTS		
Sign/Symptom	**Character**	**Causes**	**Management Issues**
Abdominal pain	Inflow pain	Excessively large volume of dwell	Reduce volume of dwell
		Low pH of infused solution	Add bicarbonate to solution (10 mEq/L)
	Diffuse/rebound	Peritonitis	Check fluid cell count and differential, culture, Gram stain, empiric antibiotics
		Bowel obstruction	
		Gastrointestinal tract pathology (e.g., appendicitis, mesenteric ischemia)	Abdominal or vascular imaging
	Focal/localized	Abdominal hernia	Surgical correction
		Constipation	Trial of stool softener and/or enema
			Avoid magnesium- and phosphate-containing products
Change in dialysate	Cloudy fluid	Peritonitis	Check fluid cell count and differential (eosinophils for allergic process), culture, Gram stain, empiric antibiotics
		Allergic reaction to solution or dialysis equipment	
		Chylous leak/superior vena cava syndrome	Check triglyceride level
		Pancreatitis	Check serum lipase
		Gastrointestinal tract pathology (e.g., appendicitis, mesenteric ischemia)	Abdominal or vascular imaging
		Fibrin strands	Add heparin (200–500 units/L) into dialysis solution for fibrin strands
	Bloody fluid	Malignancy	Check dialysate fluid cytology
		Sclerosing encapsulating peritonitis	Abdominal imaging, with possible need for biopsy
		Gynecologic source (e.g., retrograde menstruation, cyst rupture)	
		Tuberculous peritonitis	*Mycobacterium tuberculosis* polymerase chain reaction

(continued)

TABLE 21-4	COMMON SIGNS AND SYMPTOMS IN PERITONEAL DIALYSIS PATIENTS (*Continued*)		
Sign/ Symptom	Character	Causes	Management Issues
Fever	Temperature >38°C	Peritonitis	Check fluid cell count and differential (eosinophils for allergic process), culture, Gram stain, empiric antibiotics
		Allergic reaction to solution or dialysis equipment	
		Gastrointestinal tract pathology (e.g., appendicitis, mesenteric ischemia)	
		Exit-site or tunnel infection	Abdominal or vascular imaging
		Nonabdominal infectious source	General fever workup as in nondialysis patients

- Peritonitis remains a common and potentially serious complication in the PD population. Approximately 20% of peritonitis episodes result in catheter removal and initiation of HD.
- Although many cases can be treated in the outpatient setting, recurrent episodes threaten the long-term integrity of the peritoneal membrane.
- Most common causes include **inadvertent breaks in sterile technique,** migration of pathogens from the catheter site, or transvisceral passage of bacteria from gut pathology such as diverticulitis or constipation.
- Presentation can be subtle, but the most common features are cloudy peritoneal fluid, abdominal pain, and/or fever (Table 21-4).
- For diagnosis, the spent dialysis solution should be evaluated by **Gram stain, culture** (preferably prior to antibiotics), and **white blood cell count with differential;** a white blood cell count **>100 cells per mm³, of which at least 50% are polymorphonuclear neutrophils,** is supportive of the diagnosis.
- The International Society of Peritoneal Dialysis has recommended empiric therapy for both gram-positive and gram-negative organisms. This can be achieved with intraperitoneal administration of a **vancomycin OR a first-generation cephalosporin (cefazolin) AND an aminoglycoside OR ceftazidime.**[7]
- Routine long-term use of **aminoglycoside therapy is NOT recommended** in PD patients, in order to preserve residual renal function.
- In most cases, **intraperitoneal dosing is the preferred route of antibiotic therapy.** When patients are bacteremic or overtly septic, intravenous antibiotics should be administered instead.
- Suggested intraperitoneal doses for selected antibiotics are listed in Table 21-5; the intermittent dosing schedule refers to the antibiotic being added only to the longest dwell (nighttime fill for CAPD, daytime dwell for CCPD).
- Treatment strategies that are available after the results of the Gram stain and culture are obtained are outlined in Table 21-6.

TABLE 21-5	INTRAPERITONEAL DOSES OF SELECTED ANTIBIOTICS
Antibiotic	Intraperitoneal Dose
Cefazolin	15–20 mg/kg per bag once a day
Ceftazidime	15–20 mg/kg per bag once a day
Cefepime	1000 mg once a day
Gentamicin, tobramycin	0.6 mg/kg per bag once a day
Amikacin	2 mg/kg per bag once a day
Vancomycin	15–30 mg/kg (1000–3000 mg) every 5–7 days
Fluconazole	200 mg every 24–48 hrs
Ampicillin	125 mg/L in ALL exchanges
Aztreonam	1 g/L loading, then 250 mg/L in ALL exchanges

- Gram-positive infections can frequently be treated with a single antibiotic agent, tailored once the sensitivities are known.
- Infections with **Pseudomonas** species are particularly difficult to eradicate and a second antibiotic to which it is sensitive is recommended. In up to two-thirds of cases, **catheter removal** may become necessary.
- **Fungal peritonitis** can lead to rapid deterioration and immediate catheter removal is almost always mandatory along with antifungal agents. Close monitoring in the inpatient setting is typically recommended for this situation.
- A polymicrobial or anaerobic infection suggests an abdominal abscess or perforation, requiring urgent imaging or surgical exploration.

Exit-Site and Tunnel Infection
- Catheter-site infections are suspected if **erythema or exudates are present externally.** Crust formation at the exit-site, however, does not necessarily indicate infection, and positive wound cultures in the absence of other symptoms may simply indicate colonization.[7]
- **Staphylococcus aureus** is the most common cause of exit-site infections.
- As with peritonitis, the Gram stain and culture are helpful in guiding antibiotic therapy.
- Gram-positive organisms can be treated with an **oral cephalosporin or penicillinase-resistant antibiotic.** Resistant strains may require vancomycin and rifampin.
- Gram-negative organisms can usually be treated with **oral ciprofloxacin (500 mg bid);** with *Pseudomonas aeruginosa,* addition of ceftazidime or an aminoglycoside may become necessary, as well as catheter removal.
- For infections that respond to therapy, antibiotics can be discontinued after 2 weeks; relapsing infections or those that progress to tunnel infections or peritonitis may necessitate catheter removal.
- **Meticulous exit-site care** is essential to prevent such infections, with hand washing for 2 minutes before manipulating the catheter dressings. Daily application of **0.1% gentamicin cream** has been shown to be effective in reducing the incidence of exit-site infections with *S. aureus* and *P. aeruginosa.*[8]
- Catheter anchorage with tape and gauze dressings helps prevent exit-site trauma.
- **Vigorous scrubbing at the exit-site or prolonged submersion into water should be avoided.**

TABLE 21-6	TREATMENT OF PERITONITIS			
Type	Organism	Antibiotic	Choices	Duration
Gram positive	Enterococcus	IP vancomycin or ampicillin	Can add aminoglycoside If VRE, consider daptomycin or quinupristin/dalfopristin	21 days
	Staphylococcus aureus	IP vancomycin or first-generation cephalosporin	Can add oral rifampin 450–600 mg/day for 5–7 days	21 days
	Other gram positive	IP first-generation cephalosporin	IP vancomycin if resistant	14 days
Gram negative	Pseudomonas Stenotrophomonas	IP ceftazidime with aminoglycoside if urine <100 mL/day	If urine >100 mL/day, substitute aminoglycoside with oral ciprofloxacin (500 mg bid), or IV piperacillin (4 g bid), or oral TMP/SMX (double strength bid), or IP aztreonam	21–28 days
	Other single gram negative	IP aminoglycoside if urine <100 mL/day	IP ceftazidime if urine >100 mL/day	14 days
	Multiple gram negatives or anaerobes	IP cefazolin, IP ceftazidime, and oral metronidazole (500 mg tid)	Abdominal imaging and/or surgical intervention	14–21 days
Fungal	Yeasts or other fungi	Immediate catheter removal; IV amphotericin B and flucytosine until sensitivities available	Continue oral flucytosine (1000 mg daily) and fluconazole (100–200 mg daily) an additional 10 days after catheter removal if patient is stable	Variable

bid, twice daily; IP, intraperitoneal; IV, intravenous; tid, three times daily; TMP/SMX, trimethoprim/sulfamethoxazole; VRE, vancomycin-resistant *Enterococcus*.

Mechanical Complications

Outflow Failure

- Outflow failure is defined as a drain volume that is consistently and substantially less than the volume being infused in the absence of an obvious fluid leak.
- The most common cause by far is **constipation** and resolves with laxative administration. Other causes include **catheter migration, kinking** of the catheter, **adhesion formation, omental wrapping, or fibrin plugging.**
- Tracking of fluid along the abdominal wall can cause an apparent outflow failure and may manifest as abdominal wall or genital edema. This will often resolve with rest.
- A systematic approach can be used to investigate and correct the problem:
  - Check a plain film of the abdomen to evaluate the course of the catheter, which should ideally be directed toward the pelvis to avoid contact with the omentum.
  - **Constipation should be treated aggressively** and can resolve about 50% of cases of outflow failure (mechanism unclear).[9] **Magnesium and phosphate products should be avoided** in the treatment of constipation in end-stage renal disease. Lactulose is an acceptable choice.
  - Heparin can be added to the PD solution (250 to 500 units/L), especially if fibrin strands are evident in the discarded fluid. Heparin is not systemically absorbed from the peritoneal cavity, thus minimizing the risk of anticoagulation.
  - Thrombolytic agents (tissue plasminogen activator, 1 mg/mL for 1 hour) may also help break up fibrin strands.
- If these conservative measures fail to correct the problem, surgical consultation with catheter repositioning or replacement may be necessary.

Back Pain

- In the PD population, the infused solution causes a shift in the center of gravity, producing excess stress on the lumbar spine.
- Management includes bed rest in the acute situation, along with decreasing the volume of the dwells.
- A concomitant increase in the number of exchanges may be needed to maintain adequate solute clearance.
- When applicable, physical therapy with muscle-strengthening exercises may help alleviate symptoms.

Hernias

- Abdominal hernias develop in **10% to 20%** of PD patients, resulting from the increased intra-abdominal pressure created by the infused fluid, although there is no direct correlation between the magnitude of intra-abdominal pressure and hernia development.
- Risk factors include large-volume dwells, a sitting position during dwell carriage, obesity, and multiparity. Any condition that weakens the abdominal musculature, such as deconditioning, can also pose a risk for hernia formation.
- Diagnosis is clinical and treatment is typically with surgical repair.
- Small abdominal hernias carry the greatest risk of bowel incarceration, which can present with worsening abdominal pain and loss of reducibility at the hernia site.
- After surgical repair, intra-abdominal pressures must be kept as low as possible to facilitate healing. Patients with good residual renal function may be able to discontinue PD for 1 week, then gradually reinitiate with small volumes (1 L exchanges) for another week.
- Supine dialysis also helps reduce the intra-abdominal pressure.
- Patients with little residual renal function may need to temporarily switch to HD until the wound is completely healed.

Fluid Leakage

- Risk factors for fluid leakage are similar to those for hernia formation.

- Early leaks are those that occur within 1 month of catheter placement and typically occur at the exit-site.
- Late leaks can extend into the subcutaneous tissue or into the pleural space (hydrothorax), presenting more subtly with weight gain, shortness of breath, or apparent outflow failure.
- Hydrothoraces are almost exclusively found on the right side, as the left hemidiaphragm has additional coverage by the heart and pericardium. A diagnostic thoracentesis reveals markedly elevated glucose levels when the pleural fluid originates from the peritoneal solution.
- Treatment of fluid leakage entails draining the peritoneal cavity dry for 24 to 48 hours. If the leak recurs, longer periods off PD may be needed with temporary support on HD.
- A hydrothorax that is symptomatic requires medical or surgical pleurodesis, although some hydrothorax episodes resolve spontaneously with the proposed inflammatory reaction to PD fluid as the reason for resolution.
- Genital edema is a specific form of fluid leakage that can occur via a patent processus vaginalis that results in a hydrocele. This can also occur through a defect in the abdominal wall at the catheter site, allowing fluid to track down through subcutaneous tissue.
- As with abdominal hernias, reduction in the intra-abdominal pressure with small-volume or supine PD may alleviate the symptoms. Anatomical defects, however, may need to be corrected surgically.

Sclerosing Encapsulating Peritonitis

- Sclerosing encapsulating peritonitis is an uncommon clinical entity where a **fibrous transformation of the peritoneal membrane entraps loops of bowel** causing symptoms of intestinal obstruction, with nausea, vomiting, and anorexia.[10]
- A **bloody dialysis fluid** drainage may alert the physician to this problem.
- The incidence is approximately 2.5% and is more common in patients receiving long-term PD (>5 to 8 years). It can even occur after patients have previously discontinued PD.
- Although the mechanism is not clearly defined, chemical irritation of the peritoneal membrane is suspected as the inciting event. Recurrent bouts of peritonitis have also been implicated as a risk factor.
- Treatment options are limited, consisting of **bowel rest and surgical lysis of adhesions** when obstruction occurs.
- Immunosuppression with prednisone in doses ranging from 10 to 40 mg/day has shown modest benefit and case series using tamoxifen (20 mg bid) has shown success.[11]
- The overall prognosis of patients with sclerosing encapsulating peritonitis is poor, with a **1-year mortality rate >50%**.

Metabolic Complications

Hyperglycemia

- As much as 75% of the dextrose in the dialysis solution may diffuse inwardly to the blood, particularly in patients with leaky high transport membranes.
- Patients with underlying diabetes mellitus or glucose intolerance are most susceptible to this complication.[12]
- The calories provided by the dextrose account for much of the 5% to 10% weight gain frequently observed in the first year on PD.

Hyperlipidemia

- An atherogenic lipid profile is frequently encountered in patients on PD.
- The inward diffusion of dextrose results in **elevated triglycerides, as well as the elevation in total cholesterol and low-density lipoprotein** (LDL). Smaller proteins, such as high-density lipoprotein, are lost in the spent dialysate further increasing cardiovascular risk.[12]

- Treatment is focused on dietary modification, exercise, and HMG-coenzyme A reductase inhibitors as first-line medical therapy.
- Specific LDL cholesterol targets in PD patients have not been defined, and in the absence of established coronary disease or coronary disease equivalents, the accepted target is <100 mg/dL.

Protein Loss and Malnutrition

- Protein loss of approximately 0.5 g/L of drainage occurs in PD and the rate of loss may be even greater in patients with high transport membranes.
- The major protein lost is albumin.
- Factors that increase membrane permeability, such as peritonitis, can significantly magnify the rate of protein loss.
- The KDOQI guidelines recommend a **dietary protein intake of 1.2 to 1.3 g/kg/day** for PD patients.[13]

Hypokalemia

- **Approximately one-third of PD patients experience hypokalemia.**
- Patients are typically in a negative potassium balance, as standard PD solutions lack this electrolyte, and increased endogenous insulin release (stimulated by the sugar load) leads to an intracellular potassium shift.
- Poor nutritional status in hospitalized patients (particularly when placed on a low-potassium renal diet) may further exacerbate hypokalemia.
- With mild hypokalemia it is recommended that patients liberalize their potassium intake or oral supplements are initiated.
- In severe hypokalemia addition of potassium to the PD solution may be required.

INDICATIONS FOR CHANGE TO HD

- Despite the safety and effectiveness of PD, patients are sometimes required to switch to HD temporarily or permanently.
- **Common reasons for a permanent switch** include the following:
  ○ Consistent failure to achieve adequacy targets (Kt/V_{urea} <1.7)
  ○ Inadequate fluid removal (ultrafiltration failure)
  ○ Severe hypertriglyceridemia that is resistant to therapy
  ○ Frequent peritonitis or other infectious complications
  ○ Irreparable mechanical problems, including sclerosis encapsulating peritonitis
  ○ Severe protein malnutrition resistant to aggressive management
- Patients may occasionally require a temporary switch to HD for the following reasons.
  ○ Surgical operations involving the peritoneal cavity (e.g., perforated ulcer, bowel obstruction, rarely renal cell cancers)
  ○ Peritoneal fluid leaks
  ○ Infectious complications requiring temporary catheter removal
- The presence of a PD catheter does not preclude renal transplantation and the catheter can be surgically removed at the time of transplantation or at a later date.
- As with other forms of renal replacement therapy, the leading causes of death for patients on PD are cardiovascular disease and infections.
- A significant association between the loss of residual renal function and mortality has been described, stressing the importance of preserving kidney function whenever possible.[5,14,15]

Home Hemodialysis

- Home hemodialysis (HHD) is a form of renal replacement therapy that utilizes the same concepts of HD but offers treatment flexibility and self-care. Many patients and physician choose to increase the dialysis frequency and/or time beyond what is able to be done in dialysis centers.

- HHD was a predominant form of dialysis in the 1960s and 1970s but is now utilized by less than 3% of patients in the United States, although the prevalence of HHD among all home dialysis patients (HHD and PD) has increased 2.5-fold in the last decade.[16]

- In 1969 DePalma was the first to report on the successful use of short daily HD. The rationale was that shorter dialysis sessions 5 to 7 times per week would improve patient outcomes.[17]

- Only one randomized trial has examined this hypothesis and utilizing surrogate endpoints demonstrated that 5.2 treatments were superior to three HD treatments per week.[18]

- Regardless of the early successes with HHD, use of it quickly declined in the United States following passage of the Social Security Act of 1972, which allowed for rapid expansion of outpatient dialysis centers.[19]

- Patients often report greater satisfaction and quality of life with HHD as compared to those on center-based HD.

- Some dialysis databases suggest that the elimination of the 2-day interdialytic gap may be the largest benefit of the flexibility of HHD.[20,21]

- Although multiple dialysis machines have been used for HHD, two machines have been studied and given an indication for HHD by the Food and Drug Administration (FDA).

- HHD treatment regimens can vary from center to center and are outlined in Table 21-7.

- The basic mechanisms of HD at home are the same as center-based HD and will not be reviewed but differences between HHD and traditional HD will be discussed.

- **Patient selection**
  ○ Staff-assisted HHD is rarely performed largely due to financial considerations but is well received by most patients.
  ○ Patients need to understand the commitment to self-care and be capable of training or have a caregiver willing to be trained. Often, patients and a caregiver will split the responsibilities of the treatment. Patients who perform a majority of the treatment responsibilities themselves have a lower therapy discontinuation rate. Caregiver burn-out is one of the leading reasons for therapy discontinuation.
  ○ Although performing dialysis unobserved is not the usual method, the FDA has approved unobserved HD in a patient's home for appropriately trained patients.
  ○ Training typically takes 4 weeks or approximately 20 HD sessions.

- **Water supply**
  ○ Several methods of producing water for dialysis are available at home.
  ○ Traditional dialysis machines can use water produced from a small reverse osmosis machine, similar to acute dialysis, or installation of deionized water tanks in the patient home.
  ○ Other machines use a batched system of producing water and subsequent dialysate.
  ○ Bagged dialysate is also available for some dialysis systems, similar to PD.
  ○ Water testing in the home is required for source water. Numerous dialysate water contaminations have occurred in patients home over time.

- **Dialysis prescription**
  ○ Without the limitations of a dialysis center, different dialysis prescriptions are available in the patient's home.
  ○ Dialysate is often a limiting product in HHD due to supply and cost issues. Thus, the dialysate flow and dialysate volume may be markedly reduced. In this case, saturation of the dialysis is critical by having the blood flow (Qb) much greater than the dialysate flow (Qd). The highest practical dialysate saturation is achieved at a Qd/Qb of approximately 0.3.

TABLE 21-7 CHARACTERISTICS OF VARIOUS HOME HEMODIALYSIS REGIMENS

Characteristic	Dialysis Regimen				
	Conventional Hemodialysis	NxStage System One®	Short Daily Hemodialysis	Nocturnal Hemodialysis	Nocturnal Frequent
Frequency (sessions/week)	3	4–6	4–6	3–4	4–6
Duration (hours/session)	3–4	2.5–4	2.5–4	>5.5	>5.5
Dialysate flow (mL/min)	500–800	100–300	300–800	100–500	100–500
Blood flow (mL/min)	200–400	350–500	350–500	200–400	200–300
Weekly standard Kt/V_{urea}	>2.1	>2.1	>3	>3.5	>3.5

- ○ When lower dialysate volumes (and flows) are utilized, the gradient within the dialyzer is not maintained and dialysate baths will be different to maintain total mass balance. For example, with a dialysate volume of 30 L and Qd of 200 mL/min, the typical potassium concentration will be 1 mEq/L to achieve the same potassium removal as a 2 mEq/L bath with a standard high efficiency treatment.
  - ○ Both bicarbonate and lactate buffers have been utilized in HHD. In general, on demand systems use bicarbonate whereas batched and bagged systems use lactate due to stability.
  - ○ Patients who perform more than 3 times weekly HD measure adequacy with a standardized Kt/V_{urea} rather than a single pool Kt/V_{urea} to ensure equivalent or better solute clearance than achieved with 3 times weekly HD.
- **Access training and care**
  - ○ If patients are in-center dialysis patients, attempts at self-cannulation prior to the initiation of HD training decreases training time and eliminates anxiety.
  - ○ **Sterile technique cannot be overemphasized.** Infectious complications have been observed at greater rates in HHD patients.
  - ○ Many patients prefer single-site cannulation of a fistula (the so-called buttonhole cannulation) rather than the more common rotating site cannulation. This is achieved by repeated cannulation with a sharp needle in the same site creating a tract. After development of the tract, a blunt needle is utilized in the tract. Buttonhole cannulations are associated with less mechanical complications (e.g., aneurysm formation, pain) but they are associated with higher risk for infections.[22]
  - ○ Clinical monitoring of the access is critical, including careful observations of changes in hemostasis time, venous pressures, access appearance, and difficulty with cannulation.
  - ○ Patients who perform unobserved treatments (e.g., nocturnal HD) should have moisture detectors present at the venous needle to reduce the risk of harm of a venous needle disconnection.

REFERENCES

1. Moncrief JW, Popovich RP, Nolph KD. The history and current status of continuous ambulatory peritoneal dialysis. *Am J Kidney Dis.* 1990;16:579–584.
2. Mehrotra R, Ravel V, Streja E, et al. Peritoneal equilibration test and patient outcomes. *Clin J Am Soc Nephrol.* 2015;10:1990–2001.
3. Churchill DN, Thorpe KE, Nolph KD, et al. Increased peritoneal membrane transport is associated with decreased patient and technique survival for continuous peritoneal dialysis patients. The Canada-USA (CANUSA) Peritoneal Dialysis Study Group. *J Am Soc Nephrol.* 1998;9:1285–1292.
4. Lo WK, Ho YW, Li CS, et al. Effect of Kt/V on survival and clinical outcome in CAPD patients in a randomized prospective study. *Kidney Int.* 2003;64:649–656.
5. Paniagua R, Amato D, Vonesh E, et al. Effects of increased peritoneal clearances on mortality rates in peritoneal dialysis: ADEMEX, a prospective, randomized, controlled trial. *J Am Soc Nephrol.* 2002;13:1307–1320.
6. Brown EA, Davies SJ, Rutherford P, et al. Survival of functionally anuric patients on automated peritoneal dialysis: the European APD Outcome Study. *J Am Soc Nephrol.* 2003;14:2948–2957.
7. Li PK, Szeto CC, Piraino B, et al. ISPD peritonitis recommendations: 2016 update on prevention and treatment. *Perit Dial Int.* 2016;36:481–508.
8. Bernardini J, Bender F, Florio T, et al. Randomized, double-blind trial of antibiotic exit site cream for prevention of exit site infection in peritoneal dialysis patients. *J Am Soc Nephrol.* 2005;16:539–545.
9. Leehey DJ, Ash SR, Daugirdas JT. Peritoneal access devices. In: Daugirdas JT, Blake PG, Ing TS, eds. *Handbook of Dialysis.* 4th ed. Philadelphia, PA: Lippincott Williams & Wilkins; 2007:356.

10. Brown EA, Bargman J, van Biesen W, et al. Length of time on peritoneal dialysis and encapsulating peritoneal sclerosis – position paper for ISPD: 2017 Update. *Perit Dial Int.* 2017;37:362–374.

11. Korte MR, Fieren MW, Sampimon DE, et al. Tamoxifen is associated with lower mortality of encapsulating peritoneal sclerosis: results of the Dutch Multicentre EPS Study. *Nephrol Dial Transplant.* 2011;26:691–697.

12. Davies SJ. Peritoneal dialysis—current status and future challenges. *Nat Rev Nephrol.* 2013;9:399–408.

13. National Kidney Foundation. KDOQI clinical practice guidelines for nutrition in chronic renal failure. Guideline 16. Dietary Protein Intake (DPI) for Chronic Peritoneal Dialysis (CPD). Available at https://kidneyfoundation.cachefly.net/professionals/KDOQI/guidelines_nutrition/doqi_nut.html (Last Accessed December 19, 2018).

14. Bargman JM, Thorpe KE, Churchill DN, CANUSA Peritoneal Dialysis Study Group. Relative contribution of residual renal function and peritoneal clearance to adequacy of dialysis: a reanalysis of the CANUSA study. *J Am Soc Nephrol.* 2001;12:2158–2162.

15. Termorshuizen F, Dekker FW, van Manen JG, et al. Relative contribution of residual renal function and different measures of adequacy to survival in hemodialysis patients: an analysis of the Netherlands Cooperative Study on the Adequacy of Dialysis (NECOSAD)-2. *J Am Soc Nephrol.* 2004;15:1061–1070.

16. Yu JZ, Rhee CM, Ferrey A, et al. There's no place like home: 35-year patient survival on home hemodialysis. *Semin Dial.* 2018;31:300–304.

17. DePalma JR, Pecker EA, Maxwell MH. A new automatic coil dialyser system for 'daily' dialysis. *Proc EDTA.* 1969;6:26–34.

18. FHNT Group, Chertow GM, Levin NW, et al. In-center hemodialysis six times per week versus three times per week. *N Engl J Med.* 2010;363:2287–2300.

19. Rettig RA. Origins of the Medicare kidney disease entitlement: The Social Security Amendments of 1972. In: Hanna KE, ed. *Biomedical Politics.* Washington, DC: Division of Health Sciences Policy: Committee to Study Biomedical Decision Making, Institute of Medicine; 1991;176–214.

20. Suri RS, Kliger AS. When is more frequent hemodialysis beneficial? *Semin Dial.* 2018;31:332–342.

21. Foley RN, Gilbertson DT, Murray T, et al. Long interdialytic interval and mortality among patients receiving hemodialysis. *N Engl J Med.* 2011;365:1099–1107.

22. Nesrallah GE, Cuerden M, Wong JH, et al. Staphylococcus aureus bacteremia and buttonhole cannulation: long-term safety and efficacy of mupirocin prophylaxis. *Clin J Am Soc Nephrol.* 2010;5:1047–1053.

Continuous and Prolonged Intermittent Renal Replacement Therapies

22

Fahad Edrees and Anitha Vijayan

MODALITIES OF RENAL REPLACEMENT THERAPY

- The available modalities for renal replacement therapy (RRT) in the hospital are:
  - ○ **Intermittent hemodialysis** (IHD)
  - ○ **Continuous RRT** (CRRT)
  - ○ **Prolonged intermittent renal replacement therapy** (PIRRT) or **sustained low-efficiency dialysis** (SLED)
  - ○ **Peritoneal dialysis** (PD)
- The choice of modality depends on the availability of therapies at the institution, physician preference, the patient's hemodynamic status, and the presence of comorbid conditions. Table 22-1 illustrates the advantages and disadvantages of different modalities.
- Patients with sepsis or hepatic failure may have potential benefits with continuous therapies.
- The Kidney Disease Improving Global Outcomes (KDIGO) clinical practice guidelines for acute kidney injury (AKI) in 2012 suggested that CRRT is preferred in hemodynamically unstable patients and in patients with acute brain injury or other causes of increased intracranial pressure or brain edema.[1]
- Intermittent modalities are generally accepted to cause greater fluctuations in blood pressure and produce greater fluid shifts in a short amount of time.
- Continuous modalities allow for the same solute clearance and fluid removal, but spread out over a 24-hour period, and thus are favored in hemodynamically unstable patients.
- In the United States, CRRT is performed in approximately 30% of patients with AKI and has almost completely replaced PD in the treatment of AKI.
- CRRT has not shown improved survival over IHD in critically ill patients.
- Likewise, randomized trials have not shown a difference in time to renal recovery or length of intensive care unit (ICU) or hospital stay between groups treated with IHD versus CRRT.
- The principles of hemodialysis and PD are discussed in other chapters. This section will focus primarily on CRRT and PIRRT, and how these modalities compare with IHD in AKI.

DOSING OF RRT

- Evidence from end-stage renal disease patients suggests that a thrice-weekly regimen for IHD, a **urea reduction ratio (URR)** of approximately 65% to 68% per session, is considered adequate dialysis. This correlates to a **fractional urea clearance (Kt/V_{urea})** of 1.2, where K is the dialyzer efficiency, t is the time of treatment, and V is the volume of distribution of urea.
- Given the acuity of the AKI population, urea clearances are notoriously unreliable, with frequent volume shifts, sepsis, high catabolic state, and so forth.
  - ○ The acute renal failure trial network (ATN) study published in 2008, compared intensive RRT (IHD/SLED six times per week with single-pool Kt/V_{urea} of 1.3 per session or

TABLE 22-1	ADVANTAGES AND DISADVANTAGES OF RENAL REPLACEMENT THERAPIES

Modality	Advantages	Disadvantages
IHD	• High-efficiency transport of solutes when rapid clearance of toxins or electrolytes is required • Allows time for off-unit testing	• Hemodynamic intolerance secondary to fluid shifts • "Saw-tooth" pattern of metabolic control between sessions
CRRT	• Gentler hemodynamic shifts than IHD • Steady solute control	• Continuous need for specialized nursing • Requires continuous anticoagulation (heparin vs. citrate)
PIRRT	• Fewer hemodynamic shifts compared to IHD • Less work for intensive care nursing staff compared to CRRT • Can be performed at night, avoiding cessation of therapy for procedures • No need for expensive dialysate and replacement fluids	• Needs to be performed 5–6 days per week to achieve adequate clearance • Insufficient data on drug dosing
PD	• Gentler hemodynamic shifts than IHD	• Requires invasion of peritoneal cavity, which may not be possible in postoperative patients • Less predictable fluid removal rates • Efficiency of urea removal low compared with other therapies

CRRT, continuous renal replacement therapy; IHD, intermittent hemodialysis; PD, peritoneal dialysis.

continuous venovenous hemodiafiltration [CVVHDF] at 35 mL/kg/hr) to less intensive RRT (IHD/SLED three times per week or CVVHDF at 20 mL/kg/hr). There was no difference in 60-day mortality or renal recovery between the two groups.[2]
- ○ The randomized evaluation of normal versus augmented level replacement therapy (RENAL) study evaluated CVVHDF with effluent flow rates of 40 mL/kg/hr in the high-dose group versus 25 mL/kg/hr in the low-dose group. There was no difference in 90-day mortality between the two arms.[3]
- Based on current data, our recommendation is to prescribe CRRT at 20 to 25 mL/kg/hr of effluent flow rate.
- If prescribed therapy is not being delivered at least 80% of the time, because of interruptions (machine malfunction, catheter malfunction, patient interruption for procedures), then the prescription dose can be increased to ensure delivery of effluent flow rate of at least 20 mL/kg/hr per day.

- IHD should be prescribed to achieve a URR of 70% (Kt/V_{urea} of 1.3) per treatment, three times per week.
- URR should be performed during each treatment, and subsequent dialysis treatment should be adjusted (change of duration, dialysis filter, blood flow, and so forth, to improve adequacy) accordingly.[4]

CONTINUOUS RRT

Principles of CRRT

- CRRT utilizes the principles of **diffusion, convection,** or **both,** depending on the modality.[5]
- The nomenclature of CRRT is outlined in Table 22-2.
- **Diffusion:**
  - This involves the same principles as dialysis and drives solutes such as urea across the dialysis membrane from the blood (higher concentration) to the dialysate (lower concentration), which is running countercurrent to the blood.
  - The dialysate flow rate is approximately 15 to 40 mL/min compared with dialysate flow rate in IHD of 400 to 800 mL/min.
  - This process is called **continuous venovenous hemodialysis** (CVVHD).
- **Convection:**
  - During convection, solute movement across the membrane is driven by solvent drag.
  - The plasma water is pushed across the membrane by filtrating pressure and takes solutes with it, similar to glomerular ultrafiltration.
  - This large volume loss has to be restored with necessary solutes, and therefore convection requires the addition of **replacement fluid solution** to the CRRT setup.
  - This is called **continuous venovenous hemofiltration** (CVVH).

TABLE 22-2	NOMENCLATURE OF CONTINUOUS RENAL REPLACEMENT THERAPY MODALITIES
Abbreviations	
A	Arterio-
V	Veno-
C	Continuous
HD	Hemodialysis
H	Hemofiltration
HDF	Hemodiafiltration
UF	Ultrafiltration
Modalities	
CVVH/CAVH	Continuous venovenous/arteriovenous hemofiltration
CVVHD/CAVHD	Continuous venovenous/arteriovenous hemodialysis
CVVHDF/CAVHDF	Continuous venovenous/arteriovenous hemodiafiltration
SCUF	Slow continuous ultrafiltration
PIRRT	Prolonged intermittent renal replacement therapy
SLED	Sustained low-efficiency dialysis

- **Diffusion and convection:** The combination of the two processes utilizes both dialysate and replacement fluid solutions and is termed **continuous venovenous hemodiafiltration** (CVVHDF).
- **Ultrafiltration:** CRRT also can be used without dialysate or replacement fluid to treat volume overload with minimal solute clearance. This process is called **slow continuous ultrafiltration** (SCUF).
- Some of the membranes used for CRRT also have adsorptive properties but it is unclear to what extent this results in significant clearance of substances.
- Studies have suggested that adsorption with polysulfone membranes might result in clearance of cytokines but, to date, this has not been demonstrated to have clinical benefit.

Fluids in CRRT

- **Bicarbonate-based solutions** have essentially replaced lactate-based solutions in CRRT.
- Bicarbonate-based solutions are either prepared at individual institutions by the pharmacy or supplied premixed by various manufacturers.
- Even if they are provided by manufacturers, the final constitution of the fluid is conducted by the local pharmacy as various products have different compositions and mixing instructions.
- **The typical concentrations of solutes** in the solution are given below:
  - Bicarbonate concentration is approximately 35 mEq/L.
  - Sodium is 140 mEq/L.
  - Chloride is approximately 106 to 109 mEq/L.
  - Magnesium is approximately 1.0 to 1.5 mEq/L.
  - Potassium concentrations vary and the prescription should reflect the patient's serum levels.
  - Calcium is approximately 2.0 to 3.5 mEq/L. Calcium concentration should be zero if citrate anticoagulation is used and calcium should be replaced through a central venous catheter.

Anticoagulation in CRRT

- Slow continuous blood flow through extracorporeal circulation mandates the use of anticoagulation to prevent platelet activation and thrombosis of the circuit.
- The primary goal of anticoagulation is to prevent clotting of the tubes and filters, thereby ensuring the delivery of prescribed therapy.
- Currently, the **two primary methods of anticoagulation** utilized in the United States are:
  - **Intravenous heparin** (either provided through the circuit or systemically) to maintain activated partial thromboplastin time (aPTT) between 60 and 80 seconds.
  - **Citrate anticoagulation:**
    - There are different ways of administering citrate but the principles remain the same.[6]
    - Citrate administered prefilter chelates the ionized calcium extracorporeal circuit.
    - Calcium is an essential cofactor for the coagulation cascade and its deficiency prevents coagulation in the circuit.
    - To counteract the effect of citrate in the systemic circulation, calcium is given via a **central venous catheter** to maintain blood-ionized calcium in the normal range.
    - It is of utmost importance to closely monitor ionized calcium levels during citrate anticoagulation.
- Other methods of anticoagulation used include argatroban and bivalirudin, usually reserved for patients who develop heparin-induced thrombocytopenia (HIT).

Typical Regimen for CRRT

An example of CVVHDF orders for a 70-kg patient, assuming 20 mL/kg/hr of replacement fluid and dialysate, serum potassium of 4 mEq/L, is given below:

- **Blood flow 300 mL/min.** If using citrate anticoagulation, recommended blood flow is lower, usually 150 to 200 mL/min.
- **Dialysate flow rate 700 mL/hr and replacement fluid flow rate 700 mL/hr** (20 mL/kg/hr, divided between replacement fluid and dialysate).
- **Heparin bolus** XX units loading dose IV, then **infusion** (1000 units/mL) at XX mL/hr. Heparin should be individualized for the patient. Patients at high risk for bleeding should not receive heparin or target aPTT should be lower.
- **Dialysate** (bicarbonate-based solution), 3 K, 3.5 Ca.
- **Replacement fluid** (bicarbonate-based solution), 3 K, 3.5 Ca.

Drug Dosing in CRRT

- Total clearance of any compound depends on its elimination by nonrenal route, residual renal function, and CRRT.
- Unlike IHD, the clearance of medications is continuous, controlled, and somewhat predictable if the patients remain on continuous therapy.
- Patient, drug, and dialysis characteristics determine appropriate dosing schedules to be used.
- Generally, the nonrenal clearance is taken to be constant, although in critically ill patients with multiorgan system failure, this component may be less than predicted.
- The CRRT clearance relies on convection, diffusion, and adsorption.
- **Convective** elimination is determined primarily by the protein-bound fraction of the drug.
- In **diffusive** elimination, the saturation of the drug in the dialysate (and filtrate) becomes important, and decreases as flow rates increase.
- By taking these guidelines into consideration, therapeutic doses have been calculated for a variety of drugs used in the ICU. Drug dosing during RRT will be discussed elsewhere. It is important to collaborate with pharmacists to prevent underdosing or overdosing of essential medications.

Complications of CRRT

- As with any procedure, there are certain complications and adverse events that can be associated with RRTs. Vigilance for such complications and their immediate rectification are essential to prevent life-threatening situations, especially in the vulnerable population of the ICU.
- Some complications are related to the procedure itself, whereas others are a result of fluid removal or electrolyte and acid–base disturbances.
- In addition, the necessity for a central venous catheter places the patient at risk for infectious complications.
- **Hypotension:**
  - Hypotension can occur in all clinical settings with all modalities, although it is more commonly seen with IHD and its rapid fluid shifts.
  - Volume-depleted and septic patients are at heightened risk; careful attention to the physical examination and invasive hemodynamic monitoring when indicated can help ensure adequate volume resuscitation prior to initiating the dialysis session.
  - Several ways to monitor volume status can be used to dictate a reduction or stoppage of fluid ultrafiltration such as central venous pressure of 8 to 12 mm Hg, stroke volume variation, and inferior vena cava collapsibility and its variation with respiration.
  - Alternatively, if pulmonary edema or acute lung injury is complicating the picture, then pressor support can be used to maintain blood pressure while continuing

ultrafiltration with CRRT. However, this must be done with extreme caution given the risk of peripheral ischemia.

- **Arrhythmias:**
  - Cardiac arrhythmias can occur in the setting of RRT and electrolyte shifts.
  - Although generally seen with IHD, arrhythmia can also be seen in CRRT.
  - Potassium, magnesium, and calcium levels must be monitored every 12 to 24 hours during CRRT. If 0.0 or 1.0 mEq/L of potassium concentration is being used, then potassium should be monitored every 6 to 8 hours to ensure stable potassium plasma concentration.
  - Patients on digitalis are especially sensitive to hypokalemia. Potassium competes with digitalis for binding at the Na^+/K^+-ATPase pump and reduced serum levels can enhance the medicine's toxicity.
  - Supraventricular arrhythmias can also be triggered during the placement of the dialysis catheter or by a malpositioned dialysis catheter.
  - If the arrhythmia is resulting in hemodynamic compromise, then therapy is discontinued immediately and appropriate measures to treat the arrhythmia should be started.

- **Central venous catheter problems:**
  - CRRT requires the insertion of a nontunneled, large-bore, dual-lumen, central venous catheter into either the internal jugular, subclavian, or femoral veins.[7]
  - Nontunneled catheters are typically placed at the bedside into a central vein and **ultrasound guidance is the standard of care and strongly recommended** to reduce complications such as bleeding, pneumothorax, and arterial cannulation and infections.
  - Sterile precautions are mandatory during placement of central venous catheters.
  - Immediate risks include bleeding, injury to other organs or vessels (e.g., pneumothorax, carotid artery injury), and malposition of the catheter.
  - Infection risks increase after 3 weeks for internal jugular vein catheters and after 1 week for femoral vein catheters in bedbound patients.
  - When infection and bacteremia occur, prompt catheter removal is generally recommended, unless vascular access is especially difficult. Persistent bacteremia, fever, or an elevated white blood cell count should prompt a search for bacterial endocarditis in this particularly susceptible population.
  - Thrombus or fibrin sheaths can form around or inside the catheters, causing inadequate blood flows for dialysis. Although heparin is usually instilled into the hub of the catheter after each dialysis, this does not necessarily prevent clot formation. An attempt at clot lysis can be made by the local instillation of alteplase (2 mg). Alteplase should not be administered systemically for this purpose.
  - If the catheter malfunctions, then it may be changed over a guidewire or replaced, preferably at a different site.
  - In patients with chronic kidney disease (CKD), subclavian veins are not used for dialysis catheters, as there is a high risk of subclavian venous stenosis, which can prevent the future placement of an arteriovenous fistula for dialysis in that extremity.
  - Tunneled catheters maybe more beneficial in reducing infection rates, but nontunneled catheters are considered first line due to the ease of placement. Tunneled catheters are typically used in patients with multiple malfunctioning temporary catheters, or in those with poor chance for early renal recovery, or in those being transferred out of the institution to a different facility.
  - Interventional radiology or nephrology consultation is required to perform endoluminal brushing to dislodge thrombi and fibrin sheaths in malfunctioning tunneled catheters.

- **Electrolyte disturbances:**
  - Standard CRRT solutions do not contain phosphate, and uninterrupted CRRT can cause dramatic **hypophosphatemia,** especially during high-dose therapy. This

problem is aggravated by an intracellular shift that occurs during dialysis secondary to alkalemia.

■ Hypophosphatemia can be corrected by intravenous or oral repletion. Alternatively, phosphorus can be added to the dialysate solution, although this technique is not employed widely at this time.

■ To prevent severe hypophosphatemia, we recommend initiation of oral phosphorus supplementation. At our center, we typically start Neutra-Phos 1 packet three times daily PO when serum phosphorus is approximately 3 mg/dL. If PO supplementation is not feasible or if patient develops severe hypophosphatemia, <1.2 mg/dL, then IV supplementation is required.

○ **Hypokalemia and hypomagnesemia** can also result from CRRT, and serum electrolytes need to be monitored at least twice a day to avoid such complications.

■ Hypomagnesemia is usually replaced intravenously or orally.

■ Hypokalemia can be treated by increasing the concentration of potassium in the dialysate and replacement fluid. The typical concentration of potassium in the solution is 2 mEq/L. However, potassium can be added by the pharmacist to make the final concentration 3 or 4 mEq/L, depending on serum potassium levels.

- **Anticoagulation problems:**
  ○ The use of anticoagulant increases the risk for hemorrhagic episodes.
  ○ Studies have shown higher incidence with heparin compared with citrate; therefore, citrate should be used preferentially in patients who are at higher risk for bleeding.
  ○ If a major bleed occurs, then use of heparin or other systemic anticoagulants should be immediately discontinued. Citrate anticoagulation can be continued, with close attention to bleeding parameters and ionized calcium levels.
  ○ Heparin can also be associated with HIT. If HIT is suspected, heparin should be discontinued and alternative agents such as argatroban, bivalirudin, or citrate should be used. The direct thrombin inhibitor, argatroban, can be initiated at 2 μg/kg/min and adjusted to maintain an aPTT of 1.5 to 3 times the baseline value.
  ○ Citrate anticoagulation can result in metabolic alkalosis, and in the setting of hepatic dysfunction, can lead to life-threatening hypocalcemia. The ratio of total calcium to ionized calcium can be used to monitor for toxicity. The titration protocol for addressing changes in serum and machine-ionized calcium levels must be closely followed to prevent adverse events.
  ○ Metabolic alkalosis can be treated by changing the replacement fluid to sodium chloride from a bicarbonate-based product and hypocalcemia is treated by adjusting the calcium rates.

- **Hypothermia:**
  ○ Hypothermia is a frequent complication of CRRT, especially at higher flow rates of dialysate and replacement fluid, with an incidence as high as 60% to 70%.
  ○ Significant amounts of heat are lost from the slow-flowing extracorporeal circuit and can cause decreases in body temperature of 2 to 5°C.
  ○ Hypothermia can result in cardiac arrhythmias, hemodynamic compromise, increased risk for infections, and coagulation problems.
  ○ This can be **addressed by encasing the venous tubing** (blood returning to the patient) **with specialized warming devices** that can be attached to the machine.

PROLONGED INTERMITTENT RENAL REPLACEMENT THERAPY

- PIRRT is a hybrid modality which combines the benefits of CRRT and IHD.[8]
- The **dialysate flow rates** are usually approximately 100 to 200 mL/min, similar to the blood flow rates, and the procedure lasts anywhere from 6 to 12 hours.

- PIRRT is performed by the dialysis nursing staff and utilizes a modified dialysis machine. It typically does not require replacement fluids or special filters or machines. However, it can also be performed by certain machines that are typically considered as CRRT machines. In these cases, bicarbonate-based solutions are used as dialysate.
- Anticoagulation is usually required, although in our experience, during SLED therapy with NxStage®, anticoagulation is not required in about 75% of the cases.
- The therapy is **associated with fewer hemodynamic alterations compared with IHD,** and because the procedure can be performed at night in the ICU, it leaves the day for various procedures such as imaging studies, surgeries, or physical therapy. This is a clear advantage over CRRT, where stopping the therapy for various reasons prevents adequate delivery of dialysis.
- PIRRT has been shown to provide adequate urea clearance and has been successfully used in critically ill patients with AKI. More centers are using this option in addition to CRRT and IHD in the treatment of critically ill patients with AKI.
- The clearances of various drugs during PIRRT have not been established. It is recommended to give drugs after the procedure and levels, whenever available, should be monitored closely.

REFERENCES

1. Palevsky PM, Liu KD, Brophy PD, et al. KDOQI US commentary on the 2012 KDIGO clinical practice guideline for acute kidney injury. *Am J Kidney Dis.* 2013;61(5):649–672.
2. VA/NIH Acute Renal Failure Trial Network, Palevsky PM, Zhang JH, O'Connor TZ, et al. Intensity of renal support in critically ill patients with acute kidney injury. *N Engl J Med.* 2008;359(1):7–20.
3. Renal Replacement Therapy Study Investigators, Bellomo R, Cass A, Cole L, et al. Intensity of continuous renal-replacement therapy in critically ill patients. *N Engl J Med.* 2009;361(17): 1627–1638.
4. Vijayan A, Palevsky PM. Dosing of renal replacement therapy in acute kidney injury. *Am J Kidney Dis.* 2012;59(4):569–576.
5. Tolwani A. Continuous renal-replacement therapy for acute kidney injury. *N Engl J Med.* 2012;367(26):2505–2514.
6. Morabito S, Pistolesi V, Tritapepe L, et al. Regional citrate anticoagulation for RRTs in critically ill patients with AKI. *Clin J Am Soc Nephrol.* 2014;9(12):2173–2188.
7. Vijayan A. Vascular access for continuous renal replacement therapy. *Semin Dial.* 2009;22(2): 133–136.
8. Edrees F, Li T, Vijayan A. Prolonged intermittent renal replacement therapy. *Adv Chronic Kidney Dis.* 2016;23(3):195–202.

Therapeutic Plasma Exchange

Brittany Heady and Tingting Li

23

GENERAL PRINCIPLES

- Therapeutic plasma exchange (TPE) is an extracorporeal blood separation procedure in which a large volume of plasma is separated from the cellular components of blood, removed from the patient, and replaced with a colloid solution such as fresh frozen plasma (FFP) or albumin.[1]
- **Rationale** for TPE
  - Removal of high-molecular weight, circulating pathogenic substances such as autoantibodies, alloantibodies, immune complexes, paraproteins, nonimmunoglobulin proteins (such as permeability factor in primary focal segmental glomerulosclerosis), and possibly proinflammatory cytokines and other inflammatory mediators.
  - Replacement of deficient plasma factor, such as ADAMTS13 (a disintegrin and metalloproteinase with a thrombospondin type 1 motif, member 13) in thrombotic thrombocytopenic purpura (TTP).
  - Modulation of immune system which has been shown to lead to improved macrophage/monocyte function and increased susceptibility of antibody-producing cells to cytotoxic therapies.

CURRENT RENAL INDICATIONS FOR TPE

- TPE has been used in a variety of renal disorders, most often as an adjunct therapy, to rapidly remove existing pathogenic factors with the goals of ameliorating inflammation and achieving early disease control.[2]
- However, the role of TPE in the management of certain renal disorders remains controversial, mainly due to lack of high-quality data.[3] Table 23-1 lists the renal disorders for which TPE is recommended by the American Society for Apheresis as first-line therapy (category I indication), either as initial monotherapy or as adjunct therapy to immunosuppression.
- Evidence supporting the use of TPE for specific renal disorders is presented in the treatment section of each disease entity discussed in this book.

METHODS OF PLASMA EXCHANGE

- TPE can be performed using one of two technical methodologies: centrifugation or membrane plasma separation.[4]
- In both approaches, whole blood is passed through a separation device in which plasma is removed and cellular components of blood are returned to the patient along with replacement solution.
- Centrifugal separation is the more widely employed method in the United States.

TABLE 23-1	AMERICAN SOCIETY FOR APHERESIS 2016 CATEGORY I RENAL INDICATIONS AND TARGET MOLECULES FOR THERAPEUTIC PLASMA EXCHANGE		
Renal Disease	Indication	Pathogenic Molecule
Anti-GBM disease	Diffuse alveolar hemorrhage Dialysis independence	Anti-GBM antibody
ANCA-associated vasculitis	Diffuse alveolar hemorrhage Dialysis dependence	ANCA
Focal segmental glomerulosclerosis	Recurrence in transplanted kidney	Permeability factor(s)
Thrombotic microangiopathy, complement mediated	Factor H autoantibody	Factor H autoantibody
Thrombotic thrombocytopenic purpura	Autoantibody to ADAMTS13 protease or deficiency of ADAMTS13	Autoantibody to ADAMTS13 protease
Renal transplantation, ABO compatible	Antibody mediated rejection Desensitization, living donor	Alloantibodies to HLA
Renal transplantation, ABO incompatible	Desensitization, living donor	Alloantibodies to HLA

GBM, glomerular basement membrane; ANCA, antineutrophil cytoplasmic antibody; ADAMTS13, a disintegrin and metalloprotease with a thrombospondin type 1 motif, member 13; HLA, human leukocyte antigen.

Adapted from Schwartz J, Padmanabhan A, Aqui N, et al. Guidelines on the use of therapeutic apheresis in clinical practice-evidence-based approach from the writing committee of the American Society for Apheresis: The seventh special issue. *J Clin Apher.* 2016;31:149–162.

Centrifugation

- This approach uses centrifugal force to separate blood components based on their density or specific gravity.
- This is usually a continuous-flow method where blood from the patient is delivered into a spinning chamber (the centrifuge) and different components of blood are separated into layers based on their densities.
- Plasma, being the least dense, forms the innermost layer. Of the cellular elements, red blood cells are the heaviest and settle on the outside of the chamber and platelets are the lightest and layers next to plasma, while white blood cells are in between. In TPE, plasma is collected from the chamber and discarded. The cells are returned to the patient with replacement fluid.
- If desired, individual cellular component can also be collected with this method (cytapheresis).
- Given the proximity of platelets to the plasma layer, loss of platelets can occur with removal of plasma with ensuing thrombocytopenia.

Membrane Plasma Separation

- This method adopts the hemodialysis technology and is largely performed by dialysis nurses and supervised by nephrologists who are experts in extracorporeal blood purification.
- Membrane plasma separation uses hollow-fiber filters to separate plasma from the cellular elements of whole blood by filtration based on the molecular weight of proteins.
- The filters are highly permeable, with a molecular weight cut-off of up to 3 million Daltons, allowing the passage and removal of essentially all pathogenic molecules listed in Table 23-1, as well as larger molecules such as IgM and cryoglobulins. Blood cells are retained due to their significantly larger sizes.
- This procedure is performed using the standard hemodialysis machines in the ultrafiltration mode. Both PrismaFlex and NxStage System One have been used at our center with success.
- Membrane plasma separation uses higher blood flow rates compared to centrifugation to prevent filter clotting. This in turn leads to faster plasma removal and exchange rates and generally shorter duration of treatment (1 to 2 hours per TPE session).
- Transmembrane pressure needs to be monitored closely and kept below 75 mm Hg to prevent hemolysis.

KINETICS OF SUBSTANCE REMOVAL IN TPE

- Removal of pathogenic molecules by TPE is determined by several factors, including the half-life of the molecule, volume of distribution, equilibration between the intravascular and extravascular space, rate of synthesis, and volume of plasma exchanged.[5]
- The majority of the pathogenic targets that are of interest to nephrologists are immunoglobulins. Given that, the focus will mainly be on immunoglobulins in this section on kinetics.

Plasma Half-Life of Immunoglobulins

- The half-life is about 22 days for IgG and 5 days for IgM. The relatively long half-lives indicate that the pathogenic effects of these immunoglobulins can last for weeks.
- Removal of the pathogenic molecule by TPE early in the disease course can hopefully help with early disease control and reduce tissue damage. Multiple sessions of TPE can lead to a period of low plasma concentration before the effect of cytotoxic therapy takes place.

Volume of Distribution

- Immunoglobulins are mainly distributed in the extracellular space. About 45% of IgG (except for IgG3) and 80% to 90% of IgM are distributed intravascularly.
- Because of their large molecular sizes (IgG 150,000 Daltons, IgM 950,000 Daltons), immunoglobulins equilibrate very slowly between the intravascular and extravascular space. As a result, during the course of a TPE session, the removal of immunoglobulins can be calculated based on first-order kinetics (removal from a single compartment which is the intravascular space). This is assuming the production of new immunoglobulins is negligible.

Removal of Immunoglobulin in Relation to Volume of Plasma Exchanged

- The percent of immunoglobulin removed is related to the volume of plasma exchanged in an exponential manner.
- The first plasma volume exchange leads to the largest reduction in the immunoglobulin concentration in the plasma, decreasing the initial plasma concentration by 63%.

- Removal during subsequent plasma volumes in the same TPE treatment is gradually less effective, with reduction of 78% of initial immunoglobulin concentration after 1.5 plasma volume exchange, 86% after 2 plasma volume exchange, and 95% after 3 plasma volume exchange.
- Given the decreased efficiency of additional plasma volume exchanges as well as associated increased procedure time, cost, and potential complication rates, we do not recommend providing more than 1.5 plasma volume exchanges per TPE session.

THERAPEUTIC PLASMA EXCHANGE PRESCRIPTION

Dose of TPE

- **Estimation of plasma volume**
  - Plasma volume can be estimated using this formula[5]:
  - Estimated plasma volume = $0.07 \times$ weight (kg) $\times$ (1 – hematocrit)
  - For a quick bedside calculation, one can also use 35 to 40 mL/kg to estimate plasma volume. Use 40 if hematocrit is low and 35 for a normal hematocrit.
  - As above, a 1.0 to 1.5 plasma volume exchange per TPE session is usually recommended.
- **Number of TPE sessions**
  - The number of TPE sessions needed is dependent on many factors, including the disease condition and the type of pathogenic molecule removed.
  - For IgG, assuming there is very little new production of immunoglobulins (usually due to concomitant use of immunosuppression), five TPE sessions will be adequate to reduce the initial plasma concentration by 90%. Every-other-day treatment is frequently the approach to allow redistribution of the molecule from the extravascular space to the intravascular space. More sessions will be needed if there is ongoing synthesis of the IgG.
  - IgM, due to its larger molecular size, is mostly intravascular with little redistribution to the extravascular compartment. Only –two to three sessions of TPE would be required to reduce IgM to a low level, provided that there is minimal new synthesis of the molecule.

Vascular Access

- In centrifugal plasma separation, a large peripheral venous access is adequate since required blood flow rate is usually no more than 50 mL/min.
- In membrane plasma separation, required blood flow rate is at least 50 to 100 mL/min and flow rates of 150 to 200 mL/min are frequently used. Therefore, a central venous access (such as a pheresis catheter or dialysis catheter) would be necessary. Arteriovenous fistulae or grafts, if present, can also be used.

Anticoagulation

- Anticoagulation is essential with centrifugal devices to prevent clotting in the extracorporeal circuit. Usually citrate is used with this method.
- With higher blood flow rates and shorter treatment times, anticoagulation may not always be required for membrane plasma separation. The type of equipment may also be a factor in the need for anticoagulation. The absence of the air–blood interface has also been cited as the reason for decreased clotting noted when using NxStage System One.[6] If anticoagulation is required, both citrate and heparin can be used with filtration devices.
- Anticoagulation should not be used in the setting of active bleeding or if TPE is performed within 24 to 48 hours postrenal biopsy (TPE is not recommended immediately after renal biopsy due to depletion of coagulation factors).

Unfractionated Heparin

- Unfractionated heparin is used in membrane plasma separation
- The usual loading dose is 50 units/kg, followed by maintenance rate of 500 to 1,000 units/hr.
- Activated clotting time (ACT) should be checked at TPE initiation, prior to loading dose and every 15 minutes for the duration of the procedure. The goal is to maintain ACT between 180 and 220 seconds.

Regional Citrate

- Regional citrate can be used with both centrifugal TPE and membrane TPE.
- Citrate provides an anticoagulant effect by binding to ionized calcium in the extracorporeal circuit which in turn prevents the activation of the coagulation cascade.
- Citrate that enters the systemic circulation is rapidly metabolized by the liver to bicarbonate so that chelation of calcium in the systemic circulation usually does not occur to a significant degree.
- Calcium that is removed from the extracorporeal circuit must be replaced intravenously to prevent hypocalcemia.
- Although the use of regional citrate is relatively safe without bleeding risks, close monitoring of the patient is vital in preventing citrate toxicity.
- Citrate toxicity can occur when the rate of citrate accumulation exceeds the rate of metabolism and excretion. Toxicity is manifested by:
  - Severe hypocalcemia, sometimes life-threatening, can occur. This is associated with high total serum calcium level and disproportionately low ionized calcium.
  - Metabolic alkalosis.
  - Increased anion gap.
- Patients with hepatic and renal dysfunction are particularly at risk for citrate toxicity. If citrate is used in these patients, citrate infusion rate should be greatly reduced and patient closely monitored.
- If FFP is used as a replacement solution, the rate of citrate infusion should also be adjusted as FFP has a high citrate content (about 14% by volume).
- Citrate is given in a fixed ratio to blood flow. Higher blood flow rates require increased citrate infusion rates. One way to minimize citrate toxicity is to reduce blood flow rate. At our center, the initial citrate infusion rate (in mL/hr) is 1.5 × blood flow rate (in mL/min). For example, if the blood flow rate is 100 mL/min then citrate infusion rate is 150 mL/hr of ACD-A (anticoagulant citrate dextrose solution A). This may be adjusted based on various factors mentioned above.
- Plasma calcium levels should be measured pre-, intra-, and post-TPE and hypocalcemia should be corrected aggressively with calcium infusion, sometimes with additional oral calcium.

Replacement Solution

- During TPE, the removed plasma needs to be replaced to prevent volume depletion. Replacement volume should be at least 85% of plasma volume removed to avoid hemodynamic compromise.
- The most common choices for replacement solution are 5% albumin and FFP. Sometime a combination of colloid and crystalloid solutions is used.
- Given its better safety profile than FFP, albumin is generally recommended for most clinical situations.
- FFP is used in selected settings:
  - Active bleeding.
  - High risk of bleeding: combination of albumin and FFP can be used with FFP given toward the end of the TPE session.
  - Need to replace a deficient plasma factor (such as in TTP).
- Table 23-2 lists the pros and cons of different replacement solutions.

TABLE 23-2 PROS AND CONS OF DIFFERENT REPLACEMENT SOLUTIONS

Replacement Solution	Pros	Cons
Albumin	No risk of viral transmission Minimal risk of anaphylaxis No need for ABO compatibility No need to thaw	Higher cost Depletion of coagulation factors and immunoglobulins Risk for dilutional hypokalemia
Fresh frozen plasma	No depletion of coagulation factors or immunoglobulins Supplies needed factor in thrombotic thrombocytopenic purpura	Increased risk of viral transmission Higher risk of anaphylaxis Citrate load Needs to be thawed
Crystalloid	Low cost No infectious risk	Hypo-oncotic with risk of hemodynamic instability No coagulation factors or immunoglobulins

COMPLICATIONS OF TPE

- The reported frequencies of complications associated with TPE vary by studies and the underlying disease condition. The more commonly encountered complications are listed below. Death is rare, occurring in 0.03% to 0.05% of TPE treatments.[7]
- **Anticoagulation-related complications**
  - Adverse events associated with citrate toxicity, particularly signs and symptoms related to hypocalcemia. See Regional Citrate above for more details on citrate toxicity.
  - Bleeding: Mostly due to heparin use.
  - Heparin-induced thrombocytopenia and associated thrombotic events.
- **Replacement solution-related complications**
  - Hypotension due to inadequate replacement fluid volume or use of hypotonic solution.
  - Hemolytic anemia due to hypotonic solution.
  - FFP-associated adverse events may also occur (see Replacement Solution above and Table 23-2).
- **Vascular access–related complications:** bleeding, thrombosis, infection, pneumothorax, and hemothorax.
- **TPE procedure–related complications**
  - Hypotension
  - Depletion coagulopathy
    - Increased prothrombin time (PT) and activated partial thromboplastin time (aPTT) and decreased fibrinogen level as a result of clotting factor removal and use of non-FFP replacement solution.
    - This can increase the risk of clinically significant bleeding.
    - Prior to initiation of TPE, it is important to get a baseline assessment of coagulation status by checking a fibrinogen level, PT, and aPTT. This should be repeated daily or every other day if consecutive treatments are performed.

○ Immunoglobulin depletion
  ■ Low serum IgG levels will occur with use of a non-FFP replacement fluid and there may be an increased risk for infection.
  ■ With treatment of acute rejection in renal transplant patients, intravenous immunoglobulin (IVIG) is often given following TPE.
○ Thrombocytopenia (in centrifugal TPE)
○ Hemolysis (in membrane TPE in setting of high transmembrane pressure)
○ Anaphylactoid reactions due to ethylene oxide sterilization of filters in membrane TPE
○ Complement mediated reactions to the filter
○ Undesired drug removal: Drugs that are highly protein-bound and have a small volume of distribution can be removed by TPE. These drugs should be administered after the TPE procedure.

- **Angiotensin-converting enzyme (ACE) inhibitor–related complications:** In patients receiving ACE inhibitors, symptoms of flushing and hypotension can occur. This is secondary to the release of bradykinin. ACE inhibitors should be held 24 to 48 hours prior to TPE and resumed after completion of TPE.[8]

REFERENCES

1. Kaplan AA. Therapeutic plasma exchange: a technical and operational review. *J Clin Apher.* 2013;28:3–10.
2. Schwartz J, Padmanabhan A, Aqui N, et al. Guidelines on the use of therapeutic apheresis in clinical practice-evidence-based approach from the writing committee of the American Society for Apheresis: The Seventh Special Issue. *J Clin Apher.* 2016;31:149–162.
3. Williams ME, Balogun RA. Principles of separation: indications and therapeutic targets for plasma exchange. *Clin J Am Soc Nephrol.* 2014;9:181–190.
4. Reeves HM, Winters JL. The mechanisms of action of plasma exchange. *Br J Haematol.* 2014;164:342–351.
5. Kaplan AA. Therapeutic plasma exchange: core curriculum 2008. *Am J Kidney Dis.* 2008;52:1180–1196.
6. Gashti CN. Membrane-based therapeutic plasma exchange: a new frontier for nephrologists. *Semin Dial.* 2016;29:382–390.
7. Mokrzycki MH, Kaplan AA. Therapeutic plasma exchange: complications and management. *Am J Kidney Dis.* 1994;23:817–827.
8. Owen HG, Brecher ME. Atypical reactions associated with use of angiotensin-converting enzyme inhibitors and apheresis. *Transfusion.* 1994;34:891–894.

Principles of Drug Dosing in Renal Impairment

Bethany Tellor and Jennifer Hagopian

24

INTRODUCTION

- One of the most significant drug-related errors in patients with renal impairment is inappropriate medication dosing leading to toxicity or ineffective therapy.[1]
- Drugs with renally eliminated active metabolites require special dosing consideration as the consequences of accumulation can be particularly dangerous.
- High degrees of precision are required when dosing medications with a narrow therapeutic index (e.g., aminoglycosides, digoxin) that rely on renal elimination.
- Deciding on the appropriate dosing strategy of medications in patients with chronic kidney disease (CKD) or acute kidney injury (AKI) requires an understanding of the basic principles of pharmacokinetics, including absorption, protein binding, metabolism, and elimination.
- Renal impairment affects glomerular blood flow and filtration, tubular secretion, reabsorption, renal bioactivation, and metabolism.
- Nonrenal drug clearance, through mechanisms that are poorly understood, may also be impaired by kidney injury.[1]
- Dosing for medications that undergo renal elimination is based primarily on an estimate of glomerular filtration rate (GFR). The Modification of Diet in Renal Disease (MDRD) study and Cockcroft–Gault equations provide useful estimates of GFR in adults. Patient-specific dosages calculated using these equations should be conducted in the presence of stable renal function and in patients not on renal replacement therapy (RRT).
- Patients who are treated with different forms of dialysis may require supplemental dosing. The ability of dialysis to remove drugs is influenced by a variety of factors discussed elsewhere in this chapter.
- Drugs that can further impair renal function in high-risk patients (heart failure [HF], liver disease, hypoperfusion) should be used with caution or avoided altogether in preference for safer alternatives.
- Nephrotoxic medications have been linked to >20% episodes of AKI. Clinicians must recognize commonly used agents in order to ensure safety of medication administration in the setting of renal dysfunction.
- Table 24-1 lists common medications that are potentially nephrotoxic.

GENERAL DOSING AND PHARMACOKINETIC PRINCIPLES

- In general, renal insufficiency makes it difficult to predict whether a medication dose will produce an adequate, supratherapeutic, or subtherapeutic effect.[2]
- Loading doses are often used to rapidly achieve a therapeutic drug concentration; they depend on the urgency with which a pharmacologic effect is needed against the half-life of the drug.
  - The time needed to reach 90% of the plateau drug concentration is 3.3 times the half-life. If this time is too long relative to the clinical urgency of the situation, a loading dose is needed.

TABLE 24-1	MECHANISMS OF NEPHROTOXICITY AND ALTERNATIVES TO SOME COMMON DRUGS

Drug	Mechanism	Alternatives/Comments
ACE inhibitors	Intraglomerular hemodynamic alteration	β-Blockers, calcium channel blockers
Acetaminophen	Chronic interstitial nephropathy	Avoid doses >4 g/day chronically
Acyclovir (intravenous)	Acute tubular injury	Hydration, oral administration, dose adjustment
Aminoglycosides	Acute tubular injury	Monitor serum concentration, alternative antibiotic
Amphotericin	Acute tubular injury	Saline loading, lipid formulation
β-Lactam antibiotics	Interstitial nephritis	Alternative antibiotic
Carboplatin	Tubular injury	Hydration, alternative chemotherapy agents
Ciprofloxacin	Interstitial nephritis	Alternative antibiotic
Cisplatin	Tubular injury	Hydration, alternative chemotherapy agents
Cyclosporine	Chronic interstitial nephritis, intraglomerular hemodynamic alteration	Monitor serum concentrations, belatacept
Foscarnet	Tubular injury, crystal nephropathy	Dose adjustment, ganciclovir
Hydralazine	ANCA-associated vasculitis	Alternative antihypertensive
Lithium	Interstitial disease, hypercalcemia, CKD	Monitor serum concentrations, alternative mood stabilizer
Loop diuretics	Interstitial nephritis	Non–sulfa-containing diuretics
Methotrexate	Tubular injury	Adjust dosage, urinary alkalinization, allopurinol
NSAIDs	Chronic interstitial nephropathy, intraglomerular hemodynamic alteration	Acetaminophen, opiate analgesic
Phenytoin	Interstitial nephritis	Alternative anticonvulsant
Phenobarbital	Interstitial nephritis	Alternative anticonvulsant
Proton pump inhibitors	Interstitial nephritis, CKD	H_2 blockers
Sulfonamides	Tubular obstruction, interstitial nephritis	Non–sulfa-containing antibiotic
Tacrolimus	Interstitial nephritis, intraglomerular hemodynamic alteration	Monitor serum concentrations, belatacept
Vancomycin	Tubular and interstitial injuries	Monitor serum concentrations, alternative antibiotic

ACE, angiotensin-converting enzyme; CKD, chronic kidney disease.

- Physiologic determinants affecting loading doses, such as an increase in total body water (e.g., edema, ascites), may warrant a higher than normal loading dose to account for change in volume of distribution (V_d), whereas dehydration may require a loading dose reduction.
  - The loading dose is a function of the V_d and the initial target blood concentration.
    Loading dose = $V_d \times C_p$
    V_d = volume of distribution in L/kg
    C_p = desired plasma concentration in mg/L
- Maintenance doses are used to achieve steady-state concentrations.
  - Dose reduction, increasing the interval, or both can be used to avoid the accumulation of renally eliminated drugs or their metabolites.
  - The best dosing option to employ depends on the properties of the medication and the disease state being treated.
  - Regimens with closer dosing frequencies and small individual doses result in less fluctuations between peak and trough concentrations. This may be particularly helpful for medications that need to be maintained within a narrow concentration range for optimal efficacy (e.g., anticonvulsants, antiarrhythmics).
- Pharmacokinetics refers to the action of drugs in the body over time, and is used to understand drug handling as a means to optimize efficacy and minimize toxicity. As noted in Table 24-2, it involves four parameters of drug activity: **absorption, distribution, metabolism, and clearance.**[1]
- It is important to identify how the pharmacokinetic profile of medications can be altered in patients with renal impairment (Table 24-2).
- Accumulation of renally excreted active metabolites may occur (Table 24-3).

DOSAGE ADJUSTMENTS OF COMMONLY USED DRUGS

Anticoagulants

Vitamin K Antagonists

- **Warfarin** metabolism and elimination is not significantly altered in renal insufficiency, however CKD is a known risk factor associated with warfarin-related hemorrhage. This is likely due to platelet dysfunction and concomitant drug interactions.
- Reduced doses should be used in patients with significant renal impairment.

Heparins

- **Unfractionated heparin** (IV, SC) is primarily metabolized in the liver and endothelium; however, there is limited evidence to ensure safety of this agent in GFRs <30 mL/min.
- **Low–molecular-weight heparins** (e.g., enoxaparin, dalteparin) administrated SC have predictable pharmacokinetic profiles and dosing curves that justify the use of these agents without routine coagulation monitoring. However, they primarily undergo renal clearance and require dose adjustment in renal insufficiency.
- Anti-Xa monitoring has been recommended for GFRs <30 mL/min.
- Use in dialysis is contraindicated and not Food and Drug Administration (FDA) approved.

Anti-Xa Inhibitors

- **Fondaparinux** (SC) is primarily excreted in the urine as unchanged drug. Use with caution for GFRs <50 mL/min. Do not use if GFR <30 mL/min.
- **Rivaroxaban, apixaban, and edoxaban** are three of the new direct oral anticoagulant agents (DOACs).[3]
- Rivaroxaban and apixaban are renally eliminated and require dose adjustments. Use is not recommended for GFRs <30 mL/min. Neither agent is dialyzable but recent

TABLE 24-2 EFFECT OF RENAL DISEASE ON VARIOUS PHASES OF PHARMACOKINETICS

Phases	Characteristics	Effects of Renal Disease	Examples of Medications
Absorption	Bioavailability refers to the fraction of medication that reaches the systemic circulation after oral ingestion. Several factors and physiologic processes influence intestinal absorption and bioavailability.	Patients with CKD and AKI exhibit changes in the gastrointestinal tract that affect bioavailability. Gastroparesis: Patients with CKD often suffer from gastroparesis. This results in delayed gastric emptying and prolongs the time to maximum drug concentrations, which can be important when rapid onset of action is desired. Gastric alkalinization: Common use of medications such as phosphate binders, antacids, H_2-receptor antagonists, and proton pump inhibitors in patients with CKD reduces the absorption of many medications requiring an acidic environment. Cationic chelation: Ingestion of common cation-containing antacids (e.g., calcium, magnesium, aluminum hydroxide, sodium polystyrene sulfonate) in patients with renal dysfunction decreases the absorption of many coadministered medications because of chelation.	Examples of medications affected by gastric alkalinization: • Furosemide • Ferrous sulfate Examples of drugs affected by chelation: • Quinolones • Warfarin • Levothyroxine • Tetracycline

Distribution

Drug distribution or volume of distribution (V_d) is the total amount of drug present in the body, divided by the plasma concentration, expressed in liters.

The V_d determines peak concentrations. Plasma protein binding, tissue binding, active transport, and body composition affect the V_d.

Albumin and other plasma proteins bind most drugs to varying degrees. Plasma drug concentrations are representative of both bound and unbound drug, but only free drug is capable of crossing cellular membranes and exerting pharmacologic effects.

Several drugs have shown changes in V_d in patients with renal dysfunction and this may mandate a change in a loading dose of a medication.

Hypoalbuminemia due to the nephrotic syndrome often leads to an increase in the free drug fraction of medications that are highly bound to albumin.

An increase in α-1-acid glycoprotein (an acute phase protein) associated with renal dysfunction will lead to increase in protein binding of medications bound to nonalbumin proteins.

In addition, accumulation of metabolites and endogenous substances increase competition for binding sites.

Digoxin: V_d that is one-half that in a patient with normal renal function.

β-Lactams: They have increased V_d and may need higher dosing in in renal dysfunction.

Examples of acidic drugs that are usually protein bound, and have higher free drug levels with decreased albumin:

- Penicillins
- Cephalosporins
- Phenytoin
- Furosemide
- Salicylates

Examples of alkaline drugs affected by increased protein binding in CKD:

- Propranolol
- Morphine
- Vancomycin

(continued)

TABLE 24-2 EFFECT OF RENAL DISEASE ON VARIOUS PHASES OF PHARMACOKINETICS (Continued)

Phases	Characteristics	Effects of Renal Disease	Examples of Medications
Metabolism	The majority of drugs in the clinical setting undergo first-order kinetics (i.e., drug concentrations decline logarithmically over time) and rates are proportional to the total body concentration of the drug present. Biotransformation at numerous sites in the body happens through phase I reactions. Phase I reactions include hydrolysis, reduction, and oxidation (cytochrome P450 reactions). These serve to increase drug hydrophilicity to prepare for excretion or further phase II metabolism. Phase II reactions or conjugation reactions include glucuronidation, sulfation, glutathione conjugation, acetylation, and methylation.	Hepatic metabolism of medications is inhibited in both CKD and AKI. Renal dysfunction significantly slows both phase I and phase II reactions. Renal dysfunction reduces P-glycoprotein activity, resulting in increased bioavailability of some medications. Changes to oxidation reactions result in reduced activity of several of the CYP450 isoenzymes (2C9, 2C19, 2D6, 3A4). All phase II reactions are slowed in renal dysfunction.	Examples of medications with narrow therapeutic index affected by decreased P-glycoprotein activity: • Cyclosporine • Tacrolimus Examples of drugs affected by decreased phase II actions: • Acetylation: dapsone, hydralazine, isoniazid, procainamide • Glucuronidation: acetaminophen, morphine, lorazepam, naproxen • Sulfation: acetaminophen, minoxidil, dopamine, albuterol • Methylation: dobutamine, dopamine, 6-mercaptopurine

Elimination	Elimination is reported as a half-life (T½), or the time needed to reduce medication plasma concentrations by 50%.	The rate of renal elimination is dependent on GFR, renal tubular secretion, and reabsorption.	Examples of drugs affected by reduced active secretion:
	T½ is influenced by both V_d and clearance and can reflect a change in either or both of these parameters.	Reduced GFR results in prolonged free drug elimination T½.	• Ampicillin
		Medication-specific characteristics (e.g., molecular weight, protein binding) determine glomerular filtration with filtration rate dependent on free fraction.	• Furosemide
	T½ and clearance of a drug are different.		• Penicillin G
	Approximately 5 T½s are required to eliminate 97% of drug from the body.	Drugs that are highly protein bound are not filtered, but actively secreted into the proximal convoluted tubule through a saturable process.	• Trimethoprim
	This parameter is especially useful for estimation of the time required to achieve steady state (approximately 4–5 T½s), and to estimate appropriate drug dosing intervals.	In the distal portion of the nephron substantial passive reabsorption occurs and this is affected by urine concentrating activities, pH, lipophilicity, and protein binding.	Examples of drugs affected by reduced passive absorption:
		Reduced GFR will decrease secretion by active transport.	• Aspirin
			• Lithium

CKD, chronic kidney disease; AKI, acute kidney injury; V_d, volume of distribution; CYP450, cytochrome P450; GFR, glomerular filtration rate.

TABLE 24-3	COMMON MEDICATIONS WITH ACTIVE METABOLITES	
Drug	Metabolite	Cumulative Toxicity
Acetaminophen	N-acetyl-p-benzoquinoneimine	Hepatotoxicity, tubular acute necrosis
Allopurinol	Oxypurinol	Bone marrow suppression
Glyburide	4-trans-hydroxyglibenclamide (M1) 3-cis-hydroxyglibenclamide (M2)	Hypoglycemia
Meperidine	Normeperidine	Seizures
Primidone	Phenobarbital	Oversedation, coma
Procainamide	N-acetyl-procainamide	Arrhythmia, hypotension, respiratory failure
Nitroprusside	Thiocyanate	Lactic hallucinations, coma, acidosis, tinnitus
Morphine	6-Morphine glucuronide	Oversedation, coma
Tramadol	O-desmethyltramadol	Respiratory depression, seizures, increased serotonin

pharmacokinetic studies suggest a dose reduction may be used safely. However, clinical efficacy and long-term safety data are lacking in this patient population. Extreme caution is advised.

- Edoxaban requires dose adjustments in renal insufficiency. Use is not recommended for GFRs <15 mL/min and is not dialyzable. In patients with nonvalvular atrial fibrillation, use is not recommended if GFR >95 mL/min as an increased risk of ischemic stroke compared to warfarin has been noted.

Direct Thrombin Inhibitors
- **Bivalirudin** (IV) undergoes minimal renal excretion (20%) and requires minor dose reductions in renal insufficiency and dialysis.
- **Desirudin** (SC) requires dose adjustment and subsequent activated partial thromboplastin time (aPTT) monitoring in renal impairment.
- **Argatroban** (IV) requires no renal dose adjustments.
- **Dabigatran** use in the presence of renal insufficiency warrants dose adjustments. Of all the new DOACs, dabigatran has the highest proportional of renal elimination. Use is not recommended in dialysis or GFRs <30 mL/min due to lack of clinical studies. However, dabigatran is approximately 60% dialyzable and dialysis may be employed as an emergent reversal strategy (Table 24-4).

Analgesics
- The safest analgesic option in renal impairment is **acetaminophen,** however higher doses used chronically have been associated with nephropathy.
- **NSAIDs** should generally be avoided. They can induce renal injury manifesting as azotemia, interstitial nephritis, nephrotic syndrome, and/or hyperkalemia. In addition, they can cause hypertension and fluid and electrolyte imbalances.[4]

TABLE 24-4	DIRECT ORAL ANTICOAGULANTS			
Parameter	Dabigatran[a]	Rivaroxaban[a]	Apixaban[a]	Edoxaban[a]
Time to max inhibition (hrs)	0.5–2	2–4	3–4	1–3
Half-life (hrs)[b]	12–17	5–13	~12	8–10
Metabolism	Hepatic	Hepatic	Hepatic	Minimal, hepatic
Active renal secretion[b]	80%	33%	27%	50%
Pharmacotherapy pearls	Caution use if ≥80 yrs old; avoid or reduce dose if used with dronedarone, ketoconazole, glycoprotein inhibitors	CYP3A4 and P-glycoprotein drug interactions	CYP3A4 and P-glycoprotein drug interactions	Dose reduction if <60 kg, concomitant P-glycoprotein inhibitors
Reversal strategies	Idarucizumab, hemodialysis, activated charcoal	Andexanet alfa	Andexanet alfa	

[a]Dosing for all agents depends on indication and renal function as listed in the package insert.
[b]It is important to consider renal function half-life as it pertains to medication clearance prior to surgery.

- **Morphine, tramadol, and meperidine** all have active metabolites that are renally excreted and can accumulate causing toxicity (Table 24-3).
- **Fentanyl and hydromorphone** are two of the safest opioid analgesics to use in the setting of renal failure in hospitalized patients. Both are metabolized in the liver and have nontoxic inactive metabolites.

Antihypertensives

Angiotensin-Converting Enzyme Inhibitors/Angiotensin-2 Receptor Blockers

- Angiotensin-converting enzyme (ACE) inhibitors and angiotensin-2 receptor blockers (ARBs) have been shown to reduce proteinuria, slow progression of kidney disease, and provide long-term cardiovascular protection.
- Many patients experience an acute decline in GFR >15% from baseline with proportional elevations in serum creatinine (SCr) in the first week.
- If the rise in SCr is <30%, these medications can be continued safely in most patients, and can be expected to return to baseline in 4 to 6 weeks.
- Common practice includes discontinuation if the SCr rises >30% or serum potassium is >5.6 mEq/L.
- ARBs are all hepatically eliminated and no renal adjustment is necessary.
- Patients with renal impairment are at an increased risk of developing severe hyperkalemia or acute renal failure (<5% overall), with the highest risk being in patients with diabetes or a history of hyperkalemia.

β-Blockers

- Hydrophilic β-blockers such as **atenolol, bisoprolol, nadolol, and acebutolol** are renally eliminated and require dose reduction with renal impairment.
- **Metoprolol, propranolol, and labetalol** do not require dose adjustments.

Diuretics

Loop Diuretics

- Loop diuretics, such as **furosemide, bumetanide, and torsemide,** are the most commonly prescribed diuretics in patients with renal impairment as they are still effective with GFR <30 mL/min.[5]
- The CKD population can be diuretic resistant needing higher doses to achieve similar intraluminal concentrations.
- Drug resistance often occurs as a result of decreased drug delivery to the nephron lumen, increased sodium reabsorption between dosages, and increased distal sodium reabsorption.
- Dose escalation, switching to a continuous infusion, and adding a thiazide diuretic to alter distal sodium absorption are strategies that can be used to overcome resistance.
- Ototoxicity with loop diuretic use is typically reversible; however, cases of permanent deafness have been reported.
- Loop diuretics are sulfonamide derivatives and can cause hypersensitivity reaction like acute interstitial nephritis and skin rashes, although rare. **Ethacrynic acid** is not a sulfonamide derivative and may be used as an alternative; however, the risk of ototoxicity is higher.

Thiazide Diuretics

- Thiazide diuretics, such as **hydrochlorothiazide and chlorthalidone,** are not recommended as sole agents with SCr levels that exceed 2.5 mg/dL or GFRs <30 mL/min.
- These agents require activity in the lumen of the nephron to produce a natriuretic effect, which is not achieved with advanced renal impairment.
- One exception is **metolazone** which continues to be effective at GFR <30 mL/min, especially in combination with a loop diuretic.

Potassium-Sparing Diuretics
- These agents inhibit the epithelial sodium channel, thereby increasing natriuresis with a potassium-sparing action.
- **Spironolactone** is commonly used in patients with severe HF as it has been shown to reduce mortality.
- Spironolactone should be used with caution in renal insufficiency as several reports have documented severe life-threatening hyperkalemia that can occur, especially if concomitantly used with an ARB or ACE inhibitor.[6]
- Sodium restriction is also used as adjunctive therapy to diuretic management of volume overload in CKD.

Hypoglycemic Agents

Biguanides
- **Metformin** is primarily eliminated as unchanged drug by active renal tubular secretion.[7] Due to concerns of lactic acidosis, use has traditionally not been recommended in patients with SCr >1.4 mg/dL in females and >1.5 mg/dL in males.
- In 2016, FDA changed its recommendation and stated that metformin can be safely used with an estimated GFR between 30 and 60 mL/min, if patients were already on the drug. It recommended against initiating the drug in patients whose eGFR were already between 30 and 45 mL/min. It recommended at least annual monitoring of eGFR.
- The American Diabetes Association has removed SCr cutoffs for appropriate metformin use and updated recommendations for use are based upon GFR (Table 24-5).

Sulfonylureas
- Several sulfonylureas, including **glyburide,** should be avoided in patients with stage 3 to 5 CKD. Glyburide has an active metabolite that is renally eliminated and accumulation can cause prolonged hypoglycemia.
- **Glipizide** does not have an active metabolite and is safe for use in renal insufficiency.

Dipeptidyl Peptidase-4 Inhibitors
- **Sitagliptin** is excreted mostly unchanged in the urine and requires dose adjustments with GFR <50 mL/min. The dose should be reduced to 50 mg daily with GFR between 30 and <50 mL/min and further reduced to 25 mg daily when the GFR falls below 30 mL/min. **Saxagliptin** is metabolized to an active metabolite that undergoes hepatic and renal elimination. Dose should be reduced to 2.5 mg daily with a GFR <45 mL/min.

TABLE 24-5	FOOD AND DRUG ADMINISTRATION RECOMMENDATIONS FOR METFORMIN USE
eGFR (mL/min/1.73 m²)	Recommendations
≥60	No renal contraindications to metformin use
<60 and ≥45	Continue metformin use; increase monitoring frequency of renal function
<45 and ≥30	Decrease dose by 50% or use half the maximum recommended dose; should not initiate a new patient on metformin
<30	Discontinue metformin use

eGFR, estimated glomerular filtration rate.

- **Linagliptin** undergoes minimal renal elimination and does not require dose reductions in renal dysfunction.

Glucagon-Like Peptide-1 Receptor Agonists
- **Exenatide** is primarily renally eliminated and undergoes degradation by the kidneys into inactive fragments. Use caution in moderate renal impairment with initiation and dose escalation and to avoid use in severe renal impairment.
- Dose adjustments are not required in mild, moderate, or severe renal impairment for **liraglutide, albiglutide, or dulaglutide.** Limited data exist for liraglutide in severe renal impairment. **Lixisenatide** does not require adjustments in mild or moderate renal impairment but should be avoided in severe renal impairment.

Sodium-Glucose Cotransporter-2 Inhibitors
- **Canagliflozin** requires a dose reduction to 100 mg daily when GFR falls within the 45 to 60 mL/min range.
- Therapy should not be initiated or discontinued when GFR is <60 mL/min for **dapagliflozin** and <45 mL/min for both canagliflozin and **empagliflozin.**

Insulin
All preparations require dose reductions due to decreased renal elimination in renal impairment.

Antimicrobials

- Many antimicrobial agents are renally eliminated and require dose adjustment.
- Dose adjustments are complex and vary based on individual medication and degree of renal dysfunction.
- Table 24-6 below lists common antimicrobial agents that require dose adjustment.

Aminoglycosides
- Aminoglycosides are completely filtered by the glomerulus and taken up by the proximal tubular epithelial cells. Progressive accumulation in the proximal tubular epithelial cells leads to tubular injury.[8]
- There are two available dosing strategies: traditional and extended-interval (EI) dosing based on dosing weight (DW).[9]
- **Traditional dosing**
  - Calculate a **loading dose** based on DW; dose may be lowered in patients with volume depletion (Table 24-7).
  - Calculate **maintenance dose.** The maintenance dose is a percentage of the loading dose (Table 24-8).
  - For therapeutic drug monitoring, obtain peak and trough concentrations with the third maintenance dose. The clinical scenario should guide the preferred peak and trough levels (Table 24-9). Recheck the level whenever there is a change in dosing regimen or change in renal function. Recheck every 1 to 2 weeks if duration of therapy is >2 weeks.
- **Extended-interval (EI) dosing**
  - EI dosing is **equally effective and may be less toxic** compared with traditional dosing.
  - This dosing technique takes advantage of concentration-dependent killing through high peak levels and the postantibiotic effect.
  - EI dosing is not generally recommended in certain clinical situations, wherein there might be alterations to renal perfusion and drug pharmacokinetics.
  - Examples of these clinical scenarios include: pregnancy, anasarca/severe HF/liver failure, end-stage renal disease (ESRD), patients on hemodialysis or peritoneal dialysis, GFR <30 mL/min, endocarditis, cystic fibrosis, mycobacterial infection, elderly or

TABLE 24-6 DOSE ADJUSTMENTS FOR RENAL FUNCTION FOR COMMONLY USED ANTIMICROBIAL AGENTS

Name Antibiotics	Usual Dose[a]/Route	GFR (mL/min) ≥50	10–50	<10
Amoxicillin PO	250–1000 mg PO q8–12 h	No change	q8–12 h	q24 h
Ampicillin PO	250–500 mg PO q6 h	No change	q6–12 h	q12–24 h
Ampicillin IV	1–2 g IV q4–6 h	No change	q6–12 h	q12–24 h
Ampicillin/sulbactam IV	1.5–3 g IV q6 h	No change	q6–12 h	q24 h
Piperacillin/tazobactam IV	3.375–4 g IV q6 h	No change	2.25–3.375 g q6 h	2.25 g q6–8 h
Cefazolin IV	1–2 g IV q8 h	No change	q12 h	q24 h
Cefepime IV	1–2 g IV q8 h	No change	q12–24 h	q24 h
Cefotaxime IV	1–2 g IV q4–8 h	No change	q6–12 h	q24 h
Cefotetan IV	1–2 g IV q12 h	No change	q12–24 h	q48 h
Cefoxitin IV	1–2 g IV q6 h	No change	q6–12 h	q24 h
Ceftaroline IV	600 mg IV q12 h	No change	300–400 mg q12 h	200 mg q12 h
Ceftazidime IV	1–2 g IV q8 h	No change	q12–24 h	q24 h
Ceftazidime/avibactam IV	2.5 g IV q8 h	No change	0.94–1.25 g q8–12 h	0.94 g q24–48 h
Ceftolozane/tazobactam IV	1.5 g IV q8 h	No change	375–750 mg q8 h	750 mg × 1 then 150 mg q8 h
Cefuroxime PO	250–500 mg PO q12 h	No change	q24 h	q48 h
Cefuroxime IV	500 mg–1.5 g IV q8 h	No change	q12 h	q24 h
Aztreonam IV	1–2 g IV q8 h	No change	50% of usual dose	25% of usual dose
Doripenem IV	500 mg IV q8 h	No change	250 mg q8–12 h	250–500 mg q24 h
Ertapenem IV	1 g IV q24 h	No change	<30 mL/min 500 mg q24 h	500 mg q24 h

(continued)

| TABLE 24-6 | DOSE ADJUSTMENTS FOR RENAL FUNCTION FOR COMMONLY USED ANTIMICROBIAL AGENTS *(Continued)* | | | |

Name		GFR (mL/min)		
Antibiotics	Usual Dose[a]/Route	≥50	10–50	<10
Imipenem IV	500 mg IV q6 h	No change	500 mg q8–12 h	500 mg q24 h
Meropenem IV	500 mg–2 g IV q6–8 h	No change	q8–12 h	q24 h
Trimethoprim/sulfamethoxazole IV	5 mg/kg IV trimethoprim component q6–8 h	No change	*<30 mL/min* 50% usual dose q12 h	Not recommended
Trimethoprim/sulfamethoxazole PO	160/800 mg PO q12 h	No change	*<30 mL/min* 80/400 mg q12 h	Not recommended
Clarithromycin	250–500 mg PO q12 h	No change	50% of usual dose	50% of usual dose
Tetracycline PO	250–500 mg PO q6–12 h	q8–12 h	q12–24 h	q24 h
Ciprofloxacin PO	250–750 mg PO q12 h	No change	q12–24 h	q24 h
Ciprofloxacin IV	200–400 mg IV q12 h	No change	q12–24 h	q24 h
Levofloxacin PO	250–500 mg PO daily	No change	q48 h	q48 h
Levofloxacin IV	250–500 mg IV daily	No change	q48 h	q48 h
Daptomycin	4–8 mg/kg IV q24 h	No change	*<30 mL/min* q48 h	q48 h
Telavancin IV	10 mg/kg IV actual body weight q24 h	No change	7.5 mg/kg q24 h	10 mg/kg q48 h
Colistin IV	2.5 mg/kg IV q12 h	No change	1.5–2 mg/kg q12–36 h	1.5 mg/kg q48 h
Antifungals				
Amphotericin B (liposomal) IV	3–5 mg/kg IV q24 h	No change	No change	No change
Fluconazole PO	200–400 mg PO q24 h	No change	50% usual dose	50% usual dose
Fluconazole IV	200–400 mg IV q24 h	No change	50% usual dose	50% usual dose

Itraconazole PO	100–200 mg PO q12 h	No change	No change	No change
Voriconazole PO	>40 kg: 200 mg PO q12 h <40 kg: 100 mg PO q12 h	No change	No change	No change
Voriconazole IV	6 mg/kg IV q12 h × 2 then 4 mg/kg IV q12 h	No change	Not recommended (toxic vehicle may accumulate, use PO route)	Not recommended (toxic vehicle may accumulate, use PO route)
Antivirals				
Acyclovir PO[a]	200–800 mg PO 5×/day	No change	<25 mL/min q8 h	200 mg PO q12 h
Acyclovir IV	5–10 mg/kg IV q8 h	No change	5–10 mg/kg q12–24 h	2.5–5 mg/kg q24 h
Amantadine PO	100 mg PO q12 h	No change	q48 h	q7 days
Famciclovir PO	500 mg PO q8 h	No change	q12–24 h	250 mg q24 h
Ganciclovir IV induction	5 mg/kg IV q12 h	2.5 mg/kg q12 h	*25–49 mL/min* 2.5 mg/kg q24 h *10–24 mL/min* 1.25 mg/kg q24 h	1.25 mg/kg 3×/wk
Ganciclovir IV maintenance	5 mg/kg IV q24 h	2.5 mg/kg q24 h	*25–49 mL/min* 1.25 mg/kg q24 h *10–24 mL/min* 0.625 mg/kg q24 h	0.625 mg/kg 3×/wk
Oseltamivir treatment	75 mg bid	No change	*31–49 mL/min* 30 mg q12 h *10–30 mL/min* 30 mg q24 h	30 mg 3×/wk
Valacyclovir	1 g q8 h	No change	q12–24 h	500 mg q24 h
Valganciclovir	900 mg q12–24 h	No change	450 mg q24–72 h	Not recommended

[a]Exact dosing may depend on specific indication and patient-specific factors.

TABLE 24-7 AMINOGLYCOSIDE LOADING DOSE CALCULATION

Intensity	Drug	Loading Dose (mg/kg)	Infection Site
Low	Gentamicin	1	Endovascular infection
	Tobramycin	1	Gram-positive infection
	Amikacin	5	Urinary tract infection
Intermediate	Gentamicin	1.5	Bone/joint infection
	Tobramycin	1.5	Skin/skin structure infection
	Amikacin	6.5	
High	Gentamicin	2	Central nervous system
	Tobramycin	2	infection, cystic fibrosis, febrile
	Amikacin	8	neutropenia, gram-negative rod bacteremia, open fracture infection, pneumonia, septic shock with acute renal failure

infants, burns covering >20% body surface area, or critically ill patients with hemo-dynamic instability.

○ Calculate the patient's DW as outlined above. The initial dosing regimen is as follows:

■ **Gentamicin,** 5 mg/kg DW (round to nearest 50 mg)
■ **Tobramycin,** 5 mg/kg DW (round to nearest 50 mg)
■ **Amikacin,** 15 mg/kg DW (round to nearest 100 mg)

○ Therapeutic monitoring can be either based on easily available nomogram-based dosing or by individualized monitoring.

○ For nomogram-based monitoring, a single serum concentration is obtained 6 to 14 hours after the first dose and then further doses are adjusted based on nomogram.

TABLE 24-8 AMINOGLYCOSIDE MAINTENANCE DOSE CALCULATION

CrCl (mL/min)	Maintenance Dose	Maintenance Interval
>90	100% of loading dose	q12 h
80–90	92% of loading dose	q12 h
70–79	88% of loading dose	q12 h
60–69	84% of loading dose	q12 h
50–59	79% of loading dose	q12 h
40–49	92% of loading dose	q24 h
30–39	86% of loading dose	q24 h
<30	Give loading dose and draw a random level 24 hrs after the loading dose; initiation of the maintenance dose should not start until the result of the 24-hr random level is known	

TABLE 24-9 AMINOGLYCOSIDE THERAPEUTIC MONITORING

Indication	Gentamicin/Tobramycin	Amikacin
	Trough	
	<1 mcg/mL	<4 mcg/mL
	Peak	
Gram-positive coccus infection Endovascular infection Urinary tract infection	3–5 mcg/mL	10–15 mcg/mL
Bone/joint infection Skin/skin structure infection	6–8 mcg/mL	20–25 mcg/mL
Septic shock Febrile neutropenia Gram-negative rod bacteremia Pneumonia Cystic fibrosis Intra-abdominal infection Central nervous system infection	8–10 mcg/mL	25–30 mcg/mL

- ○ Alternatively, peak serum aminoglycoside concentration obtained 1 hour after the dose and a level 6 to 12 hours later can be used to adjust dosing.
- ○ It is strongly recommended that aminoglycoside dosing be done with the assistance of clinical pharmacists.
- **Dialysis patients**
  - ○ Dosing frequency and monitoring levels depend on the clearance of the dialyzer and residual renal function.
  - ○ Aminoglycosides are extensively cleared during hemodialysis and continuous RRTs and close monitoring of drug levels are required to guide appropriate dosing.
  - ○ For patients on hemodialysis, aminoglycosides have to be redosed after each session.

Vancomycin
- The typical dosing regimen is 15 mg/kg every 12 hours, based on actual body weight and renal function.
- For patients with impaired renal function, a suggested initial dosing regimen is shown in Table 24-10.

TABLE 24-10 INITIAL SUGGESTED VANCOMYCIN DOSING REGIMEN

CrCl (mL/min)	Suggested Regimen	Monitoring Levels
>90		
Age ≤35 yrs	15 mg/kg q8 h	Draw trough level prior to the 4th dose
Age >35 yrs	15 mg/kg q12 h	
50–90	15 mg/kg q12 h	Draw trough level prior to the 4th dose
30–49	15 mg/kg q24 h	Draw trough level prior to the 3rd dose
<30	15 mg/kg × 1	Draw random level 24 hrs later

CrCl, creatinine clearance.

- Frequent monitoring of vancomycin levels is indicated if concomitant nephrotoxic or ototoxic agents are being used, if there is changing renal function, suboptimal response to therapy, hemodynamic instability, or extremes of body weight.
- Trough levels (every 4 to 7 days) are recommended in patients receiving longer courses of therapy (>5 days) to ensure that concentrations are adequate but not excessive.
- Desired trough levels are 10 to 15 mg/L for skin and soft tissue infections and 15 to 20 mg/L for bloodstream, bone, lung, or central nervous system infections.[10]
- **Dialysis patients**
  - Dosing frequency and monitoring levels depend on the clearance of the dialyzer being used and residual renal function.[11]
  - Pre-hemodialysis levels should be between 20 and 30 mg/L to ensure adequate drug levels post-dialysis.

Antiretrovirals
- Many antiretrovirals agents are renally eliminated and require dose adjustment.
- Antiretrovirals that require dose reductions or should be avoided in different degrees of renal dysfunction (including hemodialysis) are atazanavir, cobicistat, didanosine, emtricitabine, lamivudine, stavudine, tenofovir disoproxil fumarate, tenofovir alafenamide, and zidovudine.
- Combination products that contain the individual components should be avoided as well.

DOSAGE ADJUSTMENTS DURING RENAL REPLACEMENT THERAPY

- There are different modalities used for RRT in the setting of AKI or ESRD. These modalities are described elsewhere in this book.[2]
- In addition to removing nitrogenous and other waste products that accumulate in renal failure, they also remove drugs and active metabolites.
- The efficiency with which each procedure removes drugs from the body depends on many factors:
  - Drug characteristics (molecular weight, plasma protein binding, volume of distribution).
  - The dialyzer (membrane type, surface area, thickness).
  - Geometry of the dialysis system (countercurrent or concurrent blood and dialysate flow).
  - Dialysis conditions (blood and dialysate flow rates, duration of dialysis treatment).
  - Types of RRT, that is, intermittent hemodialysis, continuous RRT, and sustained low-efficiency dialysis.
- For medication dosing, careful consideration needs to be taken to replace drug lost, based on an estimation of the amount removed.
- There will be situations in which a clinician is unable to find any information about the removal of a medication based on the type of RRT being utilized. Here, the assessment of the drug characteristics will be important to determine the possible dialyzability of the medication.
  - A large molecular size may prevent the drug from passing across the membrane (e.g., erythropoietin alpha).
  - If a drug is highly bound to serum proteins (>90%), it will not pass across the membrane because only free, unbound drug will cross (e.g., ceftriaxone).
  - Hydrophobic drugs are not readily dialyzed (e.g., carbamazepine).
  - Drugs with large V_d are minimally dialyzed (e.g., digoxin).

REFERENCES

1. Lea-Henry TN, Carland JE, Stocker SL, et al. Clinical pharmacokinetics in kidney disease: fundamental principles. *Clin J Am Soc Nephrol.* 2018;13:1085–1095.
2. Roberts DM, Sevastos J, Carland JE, et al. Clinical pharmacokinetics in kidney disease: application to rational design of dosing regimens. *Clin J Am Soc Nephrol.* 2018;13:1254–1263.
3. Burnett AE, Mahan CE, Vazquez SR, et al. Guidance for the practical management of the direct oral anticoagulants (DOACs) in VTE treatment. *J Thromb Thrombolysis.* 2016;41:206–232.
4. Dixit M, Doan T, Kirschner R, et al. Significant acute kidney injury due to non-steroidal anti-inflammatory drugs: inpatient setting. *Pharmaceuticals (Basel).* 2010;3:1279–1285.
5. Sica DA. Diuretic use in renal disease. *Nat Rev Nephrol.* 2011;8:100–109.
6. Juurlink DN, Mamdani MM, Lee DS, et al. Rates of hyperkalemia after publication of the Randomized Aldactone Evaluation Study. *N Engl J Med.* 2004;351:543–551.
7. Inzucchi SE, Lipska KJ, Mayo H, et al. Metformin in patients with type 2 diabetes and kidney disease: a systematic review. *JAMA.* 2014;312:2668–2675.
8. Destache CJ. Aminoglycoside-induced nephrotoxicity—a focus on monitoring: a review of literature. *J Pharm Pract.* 2014;27:562–566.
9. Wargo KA, Edwards JD. Aminoglycoside-induced nephrotoxicity. *J Pharm Pract.* 2014;27:573–577.
10. Lomaestro BM. Vancomycin dosing and monitoring 2 years after the guidelines. *Expert Rev Anti Infect Ther.* 2011;9:657–667.
11. Vandecasteele SJ, De Vriese AS. Vancomycin dosing in patients on intermittent hemodialysis. *Semin Dial.* 2011;24:50–55.

Overview of Kidney Transplantation

25

Rowena Delos Santos

GENERAL PRINCIPLES

- Over 500,000 people in the United States have end-stage renal disease (ESRD), with over 100,000 new cases of ESRD yearly.[1]
- Treatment options for ESRD include hemodialysis, peritoneal dialysis, and kidney transplantation.
- **For most patients, renal transplantation is the preferred treatment for ESRD** after careful evaluation of those patients, as it improves quality of life as well as quantity of life compared with those who remain on dialysis.[2]
- These improvements in patient outcomes accompanied by the limited supply of organs have resulted in a remarkable increase in the number of patients on the waiting list for kidney transplant.
- Approximately 100,000 people are currently listed on the kidney transplant waiting list.[3]
- Highest growth of waitlisted patients is among those aged 65 to 74, with the proportion on the waitlist of approximately 22%.[4]
- The percentage of elderly patients (age ≥65) increased from 14.5% in 2005 to reach 22% in 2015.
- A third of the patients on the waiting list are African Americans and a third are Caucasians. More Hispanics were listed in 2015 (19,188 patients) compared to 2005 (10,254 patients), which represents 20% of patients in 2015 compared to 17% in 2005.
- Diabetes and hypertension are the top two diseases leading to ESRD in those who are awaiting a kidney transplant.[4]
- Indications for kidney transplant include ESRD and irreversible kidney disease with an estimated glomerular filtration rate (eGFR) ≤20 mL/min.
- Approximately 17,000 patients receive a kidney transplant annually. Roughly two-thirds of kidneys transplanted are from deceased donors, and one-third from living donors.[4]
- Wait times for a kidney transplant can vary due to ABO blood type and history of sensitization. Median wait time on the deceased donor waitlist for a patient listed for the first time is approximately 3.5 years.[1] Wait times are longer for blood type O and B patients.
- When other solid organs are affected by their own irreversible damage, then combined organ transplant is a consideration (i.e., heart–kidney for irreversible cardiomyopathy, liver–kidney for primary oxalosis, and kidney–pancreas for type 1 diabetes mellitus).
- Due to the renal side effects of chronic calcineurin inhibitor use for prevention of rejection, some people who have had other solid organ transplants may eventually require a kidney transplant.
- Preemptive transplants (transplanted before need for dialysis) are recommended when possible.

TRANSPLANT AND OUTCOMES

- As of 2015, the number of people alive with a functioning kidney allograft was over 200,000.[4]
- One-year allograft survival rates for living and deceased donor kidney transplants were 98% and 94%, respectively in 2015.
- One-year patient survival rates in 2015 were 99% for living donor kidney recipients and 97% for deceased donor kWWWWidney recipients.[1]
- Five-year allograft survival was the lowest for those whose cause of renal disease was diabetes or hypertension (approximately 70% graft survival for each).[4]
- Ten-year allograft failure rates were better among those who received a living donor kidney compared with those who received a deceased donor kidney (47% vs. 63%).[4]
- Transplant allograft median survival for a deceased donor kidney transplant has reached 9 years, while the median survival for a living donor kidney transplant has reached nearly 13 years.[3]
- Early graft loss is usually referred to graft loss in the first 12 months post-transplant. Early graft loss is largely due to technical failures, surgical compilations, primary non-function, severe rejection, or severe recurrent glomerulonephritis (e.g., recurrent focal segmental glomerulosclerosis).
- Beyond the first year, the most common reason for allograft failure is death with allograft function, with patients usually dying from cardiovascular disease, cerebrovascular disease, malignancy, or infection.
- The incidence of acute rejection within the first year decreased for both living and deceased donor transplant recipients from 10% in 2009–2010 recipients to 7.9% in 2013–2014 recipients.
- In a greater proportion of acute rejection episodes, renal function did not return after treatment to pre-rejection baseline values, and this was associated with an incremental increase in the relative hazard for graft survival.

WAITLIST MANAGEMENT

- Patients listed for transplant wait several years before they receive a deceased donor kidney transplant. Periodic review of waitlisted patients should occur including: any new medical diagnoses, hospitalizations, overall functional status, and new medications. Retesting is also done periodically depending on center protocols.
- Blood transfusions should be avoided due to the risk of human leukocyte antigen (HLA) sensitization; if required, leukocyte-depleted blood should be given.
- Immunizations for pneumococcus, influenza, hepatitis B, and varicella should be given prior to transplantation. Live vaccines are avoided after transplant due to the risk of leading to active disease.

IMMUNOLOGY OF TRANSPLANT

Human Leukocyte Antigen/Major Histocompatibility Complex

- HLA or major histocompatibility complex (MHC) genes encode for molecules that define self and the combination of them on cell surfaces differs between individuals.
- Genes that encode for HLA are on chromosome 6.
- HLA class I molecules encode for HLA A, B, C and are found on all nucleated cells.
- HLA class II molecules encode for HLA DR, DQ, DP and are found on antigen-presenting cells (e.g., B cells, macrophages, and dendritic cells).

- HLA molecules all have a peptide-binding groove, immunoglobulin-like region, transmembrane, and intracytoplasmic region. The peptide-binding region is where molecules of self or a foreign antigen are presented to T cells.
- Individuals inherit one set, or haplotype, of HLA class I and class II from each parent. The HLA genes (genotype) then encode for the HLA molecules located on the surface of cells (phenotype).
- High genetic variability of HLA and subsequently the peptide-binding area between individuals leads to uniqueness between individuals.
- Because siblings inherit one haplotype of HLA from each parent, there is a $1 - (0.75)^n$ probability that siblings could be a 2-haplotype match or HLA identical (i.e., possess the same set of HLA genes).
- Once T cells recognize foreign HLA, they can activate other T cells and B cells to incite an immune response. T cells are involved in cellular rejection; B cells are involved in antibody-mediated rejection.

Antigen Presentation by HLA Molecules to Cells of the Immune System

- Antigen-presenting cells include B cells, macrophages, and dendritic cells.
- T cells are activated either through a direct or indirect pathway (Fig. 25-1).
- The direct pathway is where donor antigen–presenting cells in the allograft circulate through the blood stream of the recipient early after transplant and present donor HLA to recipient T cells.
- The indirect pathway is where recipient donor antigen–presenting cells take up and process donor HLA peptides, then present the donor HLA peptides to recipient T cells.

HLA Typing

- Designation of HLA is through letters and numbers (e.g., HLA A2, B7, DR4).
- Determination of HLA type is done by several methods.
  ○ Sequence-specific oligonucleotide (SSO): DNA is extracted from cells, the target gene undergoes polymerase chain reaction (PCR) amplification, then is hybridized to oligonucleotide probes, which go through flow cytometry, and results in HLA type.

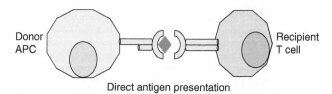

Direct antigen presentation

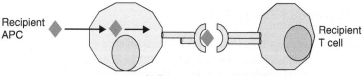

Indirect antigen presentation

◆ = donor HLA peptides

FIGURE 25-1. Donor antigen presentation to recipient cells.

○ Sequence-specific primers (SSP): DNA is extracted from cells, the target gene undergoes PCR amplification with sequence-specific primers for specific HLA, then goes through gel electrophoresis, which allows detection of HLA specificities due to known gene lengths.

• SSO and SSP provide the basic HLA designation; to get a more specific designation, sequence-based typing is done.

HLA Donor and Recipient Matching

• HLA matching is an important component of allograft survival for kidney transplantation.

• Best allograft survival is seen in 2-haplotype living-related kidney transplants, with lower survival for less well-matched living donor kidneys. Deceased donor kidneys have lower survival compared to living donor kidneys, and better-matched kidneys have higher survival compared to less well-matched kidneys (Fig. 25-2).

• For kidney transplantation, HLA A, B, and DR matching are most important. Since there are two genes each, one can match for a total of 6 HLA, best 0/6 mismatched, worst 6/6 mismatched (Fig. 25-3).

Barriers to Transplantation

• ABO compatibility is a barrier to transplant—if blood types are incompatible, transplantation is not usually done.

• Preformed HLA antibodies against a potential kidney allograft are a barrier to transplant as antibodies can lead to significant kidney allograft rejection.

• Preformed anti-HLA antibodies arise as a result of sensitization events including blood transfusions, pregnancy, and previous transplantation.

• ABO incompatibility and presence of preformed antibodies can be overcome, but is usually done at select centers with expertise in the process. This usually requires plasmapheresis

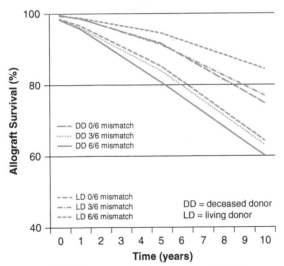

Data from: Health Resources Services Administration, U.S. Department of Health and Human Services. Organ Procurement and Transplantation Network/Scientific Registry of Transplant Patients 2010 Annual Data Report

FIGURE 25-2. Kidney allograft survival according to HLA mismatch.

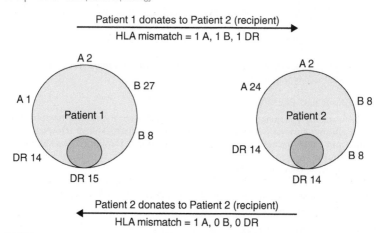

Patient 1 donates to Patient 2 (recipient)
HLA mismatch = 1 A, 1 B, 1 DR

Patient 2 donates to Patient 2 (recipient)
HLA mismatch = 1 A, 0 B, 0 DR

FIGURE 25-3. Principle of donor recipient mismatched antigens.

and administration of rituximab (monoclonal antibody against B-lymphocyte CD20) and intravenous immunoglobulin (IVIG) prior to transplantation.

Histocompatibility Testing for Kidney Transplantation

- Recipients and donors undergo HLA typing as described prior to transplantation.
- Other testing is done to determine the degree of sensitization and compatibility between kidney donor and recipient. The goal of these tests is to determine the existence of pre-formed anti-HLA antibodies against potential donors, which either precludes transplant or significantly increases the risk of allograft rejection.
- Testing for compatibility involves both serologic and solid phase methods (Table 25-1).
  - Serologic methods include complement-dependent cytotoxicity (CDC) testing with or without antihuman globulin.
  - Solid phase methods include enzyme-linked immunosorbent assay (ELISA), flow cytometry, and single antigen beads.
- Serologic methods are more specific while solid phase methods are more sensitive in detecting anti-HLA antibodies in recipient serum.

Serologic Methods for Compatibility Testing

- CDC testing is also known as NIH standard crossmatch.
- CDC crossmatch involves taking live donor cells which have HLA on the surface and mixing those cells with recipient sera which may or may not contain anti-HLA

TABLE 25-1	HISTOCOMPATIBILITY METHODS FOR KIDNEY TRANSPLANT
Serologic Testing	**Solid Phase Testing**
Complement-dependent cytotoxicity (CDC)	Enzyme-linked immunosorbent assay (ELISA)
Antihuman globulin-enhanced CDC	Flow cytometry
	Single/multiple antigen beads

antibodies. After an incubation period with complement, formalin and eosin are added to help determine if a reaction has occurred. If an antigen/antibody reaction has occurred in the presence of complement, then one sees dead cells and consequently, the donor–recipient is not a match (Fig. 25-4). The CDC crossmatch is the least sensitive of all tests but it is the most specific. It is performed for both T and B lymphocytes. B-cell crossmatch is done because it can detect both anti-class I and anti-class II antibodies, and it can detect anti-class I antibodies when the standard crossmatch is negative.

- Adding antihuman globulin to the CDC crossmatch improves sensitivity, particularly for antibodies that are present in smaller amounts, or are noncomplement binding. If this test is positive, similarly the donor–recipient pair should not undergo transplant. It is performed for both T and B lymphocytes.
- Panel-reactive antibody (PRA) represents the breadth of antibodies against HLA for an individual. This number represents the percentage of the overall population that a person is sensitized against and cannot receive a kidney transplant due to a high risk for rejection. Generally, the higher the percentage of the PRA, the harder it would be to find a match for this individual. This can be performed using CDC method or solid phase methods described below.

Solid Phase Methods for Compatibility Testing

- Solid phase methods have higher sensitivity than the CDC-based methods and are performed for T and B lymphocytes.
- Flow cytometry is used to perform compatibility testing.
- Flow PRA: Purified HLA molecules are placed onto the surface of solid surfaces, such as latex bead (Fig. 25-5).
  - HLA antigen–coated beads are incubated with patient serum and with anti-IgG attached to fluorescein isothiocyanate.
  - Laser-activated fluorochromes emit light which is detected by the machine and counted. The number of beads detected and intensity indicates the PRA.
- Flow crossmatch is done similar to the above, except instead of beads, actual donor cells are used.
  - Donor cells are incubated with patient serum and fluorochrome-tagged anti-IgG.
  - Laser-activated fluorochromes emit light when attached to anti-HLA antibodies from the recipient and the number of beads and intensity of the light leads to flow crossmatch results for both T and B cells. The resulting number is compared to positive and negative controls, and a positive test is determined by the center's cutoff points.
  - Due to the higher sensitivity of the test, the machine will be able to detect even small amounts of anti-HLA antibodies, which may or may not lead to an immune response after transplant.
  - In addition, there can be false-positive testing if a patient has autoantibodies or binding of non-HLA antibodies to other molecules on the cell surface of the lymphocytes. False-positive testing is unlikely to lead to an immune response.
- An advantage of flow crossmatch over CDC crossmatch is that CDC crossmatch requires live cells to perform the test, whereas a flow crossmatch can use live or dead cells. This can be useful if, during transportation of donor material, the lymphocytes die en route.
- Detection of donor-specific antibodies (DSA)
  - Single antigen–coated beads representing a multitude of HLA are used to detect donor-specific antibody (Fig. 25-5). Each bead has its own intrinsic color.
  - When incubated with patient serum and with fluorochrome-tagged antihuman antibody and run through a Luminex machine, the laser will detect both the intrinsic color of each bead that has antibody as well as the intensity of the antibody on the bead.

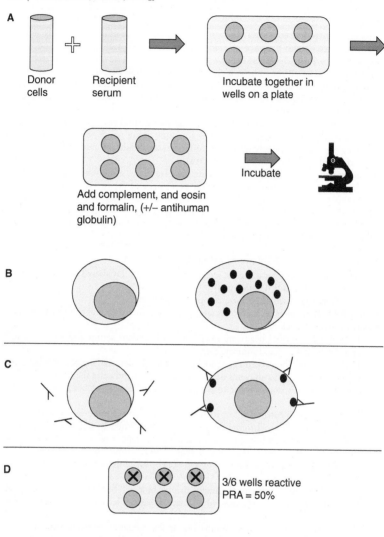

- This results in both the antigen specificity and the level of antibody present, indicated by the mean fluorescence intensity (MFI). The MFI indicates the level of antibody present.
- Antibody levels can decrease over time, and when a reintroduction of antigen occurs, can increase significantly, potentially leading to rejection.
- Depending on a center's cutoff for MFI, the center may decline potential donor kidneys for a patient if they believe that the level of antibody would lead to an unacceptable increased risk of graft rejection.
- Once a determination of unacceptable HLA is made for a patient, then these unacceptable antigens are reported to United Network of Organ Sharing (UNOS) so that donor organs with the unacceptable HLA are not offered to the recipient. Once unacceptable HLA are

FIGURE 25-4. Cytotoxic-dependent crossmatch (CDC/NIH crossmatch). Panel A: Donor cells have on their cell surface HLA antigen. Recipient serum contains antibody which may or may not be reactive to donor HLA. The donor cells and recipient serum are mixed together and incubated. After an incubation period, complement is added, as well as eosin and formalin to fix so that after another incubation period, the cells can be evaluated under a microscope. Panel B: On the **left** represents what cells would look like before the test is complete in panel A. These cells are live, small, and intact. On the **right**, what cells would look like after the test is complete in panel A. These cells are dead, will appear larger, swollen with small punched-out holes on the cell surface from the activation of complement system due to the antibody–antigen reaction between the recipient antibodies in the serum and the antigen on the donor cell surfaces. Panel C: On the **left** illustrates the live intact cell with antibody surrounding it but no complement activation. Though there are antibodies present from the recipient, they are not interacting with recipient cell surface HLA antigen. On the **right** shows the donor cell surface with attached recipient antibody, which leads to complement activation and cell death. Panel D: The panel-reactive antibody (PRA) test is not a crossmatch test. However, the PRA test can be performed using the same technique as the CDC crossmatch. The difference is that instead of one donor's cells in all the wells, each single well contains cells from one donor, so that the plate of wells provides a multitude of donors with many different possible HLA. When the test is complete, there will be a certain number of wells with dead cells. The percentage of reactive wells (wells with dead cells) is the percent PRA—the percent of the population that the recipient is sensitized and cannot receive a donor kidney. In this case, 3/6 of the wells have dead cells, depicted by the "*X*" resulting in a PRA 50%. NOTE: To increase sensitivity of the CDC test, antihuman globulin can be added during the later incubation period.

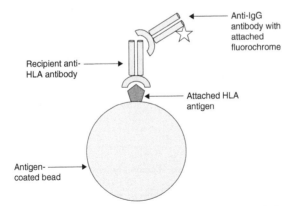

FIGURE 25-5. Depiction of solid phase testing. Solid phase testing is based on using beads that have purified HLA on the bead surface. These HLA can be to a single HLA (single antigen beads) or to multiple HLA. These beads are mixed with recipient serum and subsequently fluorochrome-tagged anti-IgG, and run through the flow or Luminex machine. This machine will detect the HLA antibody and the level of that antibody present in the recipient serum.

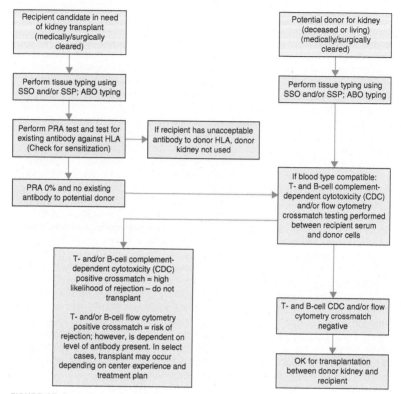

FIGURE 25-6. Compatibility and crossmatch testing flow diagram for recipient and donor prior to kidney transplant.

reported to UNOS, then a calculated PRA (cPRA) is generated from both the HLA identified and the frequency of the antigen in the population.[5] If the cPRA is a high number, this provides the patient additional points on the waitlist according to a sliding scale.

- The steps for both recipient and donor in compatibility and crossmatch testing prior to a kidney transplant are shown in Figure 25-6.

ALLOCATION OF KIDNEYS

- On December 4, 2014, a new kidney allocation system (KAS) was implemented in the United States.
- The goals of KAS were to improve equitable access to kidney transplants for those who were highly sensitized or were on dialysis the longest and to improve organ utilization through longevity matching but also having the least impact on the rest of the waitlisted patients.
- Key changes to the allocation system included:
  - Development of the Kidney Donor Profile Index (KDPI) based on key donor characteristics (Table 25-2). KDPI is calculated using 10 factors, resulting in a number 1% to 100%. The lower the number, the better quality kidney for donation.[6]

TABLE 25-2	DONOR CHARACTERISTICS IN THE KIDNEY DONOR PROFILE INDEX (KDPI)
Age	**Height**
Ethnicity (African American)	Weight
Creatinine	Donor status (DCD)
History of diabetes	HCV
History of hypertension	Cause of death (CVA)

CVA, cerebrovascular accident; DCD, donation after cardiac death.

- ○ Development of Estimated Post Transplant Survival (EPTS) score derived from four recipient characteristics (Table 25-3). Resulting number is between 1 and 100.[7]
- ○ With longevity matching, kidneys with lower KDPIs (1% to 20%) would be matched with recipients with lower EPTS scores (1% to 20%). Those who are expected to live the longest would be matched with kidneys that are thought to have the longest graft survival.
- ○ Wait time accrual begins at the time of listing, if not on dialysis. For those on dialysis, wait time begins at the initiation of dialysis.
- ○ KAS created a sliding scale of extra points that would be given to those with high calculated panel-reactive antibodies (range 0% to 100%).
- ○ As with the previous KAS, children received extra points, as do those who have matching HLA DR, as well as those who are previous live kidney donors.
- ○ Patients with antibodies against HLA had a low transplantation rate. To enhance the chances of finding a matching kidney, a sliding scale of increasing allocation points for increasing sensitization was established. Candidates with cPRA scores of 98%, 99%, and 100% receive 24.4, 50.1, and 202.1 points, respectively.[8]
- ○ Waiting times for blood type B candidates are much longer than waiting times for blood type A candidates. Blood type A2 and A2B kidneys are now offered to type B candidates at transplant programs willing to accept such organs.
- ○ Estimated allograft half-life with the new KAS is 12.5 years for kidneys from living donors, 11.4 years for kidneys with KDPI 1% to 20%, 8.9 years for kidneys of donors with KDPI 21% to 85%, and 5.6 years for kidneys with KDPI 86% to 100%.[6]
- Results of the new KAS[9]:
  - ○ The new KAS led to more patients with higher cPRA getting transplanted, which tapered after an initial bolus of patients was transplanted.
  - ○ It also led to more transplants among those patients who have been on dialysis the longest, which also tapered after an initial bolus of patients were transplanted.
  - ○ With the new KAS, there were more patients being transplanted in the younger age groups (18 to 49 years old) compared with prior.

TABLE 25-3	RECIPIENT CHARACTERISTICS IN THE ESTIMATED POST TRANSPLANT SURVIVAL (EPTS) SCORE

Age
Current diagnosis of diabetes mellitus
History of prior solid organ transplant
Time since starting dialysis

○ The downsides to the new KAS included more kidneys being transported outside their original procurement area to other states, higher cold ischemia times, and higher rates of delayed graft function.

○ The new KAS did not lead to lower discard rates for kidneys.

KIDNEY DONOR TYPES

- With donation after brain death (DBD) there is donor brain death but cardiopulmonary systems still functional; the vast majority of kidneys are donated this way.[10]
- With donation after cardiac death (DCD), the donors are those who suffered cardiac arrest after withdrawal of support (controlled DCD) or expired on arrival to the hospital with or without successful resuscitation (uncontrolled DCD). A smaller percentage of kidneys are donated this way. These DCD kidneys have a higher risk for delayed graft function but overall graft survival comparable to DBD kidneys.
- As of 2015, 82% of the kidneys were procured from DBD donors. However, the 18% use of DCD donors in 2015 represents an increase of 10% from 2005.
- A living related kidney comes from a family member such as mother, father, or sibling.
- A living unrelated kidney comes from nonblood relation such as friends, spouse, or anonymous.
- Live-donor transplantation is preferable to deceased donor transplantation as it is associated with superior long-term patient and graft survivals.
- In the last couple of years, the living donation rate has stabilized around 5600 donations/yr.
- Transplant of dual marginal kidneys is an option if the GFR of one kidney is thought not to provide adequate function.
- En bloc kidneys usually are procured together with vena cava and aorta as they come from very young donors. The donor cava and aorta are anastomosed to the recipients' vessels. Care must be taken not to allow the renal artery to torse.

SPECIAL POPULATIONS FOR TRANSPLANT

- Paired exchanged kidneys: Donor kidneys are exchanged between different donor–recipient pairs if the pairs are unable to be matched due to ABO incompatibility or positive crossmatch from HLA antibodies.
- ABO incompatible donor–recipient pair can be transplanted. The recipient receives additional treatment consisting of rituximab, plasmapheresis, IV immunoglobulin to decrease the isoagglutinin titer against the donor blood type, thus allowing transplant.
- Crossmatch-positive transplants can be transplanted at specific centers. Additional treatments such as rituximab, plasmapheresis, and IV immunoglobulin are performed on the recipient in preparation for transplant. These treatments are meant to eventually lead to a negative crossmatch between donor–recipient pair. In addition, immunosuppression doses may be higher for the recipient, who will need close follow-up to ensure no rejection occurs.
- Hepatitis C virus (HCV)-positive donor kidneys can be transplanted into HCV-positive recipients. Assuming the donor kidney has no renal disease, these kidneys have comparable graft and patient outcomes to HCV-negative donor kidneys. Additionally, recipients can be treated with newer HCV medications that can eradicate the virus post-transplant.
- HIV-positive patients are transplanted at select centers if they have an undetectable viral load and CD4 count >200 cells/μL while taking antiretroviral medications. Special evaluation is needed for malignancy and opportunistic infections in this population.

RECIPIENT AND DONOR EVALUATION FOR TRANSPLANT

- Both recipient and donor evaluations for transplantation are reviewed in detail in later chapters.
- Living donation is an elective surgery. The goal of the thorough evaluation for a donor is to determine adequate renal function for donation, no comorbidities that would preclude donation, and surgical suitability for donation.
- Recipients undergo a thorough evaluation prior to undergoing a kidney transplant. The goal of the evaluation is to determine there are no medical or surgical conditions that will prevent transplantation. Even after listing for transplant, patients will also be periodically evaluated to ensure no changes to their medical/surgical conditions have changed.

ABSOLUTE AND RELATIVE CONTRAINDICATIONS FOR TRANSPLANT

- Among the absolute contraindications to kidney transplant include active untreated malignancy, acute infection, positive T-cell cytotoxic crossmatch (Table 25-4).
- Among the relative contraindications to kidney transplant include advanced cardiopulmonary disease, extensive peripheral vascular disease, known history of noncompliance, ABO blood type incompatibility (Table 25-4).
- The risk of the likelihood of primary renal disease recurrence in the kidney allograft must be thoroughly discussed with patient. None of the described renal diseases are currently considered a contraindication to transplant.
- Evaluation of the kidney transplant candidate and donor are discussed in Chapter 26.

TABLE 25-4	ABSOLUTE AND RELATIVE CONTRAINDICATIONS FOR KIDNEY TRANSPLANT
Absolute Contraindications	**Relative Contraindications[a]**
Active, untreated, or metastatic malignancy	Advanced cardiopulmonary disease
Acute untreated infection	Extensive peripheral vascular disease
Clinically active immunologic disease leading to renal failure (i.e., lupus or vasculitis)	Severe chronic liver disease (may consider combined liver–kidney transplant)
Active substance abuse	Uncontrolled psychiatric disorder that could affect compliance
Positive T-cell cytotoxic crossmatch	Debilitating cerebrovascular disease
Reversible renal disease	History of malignancy
Well-documented treatment/medication noncompliance	Morbid obesity
	Severe malnutrition
	Estimated life span less than 5 years

[a]May vary from center to center.

TRANSPLANT SURGICAL PROCEDURE

- Most kidneys are placed extraperitoneally.
- Rutherford Morison or Gibson incision made in the right or left lower quadrant.
- Anterior rectus sheath and external oblique muscle are cut; the rectus muscle is retracted medially.
- The inferior epigastric artery and vein are exposed then ligated and divided.
- If males, the spermatic cord is moved out of the dissection area and preserved.
- Peritoneum is freed from transversus abdominis; the external oblique, internal oblique, and transversus muscles are incised.
- Lymphatics are ligated and divided; the external and internal iliac vessels are exposed.
- The bladder is prepared, including creation of submucosal tunnel for ureter anastomosis.
- The kidney allograft is prepared, including separation of the artery and vein and removal of excess tissue but leaving mesentery with the ureter.
- The donor renal artery and vein are anastomosed to recipient external iliac artery and vein.
- The donor ureter is anastomosed to the bladder (ureteroneocystostomy) using a submucosal tunnel as an antireflux mechanism. If the bladder is unable to be used for anastomosis, a ureteroureterostomy is created.
- Finally, the surgical site is closed.
- See Chapter 30 for surgical complications after transplant and Chapter 29 for immunologic complications after transplant.

REFERENCES

1. U.S. Renal Data System. *USRDS 2016 Annual Data Report: Atlas of Chronic Kidney Disease and End-Stage Renal Disease in the United States.* Bethesda, MD: National Institutes of Health, National Institute of Diabetes and Digestive and Kidney Diseases; 2016.
2. Wolfe RA, Ashby VB, Milford EL, et al. Comparison of mortality in all patients on dialysis, patients on dialysis awaiting transplantation, and recipients of a first cadaveric transplant. *N Engl J Med.* 1999;341:1725–1730.
3. Hart A, Smith JM, Skeans MA, et al. OPTN/SRTR 2017 Annual Data Report: Kidney. *Am J Transplant.* 2019;19:19–123.
4. Hart A, Smith JM, Skeans MA, et al. OPTN/SRTR 2015 Annual Report: Kidney. *Am J Transplant.* 2017;17:21–116.
5. United Network for Organ Sharing, U.S. Department of Health and Human Services, Health Resources and Services Administration. *CPRA Calculator.* Available at https://optn.transplant.hrsa.gov/resources/allocation-calculators/cpra-calculator. Accessed June 10, 2019.
6. Organ Procurement and Transplantation Network, U.S. Department of Health and Human Services, Health Resources and Services Administration. *Kidney Donor Profile Index.* Available at https://optn.transplant.hrsa.gov/resources/guidance/kidney-donor-profile-index-kdpi-guide-for-clinicians. Accessed June 10, 2019.
7. Organ Procurement and Transplantation Network, U.S. Department of Health and Human Services, Health Resources and Services Administration. *EPTS Calculator.* Available at https://optn.transplant.hrsa.gov/resources/allocation-calculators/epts-calculator. Accessed June 10, 2019.
8. Formica R, Aeder M; Organ Procurement and Transplantation Network. The new kidney allocation system: resources for protocols and procedures. Available at https://www.transplantpro.org/wp-content/uploads/sites/3/KAS_Protocols_Processes_Slides_Script.pdf. Accessed June 10, 2019.
9. Stewart DE, Kucheryavaya AY, Klassen DK, et al. Changes in deceased donor kidney transplantation one year after KAS implementation. *Am J Transplant.* 2016;16:1834–1847.
10. Rao PS, Ojo A. The alphabet soup of kidney transplantation: SCD, DCD, ECD—fundamentals for the practicing nephrologist. *Clin J Am Soc Nephrol.* 2009;4:1827–1831.

Evaluation of the Kidney Transplant Candidate

26

Sreelatha Katari

GENERAL PRINCIPLES

- Kidney transplantation improves patient survival and quality of life and reduces the total cost of medical care compared to dialysis.
- Selection of the proper transplant candidate remains a challenge due to the presence of complex medical issues and ever-increasing disparity between donor organ supply and demand.
- The transplant evaluation process includes a comprehensive assessment of patient's motivation, perioperative risk, medical history including risk of kidney disease recurrence, cardiac disease, vascular disease, infection, cancer, liver disease, gastrointestinal disease, obesity, diabetes mellitus, coagulopathy, surgical history including urinary tract abnormalities, and psychosocial situation (Table 26-1).
- In general, candidates should have a projected life expectancy exceeding 7 years.
- The initial general evaluation begins with a thorough history and physical examination, a complete blood count, chemistry panel, and coagulation studies. Other tests including blood type, serologic testing for human immunodeficiency virus (HIV), cytomegalovirus (CMV), varicella zoster virus (VZV), herpes simplex virus (HSV), Epstein–Barr virus (EBV), hepatitis B and C, and rapid plasma regain (RPR) are all essential. Immunologic testing of human leukocyte antigens (HLA) and panel reactive antibodies (PRA) of the transplant recipients is important. Other recommended testing includes ECG, chest radiograph, imaging of the kidneys, and age-appropriate cancer screening (Table 26-2).[1]
- Immunologic testing is done to assess sensitization or presence of preformed anti-HLA antibodies which can arise from prior transplantation, pregnancy, or blood transfusions.
- For details regarding HLA, PRA, and cross-match, refer to Chapter 25, Overview of Kidney Transplantation.
- Kidney transplantation should not be pursued in cases where limited life expectancy minimizes potential benefit of transplant if psychosocial barriers for posttransplant compliance exist.
- Absolute contraindications to kidney transplant are listed in Table 26-3.
- Patients with end-stage renal disease (ESRD) and other end-stage organ failure may be candidates for combined organ transplantation (e.g., kidney-liver if cirrhosis or primary

TABLE 26-1	COMPONENTS OF THE ASSESSMENT OF RENAL TRANSPLANT CANDIDATE EVALUATION
Assessment of motivation	Liver disease
Perioperative risk	Gastrointestinal disease
Recurrent disease	Obesity
Heart disease	Diabetes mellitus
Vascular disease	Coagulopathy
Infection	Age
Cancer	Psychosocial situation and support

TABLE 26-2 INITIAL TRANSPLANT CANDIDATE WORKUP

Laboratory evaluation
CMP
CBC with differential
Serologies: HIV, hepatitis B and C, CMV, EBV, HSV, RPR
PT/INR, aPTT
Urinalysis, urine culture
Blood group and cross-matching
HLA typing and HLA antibodies

Diagnostic/imaging studies
ECG
Chest radiography
Abdominal ultrasound to evaluate for gallstones in diabetes
Renal ultrasound to screen for acquired cystic disease or mass in native kidneys

Cancer screening
Colonoscopy if >50 yrs of age
Pap smear
Mammogram for women >40 yrs of age or with family history of breast cancer
PSA in men >50 yrs of age

CMP, complete metabolic panel; CBC, complete blood count; HIV, human immunodeficiency virus; CMV, cytomegalovirus; EBV, Epstein–Barr virus; HSV, herpes simplex virus; RPR, rapid plasma reagin; PT, prothrombin time; INR, international normalized ratio; aPTT, activated partial thromboplastin time; HLA, human leukocyte antigen; PSA, prostate-specific antigen.

hyperoxaluria, kidney-pancreas if type 1 diabetes mellitus, kidney-heart if severe irreversible cardiomyopathy). Refer to Chapter 31, Combined Organ Transplantation.

- Attention is given to the cause of ESRD and likelihood of recurrence, although no disease has a recurrence and graft failure rate that precludes initial kidney transplantation other than primary hyperoxaluria.
- Advanced age is not a contraindication to transplantation on its own.
- Retransplant must be carefully considered in cases of graft loss due to recurrent disease, nonadherence, or psychiatric issues.

CARDIOVASCULAR EVALUATION

- Cardiovascular complications account for nearly 30% of deaths with a functioning allograft.[2]
- Optimal screening guidelines have not been fully established.[2–4]

TABLE 26-3 ABSOLUTE CONTRAINDICATIONS TO KIDNEY TRANSPLANTATION

Active ischemic heart disease or severe cardiomyopathy
Active infection
Recent history of cancer other than non-melanoma skin cancer
Cirrhosis with portal hypertension
Active substance abuse or dependence
Active psychosis
Incorrigible nonadherence to therapy
Peripheral vascular disease with amputation of lower extremities

- All patients with advanced chronic kidney disease (CKD) are overall at high risk for cardiac disease.
- Current screening strategies for identifying cardiovascular disease in asymptomatic pre-transplant patients may include **noninvasive cardiac stress testing** with either stress echocardiography or nuclear myocardial perfusion.
- Significant risk factors for coronary artery disease include diabetes, history of ischemic heart disease, older age (age ≥45 in men and ≥55 in women), hypertension, dyslipidemia, obesity, smoking, family history of premature coronary artery disease, left ventricular hypertrophy (LVH), atherosclerotic vascular disease (peripheral arterial disease [PAD], stroke), and abnormal baseline ECG (particularly in diabetics).[2,5]
- If noninvasive cardiac testing is positive for ischemia, then the patient should undergo coronary angiography and potential revascularization procedures prior to transplantation.
- We have a low threshold to perform coronary angiography in patients older than 45 years with diabetes, or adults with diabetes for more than 25 years, or long history of tobacco.
- Most transplant centers perform noninvasive testing as the initial method of screening.
- Significant **valvular heart disease** needs to be corrected before transplantation.
- **Left ventricular ejection fraction** <35% is considered a major risk factor for complications after transplantation. In many cases, decreasing dry weight during dialysis may improve the cardiac function if patient has diastolic dysfunction or volume overload.
  - ○ In many cases, mild to moderate cardiac dysfunction could improve after kidney transplantation.
  - ○ Those with severe cardiac failure are not candidates for kidney transplant unless combined with a heart transplant.
- **Carotid imaging** is routinely done in patients with a history of transient ischemic attack, cerebrovascular accident, or presence of carotid bruit in asymptomatic patients during physical examination.
- **Lower extremity Doppler ultrasound** is indicated in patients with a history of claudication and/or signs of diminished peripheral arterial pulses on physical examination, particularly in diabetics.[6]
- Screening for **intracranial aneurysms** with either CT or MRA should be done in patients with autosomal dominant polycystic kidney disease with history of headaches, stroke, or family history of intracranial aneurysm or cerebrovascular accident.

PERIPHERAL ARTERIAL DISEASE

- PAD is a major cause of kidney allograft ischemic injury and lower extremity amputation.
- PAD is also a captured risk factor in the Scientific Registry of Transplant Recipients (SRTR) equation to measure center outcomes.[7] So it is beneficial for kidney transplant centers to detect PAD during evaluation.
- Diabetes, smoking, and CKD are major risk factors for PAD.
- We consider lower extremity amputation in the setting of PAD to be a contraindication for transplant.
- Patients with nonhealing ulcers or claudication should undergo noninvasive evaluation and possibly angiogram.
- Severe calcification in the iliac arteries needs to be reviewed by transplant surgeon for the suitability of transplant.

INFECTION

- All patients should be assessed for common latent or active infections and questioned for a history of recurrent infections.

- **Active infection must be fully treated prior to transplantation,** including diabetic foot ulcers and osteomyelitis.
- A history of **immunizations** should be obtained to assure adequate immunization for common vaccine preventable infection prior to transplantation (Table 26-4).
  - ○ Potential transplant candidates should complete all recommended immunizations at least 4 to 6 weeks before transplantation to achieve optimal immune response and to minimize the possibility of live vaccine-derived infection in the posttransplant period.
  - ○ Live vaccines should be avoided in patients on immunosuppression medications.
- Patients tested positive for **latent tuberculosis** should be evaluated clinically and radiologically for active disease. If there is no evidence of active tuberculosis, then patients can be treated with isoniazid before transplant, unless it is contraindicated due to end-stage liver disease or early transplant in whom appropriate posttransplant prophylactic therapy is acceptable.
- Patients with an established history of systemic coccidioidomycosis, histoplasmosis, or those from an endemic area should undergo appropriate antibody testing for **chronic fungal infections.**
- **CMV IgG and EBV IgG antibodies** are tested in the recipient to identify those at high risk for CMV and EBV infection posttransplant and to guide prophylaxis. CMV-positive donor to CMV-negative recipient transplantation carries the highest risk for CMV infection and usually prophylaxis is given for 6 to 9 months with valganciclovir.

Hepatitis

- In patients with positive hepatitis B virus (HBV) surface antigen or core antibody, viral load should be assessed and also referred for a liver biopsy to assess the severity of liver disease because liver enzymes may be spuriously normal despite changes on biopsy.
- Transplant candidacy should be based on both liver histology and serologic evidence of HBV replication (i.e., HBV DNA and HBeAg positivity). The presence of histologically mild liver disease does not preclude transplantation.
- In transplant candidates with active HBV replication, antiviral therapy should be initiated pretransplantation. All patients with HBV should be placed on antiviral therapy after transplantation to prevent HBV reactivation, replication, and progression of liver disease.
- In transplant candidates tested positive for hepatic C virus (HCV) antibody, further workup with HCV viral load and liver biopsy are essential.
- In selected cases, we prefer not to treat hepatitis C prior to transplant as potential recipients can get offers from donors with hepatitis C.
- HCV direct-acting antivirals are highly effective with a sustained virologic response of more than 97%. These treatments are interferon free, so it does not carry a higher risk of rejection.
- Histologic evidence of liver cirrhosis with portal hypertension is a contraindication for kidney transplantation. Selected cases of liver cirrhosis without portal hypertension could be considered for kidney transplant.
- Decompensated liver cirrhosis can be evaluated for combined kidney and liver transplant.

Human Immunodeficiency Virus

- Infection with HIV is not a contraindication for kidney transplant anymore with the advent of antiretroviral therapy (ART).
- Transplant can be considered if HIV patients are stable and achieve the following inclusion criteria[8]:
  - ○ CD4+ T-cell count ≥200 cells/mL³.
  - ○ HIV viral load <20 copies/mL or undetectable. Transient viral increases (so-called viral blips) are allowed as long as there are not consecutive measurements >200 copies/mL.

TABLE 26-4 VACCINATIONS FOR KIDNEY TRANSPLANT CANDIDATES

Vaccination	Candidates	Dosage/Timing	Comments
Inactivated influenza vaccine	All candidates	1 dose annually before influenza season	Trivalent or quadrivalent vaccine is acceptable
Pneumococcal conjugate vaccine (PCV13)	Candidates who have not yet received 1 dose of PCV13	1 lifetime dose	PCV13 should be administered at least 1 yr after PPSV23, if previously received
Pneumococcal polysaccharide vaccine (PPSV23)	Candidates who have not yet received 2 doses of PPSV23	2 doses administered at least 5 yrs apart	PPSV23 should be administered at least 8 wks after PCV13 and at least 5 yrs after previous PPSV23
			For patients who received the second dose of PPSV23 prior to age 65, a third dose is recommended after the 65th birthday (after at least 5 yrs have elapsed since the second dose)
Varicella (Varivax), live, attenuated vaccine	Candidates who are VZV IgG seronegative and have not recently received immunosuppression	2-dose series	Live varicella vaccine should only be given pretransplant
			Hold the vaccine if patient takes immunosuppressive agents
Zoster (Shingrix), non-live recombinant glycoprotein E vaccine	Candidates ≥50 yrs of age who are VZV IgG seropositive and have not previously received the 2-dose series	2-dose series	Zoster vaccine administration may be considered in patients <50 yrs of age, if allowed by insurance
			Zoster vaccine administration may be considered in candidates who are VZV IgG seronegative, if live varicella vaccine is contraindicated

- ○ Compliance with stable ART regimen for at least 3 months before transplant. For any medication change, at least 3 months is needed with stable CD4+ count (>200 cells/mL^3) and viral load (<20 copies/mL).
- ○ Absence of active malignancy (with an exception of early-stage prostate cancer and nonmelanoma skin cancers).
- ○ Absence of active opportunistic infection.
- ○ Absence of significant wasting (weight loss of at least 10% in the presence of diarrhea or chronic weakness and documented fever for at least 30 days).
- ○ No history of progressive multifocal leukoencephalopathy, primary central nervous system lymphoma, visceral Kaposi sarcoma, or chronic intestinal cryptosporidiosis.
- HIV recipients have been shown to have two- to fourfold higher rates of acute rejection (up to 30% in first year) when compared with HIV-negative recipients.[8] Therefore, thymoglobulin is recommended as an induction agent in HIV recipients.[9]
- Achieving therapeutic and nontoxic levels of the immunosuppressive drugs due to the complicated pharmacokinetic interactions of these agents with some antiretroviral agents, such as protease inhibitors, could be challenging.

RECURRENCE OF KIDNEY DISEASE

- Recurrent glomerular disease is usually a late complication after kidney transplant, except for focal segmental glomerulosclerosis (FSGS) that can clinically recur within days or even hours.
- Idiopathic membranous nephropathy recurs in 10% to 30%. De novo membranous nephropathy incidence may be higher than recurrent idiopathic membranous nephropathy.

Focal Segmental Glomerulosclerosis

- Risk of primary FSGS recurrence is estimated around 20% to 50%.
- Risk factors for FSGS recurrence are history of recurrence in a previous transplant, younger age at diagnosis, rapid progression to ESRD, presence of mesangial proliferation within native kidneys, older donors of kidney, Caucasian ethnicity, and the collapsing variant.[10]
- Factors associated with low recurrence risk are familial and sporadic form of FSGS with podocin mutation, history of slow progression to ESRD, and nonnephrotic-range proteinuria in the native kidney disease.[11]
- FSGS secondary to reflux nephropathy or obesity does not recur after transplantation.
- Podocyte fusion is the only finding that can be seen with early recurrence of FSGS.

IgA Nephropathy

- IgA nephropathy is associated with high rates of recurrence, approximately around 50%. However, it could be subclinical recurrence that, it is found in a protocol renal biopsy.
- Recipients with IgA nephropathy have a favorable outcome compared to other GNs.
- Recurrence tends to occur more frequently in younger patients and in those with a rapid progression of the original disease.
- It is rare to have a rapidly progressive renal failure caused by an underlying crescentic IgA.

Lupus Nephritis

- Clinically significant lupus nephritis recurrence occurs posttransplant in 2% to 9% of recipients.[12]

TABLE 26-5   CANCER-FREE WAITING PERIODS BEFORE TRANSPLANT

Malignancy	Waiting Period
Bladder	
Superficial lesions	<2 yrs
Localized lesions	2 yrs
All other lesions	5 yrs
Breast	
In situ, low grade, and small lesion	<2 yrs
All other lesions	2 to 5 yrs
Cervix	
Superficial lesions	<2 yrs
Localized lesions	2 yrs
All other lesions	5 yrs
Colorectal	
Dukes A or B1 (T1–T2)	2 yrs
All other lesions	5 yrs
Kaposi and other sarcomas	2 yrs
Leukemia	2 yrs
Lung	5 yrs
Lymphoma	
CML and CLL	<1 yr
Prostate	
Gleason score ≤7	No wait time
All other lesion with negative PSA	2 yrs
Renal cell carcinoma	
Incidental or noninvasive asymptomatic <7 cm	No wait time
All other lesions	5 yrs
Skin	
Melanoma	
In situ	<2 yrs
All other lesions	2 to 5 yrs
Squamous cell—localized lesion after resection	No wait time
Basal cell cancer—localized lesion after resection	No wait time
Testis	2 yrs
Thyroid	2 yrs
Uterus	2 yrs

CML, chronic myelogenous leukemia; CLL, chronic lymphocytic leukemia; PSA, prostate-specific antigen; LN, lymph node.

- The effect of recurrent lupus on graft survival is usually of minor significance.
- The overall absolute risk for allograft failure due to recurrent lupus nephritis is small.
- Risk factors for lupus nephritis recurrence are black non-Hispanic ancestry, female gender and young age.
- No difference noted in patient and graft survival rates between transplanted adults with lupus nephritis and other transplant recipients.

OBESITY

- Obesity is associated with wound-related complications, delayed graft function, lower graft survival, and higher mortality.
- Most transplant centers require candidates to have body mass index (BMI) of <40 kg/m² to be eligible for kidney transplant.
- For patients with central obesity, we require candidates to have BMI <35 kg/m².
- All obese patients should be encouraged to lose weight and follow-up with a dietitian.
- In candidates with BMI >40 kg/m² and not able to lose weight, we would consider bariatric surgery.

CANCER

- Active cancer is, in general, a contraindication to transplant.
- Among pretransplant treated cancers, the highest recurrence rates have been observed with multiple myeloma (67%), nonmelanoma skin cancers (53%), non-Hodgkin lymphoma, bladder carcinomas (29%), sarcomas (29%), symptomatic renal cell carcinomas (27%), and breast carcinomas (23%).[13]
- To reduce the frequency of cancer recurrence in the early years after transplantation, at least 2 years of cancer-free status is recommended as a requirement for most cancers, except for melanoma, breast, and colon cancer where the wait period is 5 years (Table 26-5).[14–16]
- The rapidity with which some malignancies develop after transplantation is consistent with the concept that viral oncogenesis is involved as initiation of immunosuppression may promote unchecked viral replication.

WAITLIST MANAGEMENT

- Periodic review of waitlisted patients should include review of medical history, interim illnesses and hospitalizations, and current functional status.
- Testing should be updated per center protocol. Most centers do annual labs, CXR, ECG, and sometimes cardiac stress testing.
- Annual return visits are indicated for marginal candidates.
- Blood transfusions should be avoided because of risk of HLA sensitization; if required, then leukocyte-depleted blood should be administered.
- Immunizations for pneumococcus, influenza, hepatitis B, and varicella (if antibody negative and not on immunosuppression) should be administered prior to transplant.

REFERENCES

1. Scandling JD. Kidney transplant candidate evaluation. *Semin Dial.* 2005;18:487–494.
2. Lentine KL, Costa SP, Weir MR, et al. Cardiac disease evaluation and management among kidney and liver transplantation candidates: a scientific statement from the American Heart Association and the American College of Cardiology Foundation. *J Am Coll Cardiol.* 2012;60:434–480.
3. Hart A, Weir MR, Kasiske BL. Cardiovascular risk assessment in kidney transplantation. *Kidney Int.* 2015;87:527–534.
4. Bhatti NK, Karimi Galougahi K, Paz Y, et al. Diagnosis and management of cardiovascular disease in advanced and end-stage renal disease. *J Am Heart Assoc.* 2016;5:1–14.
5. Manske CL, Thomas W, Wang Y, et al. Screening diabetic transplant candidates for coronary artery disease: identification of a low risk subgroup. *Kidney Int.* 1993;44:617–621.
6. Schold JD, Gregg JA, Harman JS, et al. Barriers to evaluation and wait listing for kidney transplantation. *Clin J Am Soc Nephrol.* 2011;6:1760–1767.

7. Scientific Registry of Transplant Recipients. Available at https://www.srtr.org/. Accessed June 11, 2018.
8. Stock PG, Barin B, Murphy B, et al. Outcomes of kidney transplantation in HIV-infected recipients. *N Engl J Med.* 2010;363:2004–2014.
9. Kucirka LM, Durand CM, Bae S, et al. Induction immunosuppression and clinical outcomes in kidney transplant recipients infected with human immunodeficiency virus. *Am J Transplant.* 2016;16:2368–2376.
10. Shimizu A, Higo S, Fujita E, et al. Focal segmental glomerulosclerosis after renal transplantation. *Clin Transplant.* 2011;265:6–14.
11. Jungraithmayr TC, Hofer K, Cochat P, et al. Screening for NPHS2 mutations may help predict FSGS recurrence after transplantation. *J Am Soc Nephrol.* 2011;22:579–585.
12. Contreras G, Mattiazzi A, Guerra G, et al. Recurrence of lupus nephritis after kidney transplantation. *J Am Soc Nephrol.* 2010;21:1200–1207.
13. Penn I. Evaluation of transplant candidates with pre-existing malignancies. *Ann Transplant.* 1997;2:14–17.
14. Chapman JR, Webster AC, Wong G. Cancer in the transplant recipient. *Cold Spring Harb Perspect Med.* 2013;3(7):a015677.
15. Penn I. The effect of immunosuppression on pre-existing cancers. *Transplantation.* 1993;55:742–747.
16. Kasiske BL, Cangro CB, Hariharan S, et al. The evaluation of renal transplantation candidates: clinical practice guidelines. *Am J Transplant.* 2001;1:3–95.

Evaluation of the Living Kidney Donor Candidate

27

Rungwasee Rattanavich

GENERAL PRINCIPLE

- Living kidney has major advantages over deceased donor kidney. In general, recipients of living kidney benefit from shorter waiting time, higher likelihood of preemptive transplantation, lower risk for delayed graft function (DGF), and has superior graft survival with a half-life of 12 to 15 years compared to 9 to 11 years for deceased donors.[1]
- A living donor evaluation is the process intended to protect the donor and to ensure that the donor is healthy enough to undergo surgery with minimal risk of developing adverse medical, psychosocial, and financial outcome after kidney donation.
- The donor's physician must balance a "do no harm" position with the autonomy of the donor, and carefully discuss the potential risks of donation.
- The Organ Procurement and Transplantation Network (OPTN) has developed policies for all U.S. transplant centers and the minimum kidney donor suitability requirements and has incorporated these within existing global policies for all living donors prior to kidney donation.
- OPTN requires informed consent, an independent living donor advocate (ILDA), blood typing report, medical evaluation, psychosocial evaluation, and a follow-up after kidney donation.[2,3]

INFORMED CONSENT

- Informed consent is a core value in living donor evaluation based on the long-standing and widely held ethical principles.
- The donor must have the ability to understand the risks, benefits, and consequences of donation and the capacity to make decision.
- The donor must be willing to donate, free from inducement and coercion.
- The donor should be informed of all of the following[3]:
  - The donor may decline to donate at any time in a way that is protected and confidential.
  - The transplant center will provide an ILDA to assist the donor during evaluation process.
  - There are alternative treatments available for the recipient such as continuation of hemodialysis and deceased donor transplantation if deceased organ may become available before completing living donor evaluation.
  - There may be health conditions that could be discovered from the evaluation process, which may be required to be shared with public health authorities.
  - There are surgical, medical, psychosocial, and financial risks associated with living donation, which may be temporary or permanent to the donor, including uncertainty in the risk estimates when it cannot be accurately quantified based on available data.
  - The donor may require long-term routine medical follow-up after donation.
  - The transplant center makes the final determination whether the donor is eligible for donation based on the results of their evaluation. Different transplant centers may evaluate the donor using different selection criteria.
  - It is a crime to receive anything of value such as money, property for their donation.

INDEPENDENT LIVING DONOR ADVOCATE

- The ILDA is a person or a team who is not involved in the potential recipient evaluation and is independent of the decision to transplant the potential recipient.[3]
- The transplant center must provide ILDA for the donor to help the donor during evaluation process and to advocate the rights of the donor.
- The ILDA must fulfill the qualification and training requirements including knowledge of living organ donation, transplantation, medical ethics, informed consent, and the potential impact of family or other external pressure on the living donor's donation.[4]

ABO BLOOD TYPING

- ABO blood typing should be drawn on two separate occasions prior to donation to reduce risk of unintended blood type incompatible transplantation.[3]
- ABO subtyping is performed to evaluate anti-A antibodies in recipients with blood type B or O receiving a kidney from donors with blood type A.
- A2 kidney has a very low A antigen expression in the renal cortex and the entire vascular bed endothelium. This low A antigen expression in A2 kidney allows recipients of blood type B or O to receive a kidney from A2 donor if recipient has low anti-A titers.
- The rhesus (Rh) factor is of little concern because it is not expressed on endothelial cells.

HUMAN LEUKOCYTE ANTIGEN TYPING

- Transplant programs routinely performed human leukocyte antigen (HLA) typing in order to counsel the patients about matching and graft survival.
- This includes HLA typing for major histocompatibility complex (MHC) class I (A, B, C) and MHC class II (DP, DQ, DR).
- HLA matching is traditionally recorded as the number of A, B, and DR mismatched antigens.
- For example, if a donor and a recipient share the same A, B, and DR antigens, this would be a 0A, 0B, 0DR mismatch.
- Poor HLA matching does not preclude living kidney transplant as it still offers better graft survival than deceased donor kidney transplant with zero antigen mismatches.
- Recipients with anti-HLA antibodies are at a higher rate of graft rejection.

PSYCHOSOCIAL EVALUATION

- Living donor psychosocial evaluation must be performed by a psychiatrist, psychologist, master's prepared social worker, or clinical social worker.[3]
- Psychosocial evaluation is performed for the following main reasons:
  - To evaluate for any psychosocial issues or the presence of behavior that may increase risk for disease transmission, smoking, alcohol, drug abuse.
  - To determine that the donor has the capacity to understand the short- and long-term medical and psychological risks of donation.
  - To assure that the decision to donate is free of inducement, coercion, or undue pressure by exploring the reasons for donating and the nature of the relationship to that transplant candidate.

- To assess the donor's ability to make an informed decision and the ability to cope with the major surgery and related stress.
- To review donor's occupation, employment, health insurance, living arrangements, and social support.
- To determine that the living donor understands the potential financial implication of living donation.
- Significant psychiatric problems are generally considered a contraindication for donation.

MEDICAL EVALUATION

- The medical evaluation must be done by a physician or surgeon experienced in living donation.
- Its purpose is to ensure that the donor is healthy enough to undergo the surgical procedure and that the donor is medically eligible for kidney donation.
- Eligibility for kidney donation includes:
  - The donor has normal kidney function appropriate with age and normal structures.
  - The donor has minimal pre-existing risk for developing future kidney disease.
  - The donor has no concurrent medical conditions that might require treatment that could deteriorate residual kidney function.
  - The donor has no risk of transmitting a disease to the recipient such as an infection or a malignancy.
- OPTN requirements for living donor medical evaluation are as listed in Tables 27-1 and 27-2.[3,5-7]
- Absolute exclusion for living kidney donation defined by the OPTN and relative exclusion criteria which may be variable between transplant centers are listed in Table 27-3.[3]

AGE

- OPTN has defined absolute exclusion criteria when donor is both less than 18 years old and incapable of making decision.
- Currently there is no absolute upper age limit for donation but the older donor has a higher likelihood of complications; therefore it is important to consider other comorbidities when evaluating older donor, particularly coronary artery disease.
- A 2007 survey reported that most programs accepted candidate without upper limit of age.[8]
- Long-term graft survival from older living donor is better than elderly deceased donor and similar to young deceased donor.

HYPERTENSION

- Hypertension is a contraindication for donation when the donor has uncontrolled hypertension or history of hypertension with end organ damage (e.g., microalbuminuria >30 mg/day, impaired renal function, cardiovascular events such as myocardial infarction or stroke, left ventricular hypertrophy).
- Selection criteria for hypertension are more flexible especially if donor is older. The decision to accept the donor with hypertension should be individualized based on lifetime predicted end-stage renal disease (ESRD) risk to take into consideration.
- Many centers allow mild hypertension that is controlled with one medication.

TABLE 27-1	GENERAL ASSESSMENT OF THE LIVING KIDNEY DONOR

Assessment	History	Physical Examination/Data
General	Hypertension Diabetes Major systems: • Lung disease • Cardiovascular disease • Gastrointestinal disease • Autoimmune disease • Neurologic disease • Genitourinary disease • Hematologic disorders, including venous thromboembolism history or risk factors (e.g., OCPs, HRT) • History of cancer, including melanoma	Vital signs Blood pressure (taken on at least 2 different occasions, or 24-hr overnight blood pressure monitoring) BMI Examination of all major organ systems Diagnostic testing: • Blood typing and subtyping (requires 2 separate samples) • CBC • BMP, calcium, phosphorous • Hepatic function panel • PT/INR, aPTT • Fasting lipid panel • Fasting glucose (perform glucose tolerance test or HbA1c in the first-degree relative of a diabetic and high-risk individuals) • HCG in females • ECG • CXR
Renal	Genetic renal disease Kidney injury Proteinuria Hematuria Stones Recurrent urinary tract infections Family history of kidney cancer	Diagnostic testing: • Urinary analysis with microscopy, urine culture if indicated • 24-hr urine collection for creatinine clearance and proteinuria • If history of stone >3 mm, do 24-hr urine for calcium, oxalate, uric, citrate, sodium, and creatinine • Specific testing per center protocol for inherited kidney disease • Renal imaging (CT scan) for anatomical assessment
Cardiac	Coronary artery disease, including family history	Diagnostic testing: • ECG for all donors • Cardiac stress test per existing guidelines for other noncardiac surgeries[6] • Echocardiogram in select donors if the history/examination suggests this will be useful

(continued)

| TABLE 27-1 | GENERAL ASSESSMENT OF THE LIVING KIDNEY DONOR (*Continued*) |

Assessment	History	Physical Examination/Data
Cancer	History of cancer and family history, including melanoma	Cancer screening should be appropriate for age, sex, and risk factors; transplant centers should develop protocols consistent with the American Cancer Society and/ or the U.S. Preventive Services Task Force to screen for: • Cervical cancer • Breast cancer • Colon cancer • Prostate cancer • Lung cancer
Family history	Coronary artery disease Cancer	
Social history	Occupation Employment status Health insurance status Living arrangements Social support Smoking, alcohol, and drug use/abuse Psychiatric illness, depression, suicidal attempts Increased risk behavior, as defined by the U.S. Public Health Services guidelines[7]	

OCPs, oral contraceptive pills; HRT, hormone replacement therapy; BMI, body mass index; CBC, complete blood count; BMP, basic metabolic profile; PT/INR, prothrombin time/international normalized ratio; aPTT, activated partial thromboplastin time; HbA1c, hemoglobin A1c; HCG, human chorionic gonadotropin.

OBESITY

• Obesity is associated with an increased risk of hypertension, diabetes, proteinuria, and kidney failure.
• Patients with a body mass index (BMI) >35 kg/m^2 should be discouraged from donation.
• Donors with BMI between 30 and 35 kg/m^2 should be carefully evaluated and encouraged to lose weight prior to donation.

CARDIAC RISK ASSESSMENT

• Perioperative cardiac events are uncommon with <5% among living kidney donors.
• Standard assessment includes CXR and ECG.

TABLE 27-2	INFECTIOUS DISEASE ASSESSMENT OF THE LIVING KIDNEY DONOR

CMV antibody

EBV antibody

HIV[a] antibody or HIV antigen/antibody
If the donor is identified as being at increased risk for HIV, HBV, and HCV transmission according to public health services guidelines, must have HIV-RNA by NAT or HIV antigen/antibody combination test[7]

Hepatitis B[a] surface antigen (HBsAg), hepatitis B core antibody (anti-HBc)

Hepatitis C[a] antibody (anti-HCV), HCV-RNA

Syphilis testing

Tuberculosis: If risk is suspected, testing must include screening for latent infection using intradermal PPD (Mantoux skin test) or IGRA

Endemic transmissible disease:
Per transplant center's protocol for testing donors at risk for transmissible seasonal or geographically defined endemic disease
Donor should avoid travel to CDC designated endemic areas between approval and donation
Repeat travel history if the time between approval and donation is prolonged

[a]HIV, HBV, HCV testing should be within 28 days prior to donation.
CMV, cytomegalovirus; EBV, Epstein–Barr virus; HBV, hepatitis B virus; HCV, hepatitis C virus; RNA, ribonucleic acid; NAT, nucleic acid testing; PPD, purified protein derivative; IGRA, interferon-gamma releasing assay; CDC, U.S. Centers for Disease Control and Prevention.

- There is no evidence to suggest that more cardiac testing than is recommended for general population decrease the risk of perioperative complications or long-term cardiovascular risk for living kidney donors. Preoperative cardiovascular assessment should follow existing guidelines for other noncardiac surgeries.[6]
- Echocardiography is recommended in cases with mild hypertension or abnormalities in CXR or ECG suggesting cardiomegaly.

RENAL ASSESSMENT

Kidney Function

- All potential donors should have renal function assessment.[3]
- An estimate of glomerular filtration rate (GFR) based on serum creatinine can be done as a screening test.
- Confirmatory methods should be performed by:
  - Measured GFR (mGFR) using exogenous filtration marker, for example, ^{99m}Tc-DTA, ^{51}Cr-EDTA, or iothalamate, is considered the gold standard.[9]
  - Measurement of creatinine clearance (mCl$_{Cr}$) with 24-hour urine collection with calculation to confirm adequacy of urine collection (estimate creatinine excretion in women 15 to 20 mg/kg/day, men 20 to 25 mg/kg/day).
  - Estimate GFR from the combination of serum Cr and cystatin C could be used if mGFR and mCl$_{Cr}$ with 24-hour urine are not available.

TABLE 27-3 EXCLUSION CRITERIA FOR KIDNEY DONATION

Absolute Exclusion Criteria According to OPTN		Relative Contraindications (variable between transplant centers)	
Both age <18 yrs and incapable of making an informed decision	Evidence of acute symptomatic infection (until resolved)	GFR <80 mL/min/1.73 m^2	Medical illness that increases risks associated with surgery
Uncontrolled hypertension or requiring multiple medications	High suspicion for donor coercion	Controlled hypertension with one medication	History of thrombotic disorders, with risk factor for future events or inherited hypercoagulable state
HIV (unless the requirements for a variance are met)	High suspicion for illegal financial exchange between donor and recipient	Microalbuminuria	Transmissible infection (hepatitis B, C)
Active or incompletely treated malignancy	Diabetes mellitus	Microscopic hematuria	Uncontrolled psychiatric conditions requiring treatment before donation
Uncontrolled, diagnosable psychiatric conditions requiring treatment before donation, including evidence of suicidality		Current pregnancy	Evidence of suicidality
		Recurrent nephrolithiasis or bilateral stones	Active substance use
		Urologic abnormalities	

OPTN, Organ Procurement and Transplantation Network; GFR, glomerular filtration rate.

- There is no absolute consensus to the level of GFR for donation but most centers use 80 mL/min/1.73 m² as a cutoff.
- The decision to approve donor candidates with mGFR 60 to 80 mL/min/1.73 m² should be individualized based on the predicted lifetime incidence of ESRD in relation to the transplant center's acceptance threshold.

Proteinuria

- OPTN requires measurement of urine protein and albumin excretion but it does not specify measurement modalities or exclusion thresholds.[3]
- Transient benign causes of proteinuria include fever, urinary tract infection, intense exercise, and orthostatic proteinuria.
- Overcollection of the urine should be excluded as a cause of mild proteinuria.
- Spot urine albumin to creatinine ratio (ACR) can be used as a screening test.
- A 24-hour urine collection for albumin excretion rate (AER) as mg/day is recommended as a confirmatory test.
- In all cases, an early morning urine sample is preferred as it minimizes variation due to diurnal variation in albumin excretion and urine concentration.
- Acceptable donor candidates should have an AER <30 mg/day.
- Persistent proteinuria with ACR >150 mg/24 hours is a major risk factor for development of kidney disease and should exclude donation.
- Persistent proteinuria between 30 and 150 mg/day should be carefully evaluated.

Microscopic Hematuria

- Microscopic hematuria could be related to infection, stones, malignancy, urologic abnormalities, or glomerular disease.
- Persistent isolated microscopic hematuria (defined as red blood cell >2–5 cells/high-power field on ≥urinalyses over 1 months) should be fully evaluated with:
  - ○ Urine culture
  - ○ Cystoscopy to rule out urologic abnormalities
  - ○ Urine stone panel to assess for nephrolithiasis
  - ○ Kidney biopsy to rule out glomerular disease
- Those ≥35 years will benefit more from cystoscopy compared to the younger donor without any risk factor for urologic malignancy.
- Some transplant centers will accept a donor candidate with hematuria if the urologic evaluation and kidney biopsy are negative.

Pyuria

- Infection should be ruled out.
- Kidney biopsy is needed if interstitial nephritis is suspected.

LIVING DONOR EVALUATION IN HEREDITARY KIDNEY DISEASE

- Knowing recipient cause of ESRD, family history of kidney disease, or any extrarenal manifestations may provide information to assess future donor risk of kidney disease if it is a living related donor.
- Living related donor may not be a suitable candidate for donation if there is a familial disease or a major risk occurrence of the same disease.[10]

Autosomal Dominant Polycystic Kidney Disease

- Autosomal dominant polycystic kidney disease (ADPKD) is the most common hereditary kidney disease.

- Donor candidate with family history of ADPKD in first degree relative may be accepted if age-specific imaging exclude ADPKD. Genetic testing may be needed.
- ADPKD2 may present later in life; therefore, genetic testing such as linkage analysis would be helpful.

Alport Syndrome

- Alport syndrome (glomerular disease, hearing loss, and ocular abnormalities) is a heterogeneous disease with X-linked, autosomal recessive, and autosomal dominant variants.
- Most cases are X-linked.
- Male siblings >20 years of age are very unlikely to have the disease if hematuria is absent.
- Sisters of affected male recipients with X-linked diseases have a 50% chance of being carriers.
- Female siblings with persistent hematuria are at risk to be a carrier, which has a 10% to 15% risk to develop chronic kidney disease (CKD). Therefore, donation is not advisable without detailed consultations with a nephrologist and geneticist.

Thin Basement Membrane Disease

- Donation from individuals with thin basement membrane disease (TBMD) is still controversial.
- Donors >40 years with TBMD without hypertension or proteinuria may be considered for donation.
- Donors should be informed that even though the disease is benign, there is risk of slow progression to CKD.

Systematic Lupus Erythematosus

- A family member of a patient with lupus should be screened with antinuclear antibodies (ANA) and complement levels.
- A family member of a patient with lupus with positive ANA carries a higher risk for developing lupus, therefore, should be excluded from donation.

Kidney Stones

- The concern with a prior history of kidney stone is that it may recur after donation, affecting the remaining kidney.
- Imaging with CT scan is recommended in donor candidates with history of stones.
- Donor candidates with remote stones (>10 year ago) without metabolic abnormalities associated with stones formation may be accepted for donation.
- A donor candidate with a one stone detected at age >50 years is unlikely to recur.
- Donor candidates aged 20 to 35 could have a higher risk of stones recurrence.
- A current stone size that is <1.5 cm or potentially removable during transplantation without evidence of metabolic abnormalities is suitable for donation.
- Presence of bilateral stones or stones recurrence despite preventive measures contradicts donation.
- Struvite stones are associated with infections that are difficult to eradicate. Thus, it may contradict donation.

Atypical Hemolytic Uremic Syndrome

- A related donor candidate might have a genetic defect that could trigger atypical HUS (aHUS) in the donor due to stress of the surgery.
- Genotyping for complement protein gene mutations should be performed in a related donor candidate to determine whether the donor shares a genetic susceptibility factor to aHUS.
- Genetic mutations of atypical HUS in a donor contradict donation.

Primary Hyperoxaluria

- Primary hyperoxaluria is a rare autosomal recessive metabolic disorder.
- Type I occurs in 0.11 to 0.26 per 100,000 births.[11]
- It is caused by a deficiency of alanine-glyoxylate aminotransferase (AGT), a hepatic enzyme that converts glyoxylate to glycine, resulting in an increase in the glyoxylate pool available for conversion to oxalate.
- Oxalate is poorly soluble and precipitates as nephrocalcinosis or nephrolithiasis.
- Living donor renal transplantation in recipient candidates with primary hyperoxaluria is controversial because of the major risk of recurrence.

Fabry Disease

- Fabry disease is an X-linked recessive lysosomal storage disease caused by a deficient activity of the lysosomal enzyme alpha-galactosidase A.
- The deficiency results in a systemic accumulation of globotriaosylceramide in the lysosomes of the vascular endothelium in multiple organs resulting in manifestations including neuropathy, angiokeratomas, gastrointestinal symptoms, corneal opacities, proteinuria, and renal dysfunction.
- Most affected males require renal therapy by the time they are 35 to 45 years of age.
- Heterozygote females have variable clinical manifestations due to random X-chromosome inactivation. Their renal manifestations may include isosthenuria, microscopic hematuria, leukocyturia, and less frequently CKD.
- Kidney transplant from a heterozygous female relative is risky as accumulation might already be present, even if there are no clinical symptoms.
- The measurement of alpha-galactosidase A activity is not sufficient since a normal value does not exclude a diagnosis because of random X-chromosome inactivation.

MEDICAL OUTCOME OF LIVING KIDNEY DONATION

Perioperative Complications

- Potential complications include wound problems, hemorrhage, pneumonia, urinary tract infection, ileus, hernia, thromboembolism, and death.
- Surgical mortality risk is very low, only 0.031% (3.1 per 10,000 donors) and did not change during the last 15 years follow-up.[12]
- Men, black, and donors with hypertension are associated with higher surgical mortality.[13]

Long-Term Medical Outcome After Donation

- Donors generally do very well after nephrectomy.
- Most studies showed no increase in long-term all-cause mortality or cardiovascular events.[12]
- Massive renal mass loss after nephrectomy causes initial reduction of GFR. Within days to weeks the remaining kidney uses hyperfiltration to increase GFR up to 75% to 85% of predonation values and stabilizes with time.
- A validated projection model can be used to expect the incidence of ESRD after donation (available at www.transplantmodels.com/esrdrisk, accessed June 12, 2019).
- Based on the above projection model, 94% of donors had a projected incidence of ESRD of less than 1%.
- Risk factors for ESRD among donors were young age, black, lower estimated GFR, albuminuria, hypertension, current or former smoking, diabetes, and obesity.[14]
- In a very large U.S. cohort study, the estimated lifetime risk of ESRD was 0.9 per 100 donors, 3.3 per 100 unscreened nondonors (general population), and 0.14 per 100 healthy nondonors.[15]

- Overall, the magnitude of the absolute risk increase of ESRD among donors is small.
- Proteinuria
  - Donors can develop small amount of proteinuria because of hyperfiltration after nephrectomy.
  - The average 24-hour urine protein was 154 mg/day on average 7 years follow-up after donation, but it is not clinically significant in most donors.[16]
- Hypertension
  - Blood pressure increase about 5 mm Hg after 5 to 10 years follow-up after donation which is greater than anticipated with normal aging.
  - Blood pressure goal in donors is similar to the general population <140/90 mm Hg.
- Gestational hypertension and preeclampsia
  - There is an increased risk of gestational hypertension (11%) and preeclampsia (5%) after donation but no significant differences in preterm birth or low birth weight.[17]
  - Pregnancy after kidney donation is overall considered safe.
- Gout
  - Reduced renal function is associated with reduced excretion of uric acid.
  - There is an increased risk of gout after kidney donation, but the absolute risk increase of gout over a median follow-up of 8 years is modest at just 1.4%.[18]

POSTDONATION FOLLOW-UP

- OPTN requires that transplant programs report follow-up clinical and laboratory data on donors at discharge, 6 months, 1 year, and 2 years after donation.[3]
- The donor should be monitored for long-term outcomes including hypertension, CKD, overall health, and should receive a healthcare maintenance similar to the general population guidelines.
- Donors should be educated on the importance and benefits of follow-up in terms of minimizing complications.
- Follow-up is imperfect and some patients are lost to follow-up, potentially due to cost and/or inconvenience.

REFERENCES

1. Hart A, Smith JM, Skeans MA, et al. OPTN/SRTR 2017 annual data report: kidney. *Am J Transplant*. 2019;19:19–123.
2. Organ Procurement and Transplantation Network, Health Resources and Services Administration, U.S. Department of Health and Human Services. Guidance for the informed consent of living donors. Available at https://optn.transplant.hrsa.gov/resources/guidance/guidance-for-the-informed-consent-of-living-donors/. Accessed June 14, 2019.
3. Organ Procurement and Transplantation Network, Health Resources and Services Administration, U.S. Department of Health and Human Services. OPTN policies, policy 14: Living donations. Available at https://optn.transplant.hrsa.gov/governance/policies. Accessed June 14, 2019.
4. Hays RE, LaPointe Rudow D, Dew MA, et al. The independent living donor advocate: a guidance document from the American Society of Transplantation's Living Donor Community of Practice (AST LDCOP). *Am J Transplant*. 2015;15:518–525.
5. Lentine KL, Kasiske BL, Levey AS, et al. KDIGO clinical practice guideline on the evaluation and care of living kidney donors. *Transplantation*. 2017;101:S7–S105.
6. Fleisher LA, Fleischmann KE, Auerbach AD, et al. 2014 ACC/AHA guideline on perioperative cardiovascular evaluation and management of patients undergoing noncardiac surgery: a report of the American College of Cardiology/American Heart Association Task Force on Practice Guidelines. *Circulation*. 2014;130:e278–e333.
7. Seem DL, Lee I, Umscheid CA, et al. PHS guideline for reducing human immunodeficiency virus, hepatitis B virus, and hepatitis C virus transmission through organ transplantation. *Public Health Rep*. 2013;128:247–343.

8. Mandelbrot DA, Pavlakis M, Danovitch GM, et al. The medical evaluation of living kidney donors: a survey of US transplant centers. *Am J Transplant.* 2007;7:2333–2343.

9. Lam NN, Lentine KL, Garg AX. Renal and cardiac assessment of living kidney donor candidates. *Nat Rev Nephrol.* 2017;13:420–428.

10. Niaudet P. Living donor kidney transplantation in patients with hereditary nephropathies. *Nat Rev Nephrol.* 2010;6:736–743.

11. Levy M, Feingold J. Estimating prevalence in single-gene kidney diseases progressing to renal failure. *Kidney Int.* 2000;58:925–943.

12. Lentine KL, Patel A. Risks and outcomes of living donations. *Adv Chronic Kidney Dis.* 2012;19:220–228.

13. Schold JD, Goldfarb DA, Buccini LD, et al. Hospitalizations following living donor nephrectomy in the United States. *Clin J Am Soc Nephrol.* 2014;9:355–365.

14. Grams ME, Sang Y, Levey AS, et al. Kidney-failure risk projection for the living kidney-donor candidate. *N Engl J Med.* 2016;374:411–421.

15. Muzaale AD, Massie AB, Wang MC, et al. Risk of end-stage renal disease following live kidney donation. *JAMA.* 2014;311:579–586.

16. Nagib AM, Refaie AF, Hendy YA, et al. Long term prospective assessment of living kidney donors: single center experience. *ISRN Nephrol.* 2014;2014:502414.

17. Garg AX, Nevis IF, McArthur E, et al. Gestational hypertension and preeclampsia in living kidney donors. *N Engl J Med.* 2015;372:124–133.

18. Lam NN, McArthur E, Kim SJ, et al. Gout after living kidney donation: a matched cohort study. *Am J Kidney Dis.* 2015;65:925–932.

Management of the Kidney Transplant Patient

28

Clarice E. Carthon and
Timothy A. Horwedel

GENERAL PRINCIPLES

- Immunosuppression is used for induction at the time of transplant to promote graft acceptance, to prevent rejection (maintenance), and for the treatment of acute rejection (AR).
- Adverse effects of immunosuppression are both immune-mediated (e.g., increased risk of infection and malignancy) and nonimmune effects.
- Immunosuppressive protocols tend to be center and organ specific, but can be individualized based on immunologic or side-effect profile.
- At present, the most commonly used regimens for recipients in the United States consist of induction with a T-cell–depleting agent (antithymocyte globulin or alemtuzumab) and maintenance immunosuppressive with a combination of tacrolimus, mycophenolate, and prednisone.

INDUCTION AND REJECTION—ANTIBODY THERAPIES

Antibody therapies have many applications in transplant medicine, including induction, treatment of acute cellular- and antibody-mediated rejection, and treatment of select recurrent diseases (Table 28-1).

Polyclonal

- Antithymocyte globulin is produced by injecting human thymocytes into animals and collecting sera containing cytotoxic antibodies against a variety of T-cell markers.
- The available preparations are horse antithymocyte globulin (ATGAM) and rabbit antithymocyte globulin (Thymoglobulin). They cause T-lymphocyte depletion and are used for induction as well as for treatment of rejection.
- Common side effects include fever, chills, arthralgias, and myelosuppression. Serum sickness and anaphylaxis (rare) can also occur.

Monoclonal

- **Alemtuzumab** is a humanized monoclonal antibody against CD52, approved for use in chronic lymphocytic leukemia (CLL). It causes rapid and profound B- and T-cell depletion and is used off-label in transplantation, desensitization protocols, and induction.
- **Basiliximab** is a humanized monoclonal antibody inhibiting the alpha subunit of the interleukin-2 receptor (CD25), thereby inhibiting IL-2 activation of T cells. Basiliximab is used for induction only. There are few side effects, although rare cases of anaphylaxis have been reported.
- **Rituximab** is a monoclonal antibody directed against CD20 on B lymphocytes, causing rapid and sustained B-cell depletion. It is used in transplantation for desensitization and ABO- and HLA-incompatible kidney transplant protocols, treatment of acute antibody-mediated rejection, certain recurrent diseases (e.g., membranous nephropathy and focal segmental glomerulosclerosis), and for CD20+ post-transplant lymphoproliferative disorders (PTLDs).

TABLE 28-1 ANTIBODY THERAPIES

Agent	Polyclonal		Monoclonal	
Agent	Antithymocyte globulin	Basiliximab	Alemtuzumab	Rituximab
Target	Numerous	CD25	CD52	CD20
Indication	Induction Rejection	Induction	Induction Rejection	Induction Rejection
Adverse effects	Moderate	Mild	Moderate	Moderate
Monitoring	CBC	None	CBC	CBC
Lymphocyte depleting	Yes	No	Yes	Yes (B-cells)

CBC, complete blood count.

MAINTENANCE IMMUNOSUPPRESSION

- Available immunosuppressive agents for maintenance immunosuppression include glucocorticoids, calcineurin inhibitors (CNIs), costimulation inhibitors, antimetabolites, and mammalian target of rapamycin inhibitors (mTORi) (Fig. 28-1).
- Owing to the different mechanisms of action, along with the renal and nonrenal toxicities of each drug, combination therapy is used to achieve the desired immunosuppressive effect while minimizing other side effects (Fig. 28-2).

Glucocorticoid (Prednisone, Prednisolone)

- Glucocorticoids are anti-inflammatory agents, which inhibit cytokine and chemokine production, and induce lymphopenia.
- Adverse side effects include development of post-transplant diabetes mellitus (PTDM), bone disease, poor wound healing, infections, cataracts, bruising, dyslipidemia, psychopathologic effects, and steroid myopathy.
- Maintenance dose is usually 5 mg of prednisone by day 30 post-transplant.
- Steroid-free or minimization protocols are offered at select centers but higher rejection rates and lack of long-term data limit general acceptance of steroid withdrawal.
- The so-called stress dose increases in steroids are generally not needed for routine surgery or illness and may only increase risk of infection, poor wound healing, or hyperglycemia.

Calcineurin Inhibitors

- Cyclosporine and tacrolimus are the two types of CNIs.
- By inhibiting calcineurin, they prevent cytokine gene expression and subsequent T-cell activation (Fig. 28-1).
- Cyclosporine and tacrolimus have similar side effects, including renal vasoconstriction, development of chronic interstitial fibrosis, hypertension, hyperkalemia, hypomagnesemia, hyperuricemia, and risk of drug-induced thrombotic microangiopathy.
- Hirsutism, hyperlipidemia, hypertension, and gingival hyperplasia are associated with cyclosporine.
- Tacrolimus is more neurotoxic and diabetogenic than cyclosporine.

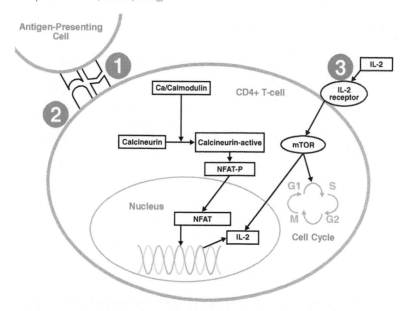

FIGURE 28-1. **Antigen-Presenting Cells of Host or Donor Origin With T cell.** Signal 1 (recognition): Antigen-presenting cells trigger T-cell receptors (TCRs). This activates several signals including the calcium–calcineurin pathway. This activates transcription factor nuclear factor of activated T cells (NFAT). Signal 2 (costimulation): CD80 and CD86 on the antigen-presenting cell engage CD28 on the T cell. Signal 3: Interleukin-2 delivers growth signals through the phosphoinositide-3-kinase (PI3K) pathway and the mechanistic target of rapamycin (mTOR) pathway, which initiates the cell cycle.

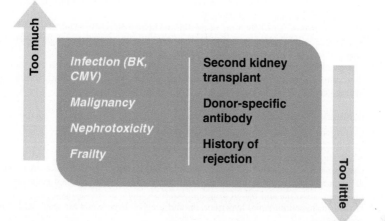

FIGURE 28-2. Rationale for individualizing immunosuppression medication.

- Cyclosporine formulations include Sandimmune (dependent on bile for absorption), microemulsion formula (Neoral), and generic (Gengraf).
  - Formulations are not interchangeable; if changes are made, then close monitoring of drug levels is needed, with dose adjustments carried out as necessary.
  - Typical starting dose is 6 to 8 mg/kg/day divided twice daily, tapered to achieve long-term maintenance troughs of 75 to 200 ng/mL or peaks of 400 to 600 ng/mL.
- Tacrolimus formulations include Prograf (available in generic formulation) dosed twice daily as well as Astagraf XL and Envarsus XR dosed once daily.
  - As with cyclosporine, a change of formulation necessitates monitoring of drug levels and allograft function.
  - Typical Prograf starting dose is 0.15 to 0.3 mg/kg/day divided twice daily, tapered to achieve maintenance trough levels of 3 to 10 ng/mL.
  - For conversion from Prograf (immediate release) to Astagraf XL, initiate treatment in a 1:1 ratio using total daily dose once daily.
  - For conversion from Prograf (immediate release) to Envarsus XR, initiate treatment with 70% to 80% of total daily dose once daily.[1]
- Intravenous administration of CNIs is almost never indicated, as tacrolimus is readily absorbed and can be given via a nasogastric tube or sublingually.
- For patients on cyclosporine, temporary conversion to tacrolimus is preferable to intravenous administration.
- Conversion from oral to sublingual should be done at a 50% dose reduction in patients with stable tacrolimus levels that are at goal.

Costimulation Inhibitors

- Belatacept is a fusion protein, which acts as a selective T-cell costimulation blocker by binding CD80 and CD86 receptors on antigen-presenting cells (APCs), blocking the required CD28-mediated interaction between APCs and T cells needed to activate T lymphocyte.
- Use only in adult Epstein–Barr virus (EBV) seropositive kidney transplant patients due to the increased risk of PTLD in EBV-seronegative patients receiving belatacept.[2]
- Belatacept is dosed as an initial phase and maintenance phase.
  - Initial phase: 10 mg/kg on day 1 and day 5, followed by 10 mg/kg at the end of week 2, week 4, and week 12 following transplant.[3]
  - Maintenance phase: 5 mg/kg every 4 weeks beginning at the end of week 16.
- Side effects include viral infections and PTLD.

Mechanistic Target of Rapamycin Inhibitors

- mTORi include sirolimus and everolimus.
- mTORi prevent cytokine- and growth factor–mediated T-cell proliferation.
- Adverse effects include potentiation of CNI-induced nephrotoxicity with standard CNI exposure, hypertriglyceridemia, hyperlipidemia, anemia, thrombocytopenia, leukopenia, poor wound healing, proteinuria, interstitial pneumonia, oral ulcers, acne, pericardial/pleural effusion (rare).[4]
- Side effects are similar between everolimus and sirolimus.
- Sirolimus is typically dosed from 2 to 4 daily and adjusted to target trough levels between 5 and 10 ng/mL.
- Everolimus is started at 1 mg bid (or 0.75 mg bid if the patient is also on cyclosporine) and titrated to levels of 5 to 10 ng/mL for patients not on CNIs or levels of 3 to 8 ng/mL for patients on CNIs.

Antimetabolites

- This category includes azathioprine, mycophenolate mofetil (MMF), mycophenolic acid (MPA).

- Azathioprine is converted to 6-mercaptopurine, which functions as a purine analog.
- Mycophenolate is converted to an active metabolite (MPA), which inhibits the de novo pathway of purine synthesis.
- Both inhibit gene replication and lymphocyte proliferation.
- Azathioprine is dosed at 1 to 2 mg/kg/day. Side effects include bone marrow suppression (especially with concomitant use of allopurinol), neoplasias, and hepatotoxicity (rare).
- Mycophenolate is typically dosed at 500 to 1000 mg bid for MMF, and 360 to 720 mg bid for MPA. Drug levels are not routinely followed.
- Important side effects include diarrhea, nausea, gastroesophageal reflux, myelosuppression, and increased risk of cytomegalovirus (CMV) infection.

Infection Prophylaxis

- Immunizations: pneumococcal, hepatitis B, and varicella (if antibody negative) vaccinations should be given prior to transplant. Live vaccines should be avoided post-transplant. Inactivated influenza vaccination is recommended yearly (see Chapter 26 for more reviewed and accurate details on vaccinations).
- Prophylaxis is given per individual center protocol at the time of transplant and reinstituted following augmentation of immunosuppression (e.g., treatment of rejection).
- Trimethoprim/sulfamethoxazole prevents *Pneumocystis jiroveci* and urinary tract infections. The most recent guidelines recommend continuing prophylaxis for 6 months to 1 year following transplant or rejection treatment.
- For those with sulfa allergies, pentamidine, atovaquone, or dapsone may be used for *P. jiroveci* prophylaxis. Guideline recommendations do not specifically state alternatives for UTI prophylaxis.
- Valganciclovir prevents CMV infection and is administered if the recipient and/or donor are seropositive pre-transplant.
- Generally, valganciclovir is most commonly used due to oral bioavailability and recommended for 3 to 6 months dependent on donor/recipient serostatus.
- Fluconazole, clotrimazole troche, or nystatin suspension is used to prevent oropharyngeal candidiasis.

Pharmacology and Drug–Drug Interactions

- Patients are instructed to notify their transplant center with any medication changes made by other providers to ensure there are no potential drug–drug interactions or effects on immunosuppressant drug levels may occur (Table 28-2).
- The following are commonly encountered interactions, but it is not meant to be an all-inclusive list. A transplant pharmacist is an invaluable resource for patient education, medication dosing, and safety issues.
- Both CNI and mTORi are metabolized by the cytochrome P450 3A microsomal enzyme systems, and therefore several potential drug–drug interactions exist that place patients at risk for either drug toxicities or rejection.
  - Drugs than **increase** levels: diltiazem, verapamil, nicardipine, azole antifungals, erythromycin, clarithromycin
  - Drugs that **decrease** levels: rifampin, rifabutin, antiepileptics (e.g., phenytoin, barbiturates, carbamazepine), St. John's wort
- CNIs have pharmacodynamic additive nephrotoxicity with amphotericin, aminoglycosides, nonsteroidal anti-inflammatory drugs, and angiotensin-converting enzyme (ACE) inhibitors/angiotensin receptor blockers (ARBs) potentiating hemodynamic effects.
- Additionally, use of cyclosporine with HMG-CoA reductase inhibitors, fibric acids, and nicotinic acid increases the risk of myopathy.

TABLE 28-2 ADVERSE EFFECTS OF MAINTENANCE IMMUNOSUPPRESSION

	Cyclosporine	Tacrolimus	Belatacept	mTORi	MMF/MPS	AZA	Steroid
Hypertension	‡‡	‡‡	∅	∅	∅	∅	‡
Hyperglycemia	+	‡‡	∅	∅	∅	∅	‡‡
Renal insufficiency	‡‡	‡‡	∅	∅	∅	∅	∅
Hyperlipidemia	‡‡	+	∅	‡‡	∅	∅	‡‡
Pancytopenia	∅	∅	∅	‡‡	+	‡‡	∅
GI toxicity	∅	+	∅	+	‡‡	+	∅

AZA, azathioprine; GI, gastrointestinal; MMF, mycophenolate mofetil; MPS, mycophenolate sodium; mTORi, mammalian target of rapamycin inhibitor; +++, severe; ++, moderate; +, mild; ∅, none.

- If initiating febuxostat or allopurinol, the dose of azathioprine must be reduced by 25% to 50% or allopurinol should be completely avoided. There is a high risk for bone marrow suppression as these drugs prevent the metabolism of azathioprine by inhibiting xanthine oxidase.

TRANSPLANT-RECIPIENT OUTCOMES

- The primary cause of graft loss is patient death with a functioning graft.
- Immunosuppressive effects contribute to post-transplant mortality, including cardiovascular and cerebrovascular risk factors, malignancy, and infection.
- Cardiovascular disease is the most common cause of death in patients with a functional allograft.
- Coronary artery disease, congestive heart failure, and left ventricular hypertrophy are more frequent in end-stage renal disease (ESRD) and transplant patients because of traditional risk factors (i.e., age, sex, diabetes, hypertension, dyslipidemia, and tobacco use) and nontraditional risk factors (e.g., dialysis duration, proteinuria, inflammation, vascular calcification, altered coagulation profiles).

HYPERTENSION

- This affects about 60% to 80% of transplant recipients.
- The etiology is often multifactorial, including medications (CNI, steroids, others), rejection, or other causes of acute/chronic graft dysfunction, transplant renal artery stenosis, and obstructive sleep apnea.
- The treatment goal is to achieve blood pressure <130/80 mm Hg.[5]
- Dihydropyridine calcium channel blockers (e.g., amlodipine, nifedipine) are considered first line for treatment of post-transplant hypertension. They are postulated to have protective effects against renal vasoconstriction mediated by CNIs.
- Transplant-specific considerations influence antihypertensive choices.
- ACE inhibitors and ARBs are associated with anemia, hyperkalemia, and are generally avoided in the immediate perioperative period because of hemodynamic effects, although they may be renoprotective in the long term.[6]
- Verapamil and diltiazem lead to increased CNI levels, and alternative dihydropyridine calcium channel blockers (e.g., amlodipine) are preferred.
- Hypovolemia can ensue with diuretic use and is usually avoided as the first line to treat hypertension.

ENDOCRINE AND METABOLIC COMPLICATIONS

Hyperlipidemia

- Occurs in over half of transplant recipients.
- Causes include medication-induced (mTORi > corticosteroids > CNI; also thiazides), renal dysfunction, proteinuria, obesity, age, diabetes, and genetic factors.
- It is essential to control hyperlipidemia with appropriate medications.
- There are some pharmacologic concerns regarding the use of statins and fibrates. There is increased risk for myopathy with cyclosporine plus HMG-CoA reductase inhibitors, fibric acids, nicotinic acid.
- Close monitoring for side effects and laboratory abnormalities should be done.
- Bile acid sequestrants may decrease immunosuppressive medication absorption.

Post-Transplant Diabetes Mellitus

- About a total of 30% to 40% of patients have pre-transplant diabetes.
- An additional 25% of patients without pre-transplant diabetes develop PTDM by 3 years from transplant.
- Diagnosis may not be made until after 45 days post-transplant.[7]
- Due to the early effects of postprandial glucose intolerance, fasting blood glucoses may be insufficient to detect PTDM and alternative methods of detection should be used.
- Hyperglycemia may worsen post-transplant because of corticosteroids, as well as decreased half-life of endogenous and exogenous insulin because of improved kidney function.
- Risk factors for PTDM include age, obesity and weight gain post-transplant, race/ethnicity (more common in African Americans and Hispanics), CNI use, hepatitis C infection, and male gender.[8]
- Diagnostic criteria for PTDM are controversial but the current American Diabetes Association guidelines may be utilized.[9]

Obesity

- Average body mass index (BMI) is increasing in transplant candidates as well as in the general population, prompting BMI cutoffs of 35 to 40 kg/m^2 at most centers.
- Although obese patients have overall improved mortality after transplant compared with maintenance dialysis, obesity causes increased risk of delayed graft function, graft loss, prolonged wound healing, and infectious complications.
- Treatment includes dietary modification, exercise and lifestyle counseling, consideration for bariatric surgery.
- Studies suggest little impact of steroid withdrawal versus continuation on post-transplant weight gain, emphasizing the importance of lifestyle modifications.

Bone Disease

- Unlike the general population, causes of bone disease in ESRD patients are multifactorial.
- They include osteitis fibrosa related to secondary hyperparathyroidism, as well as adynamic (low-turnover) bone disease, β2-microglobulin–associated arthropathies, and less commonly aluminum-related osteomalacia.
- This is compounded by the use of corticosteroids pre- and post-transplant, causing bone loss and osteoporosis.
- Bisphosphonates may worsen adynamic bone disease. Therefore, routine use of bone densitometry screening as well as the use of bisphosphonates is controversial in transplant recipients.
- Monitoring of hyperparathyroidism post-transplant and correction of vitamin D deficiency are presently advised, with consideration for parathyroidectomy in patients with persistent hypercalcemia and secondary hyperparathyroidism post-transplant.

HEMATOLOGIC COMPLICATIONS

Anemia

- Anemia is relatively common and multifactorial.
- It can be caused by perioperative or other sources of blood loss, iron, vitamin B$_{12}$, or folate deficiency.
- Decreased renal erythropoietin production is seen in the presence of renal allograft dysfunction and medications such as ACE inhibitors, ARB, and mTORi.
- Hemolytic anemia can result from recurrent, de novo, or drug-induced thrombotic microangiopathy.

- Parvovirus infection should be considered in cases of refractory anemia and may respond to intravenous immunoglobulin infusion therapy.

Post-Transplant Erythrocytosis

- Post-transplant erythrocytosis is defined by a hematocrit exceeding 50% to 52% and occurs in about 10% to 20% of renal transplant recipients.
- Secondary causes should be excluded, including transplant renal artery stenosis, smoking, renal cell, hepatocellular or breast cancers, native polycystic kidney disease, or inappropriate erythropoietin use.
- Treat if the hematocrit is >55% to avoid thrombotic complications.
- ACE inhibitor therapy is effective if tolerated.[10]
- Refractory cases or those intolerant of ACE inhibitors or ARB may require phlebotomy and hematology referral.

MALIGNANCY

- Post-transplant malignancy can be recurrent, de novo, or donor transmitted (rare).
- Immunosuppression inhibits normal immune surveillance, causes direct DNA damage, and promotes viral-mediated oncogenesis.
- Many transplant recipients have a history of pre-transplant immunosuppression exposure and cumulative exposure should be considered in assessing malignancy risk.
- Important viral/malignancy associations include hepatitides B and C (hepatocellular carcinoma), EBV (PTLD), human herpesvirus 8 (Kaposi sarcoma), and human papilloma virus (squamous cell skin cancer, vulvar, vaginal, and cervical cancer).
- Overall risk is three- to fourfold that of age-matched general population.
- Greatest risks are for nonmelanoma skin and lip cancer, PTLD, Kaposi sarcoma, renal cell carcinoma, as well as bladder, cervical, vulvar, perineal, anogenital, and liver cancers.
- Patients with toxic or obstructive nephropathies have the highest risk of renal and bladder cancers.
- PTLD accounts for one-fifth of malignancies post-transplantation, with an incidence of 1% to 2%.
  - Development of PTLD is associated with the use of antilymphocyte therapy for induction or rejection.
  - Majority of PTLD are non-Hodgkin lymphomas of B-cell origin, resulting from EBV-induced B-cell proliferation.[11]
  - Treatment options include immunosuppression reduction and possibly chemotherapy. Rituximab is utilized for CD20+ PTLD.
- General population guidelines are followed for breast, cervical, prostate, and colon cancer screening.
- Annual skin examination and use of sunscreen are advised for all recipients.
- Other screening is patient specific, for example, alpha fetoprotein (AFP) and liver ultrasound in HCV-positive recipients for hepatocellular carcinoma screening.
- Life-threatening malignancies may warrant significant or total withdrawal of immunosuppression.

PREGNANCY

- Female transplant recipients of childbearing age must be counseled regarding increased fertility and likelihood of pregnancy following successful transplant, to include contraception if desired, and medication counseling.

- Improved outcomes are seen if pregnancy occurs >12 to 24 months after a successful transplant in a recipient with serum creatinine <1.5 to 2.0 mg/dL, minimal proteinuria, no history of rejection, requiring minimal/no hypertensive therapy, with minimal comorbid conditions, and with appropriate preconception medication counseling.[12]
- Immunosuppressive practice in transplantation has arisen from clinical experience.
- All immunosuppressive drugs are Food and Drug Administration pregnancy safety class C (risk cannot be ruled out) or D (positive evidence of risk), driven by both human data and animal studies.
- However, MMF/MPA has been clearly demonstrated to be teratogenic, causing facial and ear structural malformations, and should be substituted with azathioprine.
- mTORi are avoided due to embryotoxicity and fetotoxicity in animal models. Prednisone, CNIs, and azathioprine are used during pregnancy.
- CNI levels may fall during pregnancy because of increases in maternal blood volume, and close monitoring of drug levels is needed to avoid precipitation of rejection.
- Common complications include preeclampsia, preterm delivery, and small for gestational age infants. Additionally, urinary tract infections are common and should be treated promptly in the transplant recipient with culture documentation of clearance.

REFERENCES

1. Bunnapradist S, Ciechanowski K, West-Thielke P, et al. Conversion from twice-daily tacrolimus to once-daily extended release tacrolimus (LCPT): the phase III randomized MELT trial. *Am J Transplant.* 2013;13:760–769.
2. Sam T, Gabardi S, Tichy EM. Risk evaluation and mitigation strategies: a focus on belatacept. *Prog Transplant.* 2013;23:64–70.
3. Vincenti F, Rostaing L, Grinyo J, et al. Belatacept and long-term outcomes in kidney transplantation. *N Engl J Med.* 2016;374:333–343.
4. Pascual J, Chadban S, Tedesco H, et al. Efficacy and safety of everolimus with reduced-dose calcineurin inhibitor in de novo kidney transplant recipients: results from the TRANSFORM Study. *Transplantation.* 2018;102:S367.
5. KDIGO clinical practice guideline for the management of blood pressure in chronic kidney disease. *Kidney Int Suppl.* 2012;9:370–371.
6. Cross NB, Webster AC, Masson P, et al. Antihypertensive treatment for kidney transplant recipients. *Cochrane Database Syst Rev.* 2009;(3):CD003598.
7. Sharif A, Hecking M, de Vries AP, et al. Proceedings from an international consensus meeting on posttransplantation diabetes mellitus: recommendations and future directions. *Am J Transplant.* 2014;14:1992–2000.
8. Wissing KM, De Meyer V, Pipeleers L. Balancing immunosuppressive efficacy and prevention of posttransplant diabetes—a question of timing and patient selection. *Kidney Int Rep.* 2018;3:1249–1252.
9. American Diabetes Association. 2. Classification and diagnosis of diabetes: *Standards of Medical Care in Diabetes—2019. Diabetes Care.* 2019;42:S13–S28.
10. Hiremath S, Fergusson D, Doucette S, et al. Renin angiotensin system blockade in kidney transplantation: a systematic review of the evidence. *Am J Transplant.* 2007;7:2350–2360.
11. Dierickx D, Habermann TM. Post-transplantation lymphoproliferative disorders in adults. *N Engl J Med.* 2018;378:549–562.
12. McKay DB, Josephson MA, Armenti VT, et al. Reproduction and transplantation: report on the AST Consensus Conference on reproductive issues and transplantation. *Am J Transplant.* 2005;5:1592–1599.

Immunologic Complications After Kidney Transplantation

Karthikeyan Venkatachalam and
Tarek Alhamad

GENERAL PRINCIPLES

- Acute rejection is characterized by decline in graft function with diagnostic features on a kidney biopsy after ruling out other nonimmunologic causes of graft dysfunction.
- Cellular and antibody types of rejection can be early or late and isolated or concomitant.
- There have been significant decreases in acute rejection rates during the first year of transplantation.
- The incidence of acute rejection within the first year decreased from 10% in 2009–2010 recipients to 8% in 2015–2016 recipients.[1]
- Despite available treatment, acute rejection remains a risk factor for graft loss.
- Risk factors for rejection:
  - The number of human leukocyte antigen (HLA) mismatches. Six antigen mismatches carry the highest risk for rejection in deceased donor kidney transplant
  - Younger recipient age
  - Older donor age
  - African-American ethnicity
  - Panel-reactive antibody (PRA) >30%. This can be seen with pregnancy, blood transfusion, or previous kidney transplant
  - Presence of a donor-specific antibody (DSA)
  - Blood group incompatibility
  - Delayed graft function. It is more likely to see delayed graft function with long cold ischemia time (>24 hours), donation after cardiac death (DCD), donor with acute kidney injury before donation
- Factors associated with a low risk of rejection
  - Zero HLA mismatch
  - Elderly recipient
  - Living donation
  - First kidney transplant

DIAGNOSIS

Differential Diagnosis

Based on the time of transplantation, the differential diagnosis of acute kidney injury varies. It can be classified as follows:
- **Week 1 post-transplantation:**
  - Acute tubular necrosis
  - Hyperacute/accelerated rejection
  - Urologic obstruction, urine leak
  - Vascular thrombosis of the renal artery or renal vein
- **<12 weeks post-transplantation:**
  - Acute rejection
  - Calcineurin inhibitor toxicity

- ○ Volume contraction
- ○ Urologic obstruction
- ○ Infections: bacterial pyelonephritis or viral infection
- ○ Recurrent GN disease
- **>12 weeks post-transplantation:**
  - ○ Acute rejection
  - ○ Volume contraction
  - ○ Calcineurin inhibitor toxicity
  - ○ Urologic: obstruction
  - ○ Infection: bacterial pyelonephritis, viral infections
  - ○ Chronic allograft nephropathy
  - ○ Recurrent glomerular disease
  - ○ Renal artery stenosis
  - ○ Post-transplantation lymphoproliferative disorder

Diagnostic Testing

- Causes of acute kidney injury other than rejection should be performed including renal ultrasound, urine, and serum workup.
- A renal allograft ultrasound with Doppler provides information regarding any anatomical abnormalities leading to a rise in creatinine.
- Test for urinary tract infection and pyelonephritis with urine analysis, microscopy, and culture.
- Serologic workups include cytomegalovirus (CMV) and BK viral serologies (serum PCR).
- Infection with BK virus can mimic acute cellular rejection on kidney biopsy.
- A renal allograft biopsy is the gold standard test for diagnosing acute and chronic rejection. There are other less invasive methods that are under investigation to diagnose rejection before clinical decline of renal function occurs. These include:
  - ○ T-cell reactivity assays: ELISPOT interferon-γ
  - ○ Gene expression assays: kSORT, Quest renal transplant monitoring panel
  - ○ Urine chemokine measurements: Chemokine (C-X-C motif) ligand 9 (CXCL9), this is also known as the monokine induced by interferon-γ (MIG), CXCL10 (also known as interferon-γ protein 10kDa [IP10]), C-C motif chemokine receptor 1 (CCR1), CCR5, C-X-C motif receptor 3 (CXCR3), C-C motif ligand 5 ([CCL5], RANTES)
  - ○ Donor-derived cell-free DNA

REJECTION TYPES

Hyperacute Rejection

- It occurs due to pre-sensitization mediated by antibodies against donor HLA.
- Usually evident before wound closure or manifests as primary nonfunction of the allograft.
- Clinically presents as anuria, fever, and graft tenderness.
- Can be diagnosed by a renal scan, where there is little or no uptake of the tracer.
- Prompt surgical exploration and allograft removal is the treatment in most cases.

Accelerated Acute Rejection

- Accelerated acute rejection occurs within 24 hours to a few days after transplantation.
- It may involve antibody-mediated or cellular immune mechanisms.
- HLA sensitization through repeat transplants, multiple pregnancies, or multiple transfusions are risk factors.

TABLE 29-1	HISTOLOGICAL CLASSIFICATION OF ACUTE CELLULAR REJECTION
Banff Classification of Acute Cellular Rejection	
Type IA	Cases with significant interstitial infiltration (>25% of parenchyma affected, i2 or i3) and foci of moderate tubulitis (t2)
Type IB	Cases with significant interstitial infiltration (>25% of parenchyma affected, i2 or i3) and foci of severe tubulitis (t3)
Type IIA	Cases with mild to moderate intimal arteritis (v1)
Type IIB	Cases with severe intimal arteritis comprising >25% of luminal area (v2)
Type III	Cases with "transmural" arteritis or arterial fibrinoid change and necrosis of medial smooth muscle cells with accompanying lymphocytic inflammation (v3)

- With the current sensitive flow cross-matching techniques, hyperacute or accelerated rejection have virtually been nonexistent.

Acute Cellular Rejection

- Classical signs and symptoms of acute rejection could include fever, malaise, graft tenderness, and oliguria.
- Since the advent of cyclosporine and other potent immunosuppressive agents, the classical clinical signs and symptoms of acute rejection are seen less frequently. Most rejections would present as asymptomatic elevations in serum creatinine.
- Differential diagnosis includes opportunistic infections that are common in the early and late post-transplant period.
- CMV and BK infections can histologically mimic acute rejection.
- Please see Table 29-1 for histologic classification of acute cellular rejection.

Chronic Active T-Cell–Mediated Rejection

- The historic histologic criteria of chronic active T-cell–mediated rejection are chronic allograft arteriopathy, which is arterial intimal fibrosis with mononuclear cell infiltration in fibrosis, and formation of neointima.
- A new criterion came in Banff 2017 that counted the inflammation in the areas of interstitial fibrosis or tubular atrophy (iIFTA) as a grade 1 in the diagnosis.
- Further studies are needed to evaluate the significance of iIFTA in kidney transplant outcomes.

Active Antibody-Mediated Rejection

- The major mechanism involved in antibody-mediated kidney injury is activation of the classical complement pathway by the binding of DSA to HLA.
- This binding ultimately leads to formation of the membrane attack complex (C5b–C9).
- The extent of complement activation is influenced by antibody strength, antibody isotype, epitope density, and the local concentration of complement regulatory proteins.
- IgG is the most common immunoglobulin isotype in antibody-mediated rejection.
- There is a strong association between the presence of the complement-fixing IgG3 subclass and loss of kidney graft.

- The presence of DSA, histologic findings of microcapillary injury, and diffuse (>50%) C4d deposits in the peritubular capillaries are the key components of the diagnosis.
- ABMR could be C4d negative or DSA negative if other criteria are met.

C4d

- C4d is a degradation product of the complement pathway that binds covalently to the endothelium.
- C4d has been described as a "footprint" for the presence of antibody-mediated rejection.
- C4d has a low sensitivity for the diagnosis.
- Therefore, C4d staining per se is no longer a requirement for the diagnosis if other criteria are met.
- C4d staining may not be associated with measurable DSA in the case of non-HLA antibodies, HLA antibodies absorbed by the allograft, or noncomplement-mediated rejection.

Donor-Specific Antibodies

- Antibodies may be directed against HLA or non-HLA molecules on endothelial cells.
- Non-HLA antibodies include major histocompatibility complex class I-related chain A antibody (MICA), major histocompatibility complex class I-related chain B (MICB), antibody angiotensin type 1 receptor (ATR1) antibody, or non-HLA antiendothelial cell antibodies.
- In sensitized patients with pre-existing DSA, 8-year graft survival rates were significantly worse than in sensitized patients without DSA or non-sensitized patients.[2]
- Renal transplant recipients without de novo DSA had better long-term graft survival than patients who developed de novo DSA.[3]
- Class I antibodies are associated with early ABMR, whereas class II antibodies are more commonly associated with late ABMR and graft failure.[3]
- Although DSAs are important risk factors for graft loss, the majority of patients with DSA have stable allograft function and experience no rejection.
- It is therefore important to determine the pathogenic role and specificity of anti-class I and class II HLA and non–HLA-DSA and to better understand the effect of de novo DSA compared with pre-existing DSA.
- Please see Table 29-2 for diagnostic criteria of ABMR.

TABLE 29-2	CRITERIA FOR ACTIVE ANTIBODY-MEDIATED REJECTION DIAGNOSIS (ABMR)

1. Histologic evidence of acute tissue injury, including one or more of the following:
   - Microvascular inflammation (g>0 and/or ptc>0)
   - Intimal or transmural arteritis (v>0)
   - Acute thrombotic microangiopathy, in the absence of any other cause
   - Acute tubular injury, in the absence of any other apparent cause
2. Evidence of current/recent antibody interaction with vascular endothelium, including at least one of the following:
   - Linear C4d staining in ptc (C4d2 or C4d3 by IF, or C4d>0 by IHC)
   - At least moderate microvascular inflammation ([g + ptc]≥2)
   - Increased expression of gene transcripts indicative of endothelial injury
3. Serologic evidence of DSAs (HLA or other antigens). C4d staining or expression of validated transcripts/classifiers as noted above in criterion 2 may substitute for DSA

TABLE 29-3	FEATURES OF CHRONIC ACTIVE ANTIBODY-MEDIATED REJECTION

1. **Morphologic evidence of chronic tissue injury, including one or more of the following:**
   - Transplant glomerulopathy (cg>0), if no evidence of chronic thrombotic microangiopathy
   - Severe peritubular capillary basement membrane multilayering (requires EM)
   - Arterial intimal fibrosis of new onset, excluding other causes
2. **Evidence of current/recent antibody interaction with vascular endothelium, including at least one of the following:**
   - Linear C4d staining in peritubular capillary (C4d2 or C4d3 by IF, or C4d>0 by IHC)
   - At least moderate microvascular inflammation ([g + ptc]≥2)
   - Increased expression of gene transcripts indicative of endothelial injury
3. **Serologic evidence of DSAs (anti-HLA or other antigens).**

All three features must be present for diagnosis.

Chronic, Active Antibody-Mediated Rejection

- Includes features of recurrent endothelial injury of micro- or macrovascular injury.
- Recurrent microvascular injury presents as thickness of the glomerular basement membrane (GBM), known as transplant glomerulopathy, or peritubular capillary basement membrane multilayering.
- Recurrent macrovascular injury presents as new onset of arterial intimal fibrosis.
- The presence of histologic features of chronic injury without active inflammation, DSA, or C4d is consistent with chronic antibody-mediated rejection.
- Please see Table 29-3 for features of chronic active antibody-mediated rejection.

Borderline Rejection

- The finding of inflammation in 10% to 25% of the interstitium with tubulitis of fewer than 4 cells per tubular cross section is classified as borderline rejection.
- This currently remains a pathologic definition without clear clinical significance.
- When it is identified in the setting of graft dysfunction, the risk of progression to clinical rejection on subsequent biopsies is increased, and thus treatment may be considered.

Subclinical Rejection

- Subclinical ABMR may be related to allograft outcomes and accelerated progression to chronic antibody-mediated injury.[4]
- Studies have shown that subclinical ABMR is associated with increased GFR decline, development of transplant glomerulopathy, and higher risk of graft loss, whereas subclinical T-cell mediated rejection does not have a significant effect on long-term graft outcome.[5]

TREATMENT

Acute Cellular Rejection

- Borderline and Banff IA rejections are treated with pulse corticosteroids and increase in the intensity of immunosuppression.
- Banff type IIA, IIB, and III rejections are treated more intensively with antithymocyte globulin in addition to pulse steroids and intensification of immunosuppression.

- Corticosteroid therapy is the first-line treatment for acute cellular rejection episodes. Intravenous methylprednisolone 250 to 500 mg daily for 3 days is typically used as the initial treatment option.
- Antithymocyte globulin is a polyclonal lymphocyte-depleting agent that is used for induction and treatment of rejection.
- Antithymocyte globulin is more effective in restoring kidney function and preventing graft loss than treatment with corticosteroids.[6]

Antibody-Mediated Rejection

- The primary aims of therapeutic modalities are to remove existing antibodies and inhibit their redevelopment.
- The management of ABMR is challenging and is associated with poorer outcomes compared with treatment of pure T-cell–mediated rejection.[7]
- Treatment of active antibody-mediated rejection (ABMR) has been debatable with no conclusive clinical trials done.
- Standard Treatment
  - There is no consensus on the treatment of ABMR. However, a combination of steroids, plasmapheresis, intravenous immunoglobulin (IVIG), and rituximab is considered the standard therapy.
  - IVIG is immune globulin derived from the plasmas of healthy donors.
  - IVIG has several potential anti-inflammatory and immunomodulatory effects including accelerated clearance of pathogenic IgG such as anti-HLA antibodies.
  - IVIG dose is 100 mg/kg after each session of plasmapheresis. Final dose could be between 500 and 1000 mg/kg.
  - Plasmapheresis is highly efficacious for the removal of pathogenic antibodies such as anti-HLA IgG antibodies.
  - We usually perform 1 to 1.5 plasma volume exchange at each session, with albumin or fresh frozen plasma for replacement. After biopsy, we tend to use fresh frozen plasma to prevent bleeding.
  - Rituximab single dose is administered after completion of last plasmapheresis.
  - DSA could be rechecked in a week or two after the treatment to monitor the response.
  - Further plasmapheresis can be given based on the injury and the level of antibodies. In general, we do four to five sessions of plasmapheresis with the initial diagnosis.
  - In one study, steroids, plasmapheresis, IVIG, and rituximab were associated with 85% lower risk of graft failure compared to steroids and IVIG alone.[8]
- **Tocilizumab**
  - Tocilizumab is an anti-interleukin-6 (IL-6) receptor antibody.
  - IL-6 is a key cytokine that regulates inflammation and the development, maturation, and activation of T cells, B cells, and plasma cells.
  - IL-6 is a stimulant for pathogenic IgG production.
  - Blocking IL-6 results in significant reductions of alloantibodies, direct inhibition of plasma cell anti-HLA antibody production, and induction of T-regulatory cells (Tregs) with inhibition of T-follicular helper cells.
  - Data are emerging from animal and human studies indicating a critical role for IL-6 in mediation of antibody-mediated rejection and chronic allograft vasculopathy.[9]
  - Patients with chronic active ABMR treated with tocilizumab had significant reduction of DSA and better stabilization of kidney function at 2 years compared to no tocilizumab treatment.[10]
  - Suggested dose is 8 mg/kg, monthly infusion dose for 6 to 12 months.
  - We recommend performing monthly BK and CMV PCR while on treatment.
- **Eculizumab**
  - Eculizumab is an anti-C5 monoclonal antibody, which inhibits terminal complement activation.

○ There was some early interest with the use of eculizumab as it decreased the incidence of early ABMR in HLA-sensitized patients. However, 5-year outcomes showed no improvement in graft survival.[11]

○ Eculizumab also failed to prevent chronic ABMR with similar incidence of transplant glomerulopathy.[11]

○ An ongoing study is investigating the impact of proximal complement inhibition as a therapeutic target. One pilot study showed that the plasma C1 esterase inhibitors Cinryze (Shire ViroPharma) may prevent antibody-mediated rejection in HLA-sensitized patients.[12]

REFERENCES

1. Hart A, Smith JM, Skeans MA, et al. OPTN/SRTR 2017 Annual Data Report: Kidney. *Am J Transplant.* 2019;(19 Suppl 2):19–123.
2. Lefaucheur C, Loupy A, Hill GS, et al. Preexisting donor-specific HLA antibodies predict outcome in kidney transplantation. *J Am Soc Nephrol.* 2010;21(8):1398–1406.
3. Wiebe C, Gibson IW, Blydt-Hansen TD, et al. Evolution and clinical pathologic correlations of de novo donor-specific HLA antibody post kidney transplant. *Am J Transplant.* 2012;12:1157–1167.
4. Loupy A, Suberbielle-Boissel C, Hill GS, et al. Outcome of subclinical antibody-mediated rejection in kidney transplant recipients with preformed donor-specific antibodies. *Am J Transplant.* 2009;9:2561–2570.
5. Loupy A, Vernerey D, Tinel C, et al. Subclinical rejection phenotypes at 1 year post-transplant and outcome of kidney allografts. *J Am Soc Nephrol.* 2015;26:1721–1731.
6. Webster AC, Pankhurst T, Rinaldi F, et al. Monoclonal and polyclonal antibody therapy for treating acute rejection in kidney transplant recipients: a systematic review of randomized trial data. *Transplantation.* 2006;81:953–965.
7. Lucas JG, Co JP, Nwaogwugwu UT, et al. Antibody-mediated rejection in kidney transplantation: an update. *Expert Opin Pharmacother.* 2011;12:579–592.
8. Lefaucheur C, Loupy A, Vernerey D, et al. Antibody-mediated vascular rejection of kidney allografts: a population-based study. *Lancet.* 2013;381:313–319.
9. Vo AA, Choi J, Kim I, et al. A phase I/II trial of the interleukin-6 receptor–specific humanized monoclonal (tocilizumab) + intravenous immunoglobulin in difficult to desensitize patients. *Transplantation.* 2015;99:2356–2363.
10. Jordan SC, Choi J, Kim I, et al. Interleukin-6, a cytokine critical to mediation of inflammation, autoimmunity and allograft rejection: therapeutic implications of IL-6 receptor blockade. *Transplantation.* 2017;101:32–44.
11. Cornell LD, Schinstock CA, Gandhi MJ, et al. Positive crossmatch kidney transplant recipients treated with eculizumab: outcomes beyond 1 year. *Am J Transplant.* 2015;15:1293–1302.
12. Vo AA, Zeevi A, Choi J, et al. A phase I/II placebo-controlled trial of C1-inhibitor for prevention of antibody-mediated rejection in HLA sensitized patients. *Transplantation.* 2015;99:299–308.

Nonimmunologic Complications After Kidney Transplantation

Sagar Gupta and Tarek Alhamad

30

GENERAL PRINCIPLES

- Differential diagnosis for post-transplant allograft dysfunction depends on many factors; importantly, the timing after transplantation (please see Table 30-1).
- For allograft dysfunction in the early perioperative period, urologic and vascular surgical complications should be investigated and the possibility of rejection considered; other common etiologies include hypovolemia, hyperglycemia, drug toxicity (commonly calcineurin inhibitor [CNI] toxicity), and infection.
- Acute rejection, recurrent disease, chronic allograft nephropathy, CNI toxicity, BK virus nephropathy (BKVN), and transplant renal artery stenosis are transplant-specific causes of renal dysfunction. However, it is important to recognize that renal failure can also ensue from all causes affecting nontransplant patients.

TABLE 30-1	DIFFERENTIAL DIAGNOSIS OF RENAL ALLOGRAFT DYSFUNCTION	
First Week Post-Transplant	<3 Months Post-Transplant	>3 Months Post-Transplant
Acute tubular necrosis	Acute rejection	Acute rejection
Accelerated rejection	Calcineurin inhibitor toxicity	Chronic rejection
Hypovolemia	Hypovolemia	Calcineurin inhibitor toxicity
Obstruction	Hyperglycemia, hypercalcemia	Hypovolemia
	Obstruction	Obstruction
Urinary leak	Infection	Recurrent or de novo renal disease
Vascular thrombosis	Infectious (e.g., BKVN) or drug-induced interstitial nephritis	Infection
Atheroemboli	Recurrent renal disease	Transplant renal artery or iliac stenosis
Infections	Malignancy (allograft PTLD)	Malignancy
Thrombotic microangiopathy	Thrombotic microangiopathy	Thrombotic microangiopathy

BKVN, BK virus nephropathy; PTLD, post-transplant lymphoproliferative disorder.

Surgical Complications

- Postoperative complications range between 5% and 10% (please see Table 30-2)
- Arterial surgical complications include bleeding, renal artery thrombosis, and renal artery stenosis
- Venous surgical complications include bleeding and renal vein thrombosis
- Ureteral surgical complications include urinary leak and ureteral obstruction
- Other complications are lymphocele, seromas, and infections

Infections

GENERAL PRINCIPLES

- A wide spectrum of potential pathogens infects immunocompromised hosts; many are infrequent pathogens in normal individuals.
- Fever and physical signs of infection (e.g., erythema) are often diminished.
- Risk factors for infections include:
  - Prior therapies (chemotherapy or antimicrobials)
  - Immunosuppressive therapy: type, temporal sequence, and intensity
  - Mucocutaneous barrier integrity (catheters, lines, drains)
  - Neutropenia, lymphopenia, hypogammaglobulinemia (often drug induced)
  - Technical complications (graft injury, fluid collections, wounds)
  - Underlying immune defects (e.g., genetic polymorphisms, autoimmune disease)
  - Metabolic conditions: uremia, malnutrition, diabetes, alcoholism, cirrhosis, advanced age
  - Viral infection (e.g., herpesviruses, hepatitides B and C, HIV, respiratory syncytial virus [RSV], influenza)

Cytomegalovirus (CMV)

GENERAL PRINCIPLES

- It is the human herpesvirus 5 (HHV-5).
- Seroprevalence of CMV is around 60% in the general population and it varies according to the age and race.[1]
- Transmission is through blood, sexual intercourse, and transplanted organs.
- Active infection in kidney transplant recipients is 30% to 70% without prophylaxis at 1 month from transplant with the highest rate in patients with donor CMV IgG positive into recipient CMV IgG negative.[2]
- CMV infection leads to increased morbidity, mortality, and allograft failure.
- Risk factors for CMV infection:
  - Highest risk: CMV donor positive into recipient-negative serostatus
  - Comorbid illnesses
  - Neutropenia
  - Lack of CMV prophylaxis
- CMV infection is uncommon in CMV negative into recipient-negative serostatus.
- Often considered as a disease of overimmunosuppression.

TABLE 30-2 SURGICAL COMPLICATIONS AFTER TRANSPLANTATION: CAUSES, SYMPTOMS, AND MANAGEMENT

Surgical Complication	Causes/Risk factors	Signs and Symptoms	Evaluation and Treatment
Arterial bleeding	Anastomotic leak Systemic anticoagulation Bleeding diathesis	Hypotension Tachycardia Drop in hematocrit Allograft dysfunction from compression	Blood transfusion Imaging (US/CT) Conservative management Surgical exploration and evacuation (if not a brisk or significant bleed and/or allograft dysfunction)
Venous bleeding	Anastomotic leak Systemic anticoagulation Bleeding diathesis	Hypotension Tachycardia Drop in hematocrit Allograft dysfunction from compression	Blood transfusion Imaging (US/CT) May need surgical exploration and evacuation
Renal artery thrombosis	Hypotension Hyperacute or unresponsive acute rejection Hypercoagulable state Multiple renal arteries Unidentified intimal flaps	Occurs early after transplant Sudden-onset oliguria/anuria (often complete) AKI Hyperkalemia	US Doppler shows no flow Radionuclide renal scan shows no uptake Immediate return to operation room for thrombectomy, but may need allograft nephrectomy
Renal vein thrombosis	Hypercoagulable state Hematomas or lymphoceles causing compression Anastomotic stenosis Extension of a DVT	Occurs early after transplant Tender swollen allograft Hematuria	US Doppler shows decreased flow in vein Attempt at thrombectomy, but may need allograft nephrectomy if unsuccessful

(continued)

333

TABLE 30-2	SURGICAL COMPLICATIONS AFTER TRANSPLANTATION: CAUSES, SYMPTOMS, AND MANAGEMENT (Continued)		
Surgical Complication	Causes/Risk factors	Signs and Symptoms	Evaluation and Treatment
Urinary leak	Ureteral necrosis Disrupted anastomosis	Decreased urine output Pain due to urine irritation AKI	US, nuclear scan or CT shows fluid collection If Jackson–Pratt (JP) drain is present, JP fluid Cr will be elevated (equals urine creatinine) Treat with Foley catheter, nephrostomy, or surgical revision of anastomosis
Ureteral obstruction	Extrinsic: fluid collection or mass compressing the ureter Intrinsic: ureteral stenosis, structure, renal calculi Late structuring can be seen in BK nephropathy	Decreased urine output AKI	US dilation of ureter Nuclear scan shows poor flow/retained tracer Treat with percutaneous nephrostomy with stenting and dilation, surgical revision of anastomosis
Lymphocele		Decreased urine output AKI (if compresses allograft) Suprapubic pressure Scrotal edema Unilateral leg edema Possible DVT	US or CT will show fluid collection, compression of allograft, or hydronephrosis. Drain lymphocele (percutaneous in VIR or laparoscopic) Peritoneal window to prevent recurrence
Renal artery stenosis	Difficulties in harvesting and operative techniques Atherosclerotic disease CMV infection Delayed graft function	Most commonly between 3 months and 2 years Difficult to control or acute increase in BP Fluid retention Flash pulmonary edema Allograft dysfunction which worsens with ACEI/ARB	Screening with US Doppler: shows increased velocity at stenosis site Confirmatory tests: MR/CT angiography Arteriography is ideal but invasive—diagnose and treat at same time Treat with endovascular stenting Rarely surgical redo of anastomosis may be needed

ACEI, angiotensin-converting enzyme inhibitor; AKI, acute kidney injury; ARB, angiotensin receptor blocker; BP, blood pressure; CMV, cytomegalovirus; CT, computed tomography; DVT, deep venous thrombosis; US, ultrasound; VIR, vascular interventional radiology.

DIAGNOSIS

Clinical Presentation

- Occurs 1 to 2 months after prophylaxis course is completed
- CMV viremia (also known as CMV infection) is defined as the presence of CMV replication in blood regardless of whether signs or symptoms are present
- CMV disease may manifest with either or combined:
  - CMV syndrome: fever, malaise, arthralgia, leukopenia particularly lymphopenia, thrombocytopenia with no tissue invasion
  - Tissue-invasive CMV disease: end-organ involvement like retinitis, esophagitis, enteritis, colitis, hepatitis, nephritis, encephalitis, or pneumonitis
- Diagnosis is made using nucleic acid testing using PCR for the detection of CMV DNA

PROPHYLAXIS

- Prophylactic therapy is given 3 to 9 months based on the donor and recipient serostatus (see Table 30-3).[3]
- Preemptive early detection of CMV infection is the standard approach in many kidney transplant centers.
- Valganciclovir (VGCV) is usually used for prophylaxis for medium- to high-risk transmission (recipient CMV IgG positive). Standard dose is 900 mg daily for 3 to 9 months.
- Dose should be reduced according to the estimated glomerular filtration rate (eGFR).
- For eGFR 30 to 60, the dose should be 450 mg daily. For eGFR <30, the dose should be <30 mL/min.
- For low risk of transmission, CMV-negative donor into CMV-negative recipients, acyclovir 200 mg twice a day for 3 months can be used for prophylaxis.

TREATMENT

- Treatment of CMV infection includes decreasing immunosuppression. There are two main strategies:
  - Decease antimetabolite by 50% along with a decrease in the CNIs
  - Hold antimetabolite and continue the current dose of CNIs
- At Washington University, we hold antimetabolite. For low-level CMV viremia or patients with high risk of rejection, we restart 50% of the previous dose of antimetabolite in 3 months after the resolution of CMV viremia.

TABLE 30-3	CMV PROPHYLAXIS AFTER KIDNEY TRANSPLANTATION	
Donor CMV Serostatus	Recipient CMV Serostatus	Strategy
Positive	Negative	6–9 months of prophylaxis with VGCV
Positive	Positive	3 months of prophylaxis with VGCV
Negative	Positive	3 months of prophylaxis with VGCV
Negative	Negative	3 months of prophylaxis with acyclovir

CMV, cytomegalovirus; VGCV, valganciclovir.

- In addition to titrating down the immunosuppression, we start antiviral therapy.
- For mild CMV disease, treat with oral therapy of VGCV. The treatment dose is 900 twice a day for eGFR >60.
- For severe cases, we use intravenous ganciclovir for the initial treatment then switch to oral VGCV.
- Minimum length of treatment is 3 weeks. End date depends on the resolution of clinical signs and symptoms, and the clearance of CMV viremia in two blood PCRs performed at least 1 week apart.
- For invasive or severe disease or hypogammaglobulinemia, consider adding Cytogam or pooled IVIG 100 mg/kg daily for 3 to 5 doses.
- For refractory cases, look for CMV genetic mutation (UL97 and UL54). Resistant genetic mutations are more common in the low-dose VGCV regimen. In these cases, foscarnet can be used.

BK Virus

GENERAL PRINCIPLES

- BK virus is a human polyomavirus that was identified in a transplant recipient (BK) with an associated nephropathy.
- Named after initials of a patient from whom the virus was first isolated.
- BK virus is acquired during childhood with BK seroprevalence of 90% in the pre-transplant population.
- Transmission likely occurs via the respiratory or oral route.
- BK virus colonizes the urinary tract as the principle site of latent infection.
- Replication of BK virus occurs during states of immune suppression (pregnancy, cancer, HIV infection, diabetes, and immunosuppression for transplantation).
- In healthy nontransplant patients, asymptomatic urinary shedding of BK virus is detectable in up to 10%. Therefore, viruria is not checked in the clinical practice.[4]
- Reported prevalence of BK viremia is 10% to 25% in the kidney transplant recipients.
- BK nephropathy is estimated around 8% of kidney transplant recipients.
- Studies suggest that it is a result of overimmunosuppression.
- About 50% who develop BK nephropathy lose their allograft and the other 50% have significant loss in allograft function.
- Please see Table 30-4 for risk factors for BK viremia.

DIAGNOSIS

- BK causes tubulointerstitial nephritis and could cause ureteral stenosis.
- Hemorrhagic and nonhemorrhagic cystitis may occur, but it is more commonly in hematopoietic cell transplant recipients.

TABLE 30-4 RISK FACTORS FOR BK VIREMIA	
Degree of immunosuppression	Older age
Acute rejection following treatment	Male gender
Ureteral stents	Diabetes mellitus
Prolonged cold ischemia time	Delayed graft function

- Most patients are asymptomatic and present with acute or slowly progressive rise in the serum creatinine concentration or occasionally as an unsuspected finding on surveillance renal allograft biopsy.
- Lab abnormalities include rising creatinine and rarely leukopenia. Urinalysis may reveal pyuria, hematuria, and/or cellular casts consisting of renal tubular cells and inflammatory cells.
- BK nephropathy is associated with findings on kidney biopsy which can also be observed with cellular rejection, CMV, adenovirus, and herpes simplex virus infections.
- Medullary tissue should be included because BK virus is more likely to be present in the medulla.
- *Light microscopy:* Intranuclear basophilic viral inclusions without a surrounding halo. (CMV has cytoplasmic inclusions and HHSV has both intranuclear and cytoplasmic inclusions), interstitial mononuclear or polymorphonuclear cell infiltrates, tubular injury, tubulitis.
- *Immunofluorescence (IF)/Immunohistochemistry (IH):* Positive IH tests using antibodies directed specifically against BK or against the cross-reacting SV40.
- *Electron microscopy:* intranuclear viral inclusions (diameter size of 30 to 50 nm).
- In certain situation, it is difficult to differentiate BK nephropathy from allograft rejection. Positive IF/IH and serum BK PCR are important adjunctive tools to distinguish BK nephropathy from acute cellular rejection.

TREATMENT

- Active surveillance is the key! Check BK PCR blood on a periodic basis.
- We suggest checking BK monthly in the first year.
- Targeted reduction of immunosuppression can resolve the infection with stable renal function.[5,6]
- Fluoroquinolones and leflunomide have been tried and shown to have no significant benefits.
- Cidofovir is nephrotoxic, so it needs to be given with caution; could be considered as a last resort.
- Brincidofovir is a lipid-ester formulation of cidofovir that has enhanced in vitro potency against BK and less nephrotoxicity compared with cidofovir, but efficacy is not established yet.

Epstein–Barr Virus

GENERAL PRINCIPLES

- Epstein–Barr Virus (EBV) is a member of the herpes family with a seroprevalence of 90% by age 19.[7]
- Asymptomatic low-level viremia occurs in up to 40% within the first year of transplantation.[8]
- It is the first identified carcinogenic virus in humans and has been linked to the following malignancies:
  - Burkitt lymphoma
  - Hodgkin lymphoma
  - Immune-suppressed B-cell lymphoma
  - Post-transplant lymphoproliferative disorder (PTLD) (~75% are EBV associated)[9,10]
  - Gastric carcinoma (~10% are EBV associated)[11,12]
  - Nasopharyngeal carcinoma

- For development of PTLD, no one cutoff level has high enough sensitivity, specificity, and positive predictive value to predict, hence quantification is not routinely used.
- EBV-negative PTLD does occur in up to 30% of patients with PTLD.[13]
  - Occurs at 50 to 60 months versus 6 to 10 months (EBV positive)
  - More likely to be of recipient origin
  - Tends to be monomorphic
  - Occurs at sites distant from the allograft
  - Tends not to respond to reduction in immunosuppression

DIAGNOSIS

- Usually EBV viremia is asymptomatic
- Clinical presentation of EBV viremia could include the following:
  - Unexplained fever
  - Mononucleosis-like syndrome (fever, malaise, pharyngitis, tonsillitis)
  - Gastrointestinal obstruction, perforation, or bleeding
  - Infiltrative disease of the kidney allograft
  - Infiltrative disease of the liver or central nervous system

TREATMENT

- A reduction of the immunosuppression medications may lead to regression of the PTLD, particularly if it is polyclonal.[14]
- If no response to the reduction of immunosuppression, chemotherapy and anti-CD20 antibodies are used.
- For central nervous system involvement, irradiation might be needed.

REFERENCES

1. Bate SL, Dollard SC, Cannon MJ. Cytomegalovirus seroprevalence in the United States: the national health and nutrition examination surveys, 1988–2004. *Clin Infect Dis.* 2010;50: 1439–1447.
2. Atabani SF, Smith C, Atkinson C, et al. Cytomegalovirus replication kinetics in solid organ transplant recipients managed by preemptive therapy. *Am J Transplant.* 2012;12:2457–2464.
3. Kotton CN. CMV: prevention, diagnosis and therapy. *Am J Transplant.* 2013;13(Suppl 3): 24–40.
4. Egli A, Infanti L, Dumoulin A, et al. Prevalence of polyomavirus BK and JC infection and replication in 400 healthy blood donors. *J Infect Dis.* 2009;199:837–846.
5. Hirsch H, Randhawa P; AST Infectious Diseases Community of Practice. BK polyomavirus in solid organ transplantation. *Am J Transplant.* 2013;13(Suppl 4):179–188.
6. Hirsch HH, Brennan DC, Drachenberg CB, et al. Polyomavirus-associated nephropathy in renal transplantation: interdisciplinary analyses and recommendations. *Transplantation.* 2005;79(10):1277–1286.
7. Balfour HH Jr, Sifakis F, Sliman JA, et al. Age-specific prevalence of Epstein-Barr virus infection among individuals aged 6-19 years in the United States and factors affecting its acquisition. *J Infect Dis.* 2013;208:1286–1293.
8. Bamoulid J, Courivaud C, Coaquette A, et al. Subclinical Epstein-Bar virus infection among adult renal transplant recipients: incidence and consequences. *Am J Transplant.* 2013;13:656–662.
9. Reshef R, Morgans AK, Pfanzelter NR, et al. EBV-negative post-transplant lymphoproliferative disorder (PTLD): a retrospective case-control study of clinical and pathological characteristics, response to treatment and survival. *Blood.* 2008;112:2823.

10. Parker A, Bowles K, Bradley JA, et al. Diagnosis of post-transplant lymphoproliferative disorder in solid organ transplant recipients—BCSH and BTS Guidelines. *Br J Haematol.* 2010;149: 675–692.

11. Shibata D, Weiss LM. Epstein-Barr virus-associated gastric adenocarcinoma. *Am J Pathol.* 1992; 140:769–774.

12. Tokunaga M, Land CE, Uemura Y, et al. Epstein–Barr virus in gastric carcinoma. *Am J Pathol.* 1993;143:1250–1254.

13. Leblond V, Davi F, Charlotte F, et al. Posttransplant lymphoproliferative disorders not associated with Epstein-Barr virus: a distinct entity? *J Clin Oncol.* 1998;16(6):2052–2059.

14. Fishman JA. Infection in solid-organ transplant recipients. *N Engl J Med.* 2007;357(25): 2601–2614.

Combined Organ Transplantation

Andrew Malone

31

GENERAL PRINCIPLES

- Kidney failure can occur as a consequence of pathology primary to another vital organ such as the pancreas, liver, or heart. Therefore, frequently both diseased organs are transplanted at the same time.
- Pancreas transplantation is a therapeutic option for certain diabetic patients.
- Diabetes mellitus type 1 is due to pancreatic endocrine failure resulting in the reduction or loss of insulin secretion from pancreatic beta cells.
- Diabetes mellitus type 2 is due to the reduction of insulin sensitivity in the peripheral tissues resulting in the need for increased circulating insulin levels.
- Simultaneous kidney and pancreas transplantation is the most common form of pancreas transplantation. Pancreas transplantation after kidney transplant and pancreas transplant alone represents approximately 20% of all pancreas transplantation.[1]
- The number of combined liver and kidney transplants has been increasing in recent years. In 2017, liver and kidney transplants made up 9.6% of livers transplanted.[2]
- Pancreas transplant function can be compromised for many reasons both immunologic and nonimmunologic.
- Pancreas transplant dysfunction occurs more frequently than kidney transplant dysfunction.
- Combined heart and kidney transplantation is performed less frequently than kidney-pancreas and kidney-liver transplants.
- In total 807 combined heart-kidney transplants have been performed between 1988 and 2012 according to United Network for Organ Sharing (UNOS) and in 2017 combined heart-kidney transplants made up 6.5% of all hearts transplanted.[3]
- There are currently no standardized guidelines or indications for combined heart-kidney transplantation.
- Pre-heart transplantation estimated glomerular filtration rate predicts post-heart transplant mortality and progression to end-stage renal disease (ESRD). Hazard ratio for mortality post-heart transplantation is 1.55 (95% CI 1.41–1.70) for eGFR <30 mL/min/1.73 m^2 by MDRD.[4]
- Simultaneous pancreas-kidney (SPK) transplantation is the most common combined transplant performed.
- This chapter will focus on SPK transplantation for this reason. The details of induction and maintenance immunosuppression for other combined transplants are beyond the scope of this chapter.

INDICATIONS FOR PANCREAS TRANSPLANTATION

- UNOS is a not-for-profit organization charged with overseeing the allocation of organs in the United States.
- Indications for pancreas transplantation according to UNOS policy (11.2.A); one of these is required[5]:
  - Have a diagnosis of diabetes mellitus

- ○ Have documented pancreatic exocrine deficiency
- ○ Require the procurement or transplantation of a pancreas as part of a multiple organ transplant for technical reasons (e.g., part of a multivisceral abdominal organ transplant—bowel, liver, pancreas)
- The American Diabetic Association (ADA) guidelines recommend pancreas transplantation as a therapeutic alternative to insulin in certain circumstances[6]:
  - ○ Patients with advanced chronic kidney disease or end-stage kidney disease who are eligible for or have had a kidney transplant
  - ○ In the absence of indications for kidney transplantation, pancreas-alone transplantation should only be considered a therapy in patients who fulfill these three criteria:
    - (1) History of frequent, acute, and severe metabolic complications such as hypoglycemia, marked hyperglycemia, or ketoacidosis that have required medical attention;
    - (2) Clinical and emotional problems related to exogenous insulin use that are severe and incapacitating; and
    - (3) Consistent failure of insulin-based management to prevent acute complications.

RISKS AND BENEFITS

- For each patient an assessment of the short- and long-term risk/benefit ratio must be considered before perusing pancreas transplantation.
- Simultaneous kidney-pancreas transplantation offers a survival benefit greater than deceased kidney transplant alone or remaining on dialysis in type 1 diabetic patients.
- Pancreas transplantation alone can reverse diabetic nephropathy changes after 5 years of successful pancreas function.
- It is thought that simultaneous kidney-pancreas transplantation can reduce the incidence and progression of diabetic nephropathy in the transplanted kidney compared to kidney transplantation alone in a diabetic patient.
- Diabetic retinopathy improves after 3 years of functioning SPK compared to KTA.
- Diabetic neuropathy by clinical assessment improves after pancreas transplant alone.
- Simultaneous kidney-pancreas transplant patients have higher mortality risk for the first few months post transplantation compared to living kidney transplant patients, however, the risk is equal thereafter and even gets better in patients with functional pancreas at 1 year posttransplant.
- More surgical complications are observed post SPK compared to KTA alone and tend to be more likely to increase mortality. These complications are related to the pancreas surgery, which is technically more challenging than kidney transplantation.

INDICATIONS FOR COMBINED LIVER AND KIDNEY TRANSPLANTATION

- The indications for transplanting a kidney with a liver in a patient with cirrhosis requiring a liver transplant are not well defined currently.
- Patients requiring a liver transplant that have advanced renal failure that is deemed not likely to recover should get a simultaneous liver and kidney transplant.
- Ideally assessment of chronic changes in a kidney should be assessed by kidney biopsy, however, this is frequently not feasible in a patient with cirrhosis due to coagulopathy.
- Cirrhotic patients with advanced chronic histologic kidney changes are not likely to recover renal function with liver transplant alone.
- Cirrhotic patients with decompensated cirrhosis (with ascites most frequently) may have renal dysfunction that is due to hepatorenal syndrome (HRS) physiology, reduced effective circulation, or other acute insults that can cause ATN.

TABLE 31-1	MINIMUM CRITERIA FOR LISTING FOR LIVER AND KIDNEY TRANSPLANT
If the candidate's transplant nephrologist confirms a diagnosis of:	Then the transplant program must document in the candidate's medical record:
Chronic kidney disease (CKD) with a measured or calculated glomerular filtration rate (GFR) less than or equal to 60 mL/min for greater than 90 consecutive days	At least one of the following: That the candidate has begun regularly administered dialysis as ESRD patient. That the candidate's most recent measured or calculated creatinine clearance (CrCl) or GFR is less than or equal to 35 mL/min at the time of registration on the kidney waiting list.
Sustained acute kidney injury	At least one of the following: 1. That the candidate has been on dialysis for at least 6 consecutive weeks. 2. That the candidate has a measured or calculated CrCl or GFR less than or equal to 25 mL/min for at least 6 consecutive weeks.
Metabolic disease	A diagnosis of at least one of the following: 1. Hyperoxaluria 2. Atypical HUS from mutations in factor H and possibly factor I 3. Familial nonneuropathic systemic amyloid 4. Methylmalonic aciduria

- HRS, hemodynamic insults, and ATN causing renal failure secondary decompensated liver cirrhosis usually reverse after successful liver transplant alone.
- ESRD caused by a metabolic disease of the liver is also an indication for simultaneous liver and kidney transplantation.
- The Organ Procurement and Transplantation Network (OPTN) has proposed the following minimum criteria for simultaneous liver and kidney transplantation (Table 31-1).

TREATMENT

Induction for Combined Transplantation—Pancreas

- Induction immunotherapy includes high-dose IV corticosteroids, lymphocyte-depleting antibody therapy, or nonlymphocyte-depleting antibody therapy.
- Most transplant centers in the United States use lymphocyte-depleting antibody therapy with IV corticosteroids for induction at the time of pancreas transplantation (SPK or pancreas alone).
- 87% of pancreas transplants in the United States get depleting antibody induction therapy compared to 75% of kidney transplants.[1,7]
- There are higher rejection rates in pancreas transplants compared to kidney transplants.
- Studies comparing depleting antibody therapy (thymoglobulin) with nondepleting antibody (basiliximab) showed increased acute pancreas rejection rates with basiliximab.

- Alemtuzumab is another lymphocyte-depleting antibody therapy used for induction. This has comparable efficacy with thymoglobulin with respect to graft and patient survival after pancreas transplantation.
- At Washington University we use thymoglobulin induction for all pancreas transplants. The thymoglobulin dose is 6 mg/kg divided into three doses.

Maintenance Immunosuppression for Combined Transplantation—Pancreas

- Following induction therapy maintenance immunosuppression therapy is used for the life of the transplant(s).
- Most centers in the United States use triple immunosuppression of calcineurin inhibitor (tacrolimus), antimetabolite (mycophenolic acid), and corticosteroids.
- The vast majority of centers in the United States used tacrolimus as the preferred calcineurin inhibitor.
- Study data have shown that tacrolimus is a better calcineurin than cyclosporine in terms of pancreas rejections rates and severity and pancreas thrombosis.
- At Washington University we use LCP-tacrolimus targeting trough levels of 7 to 10 ng/mL for the first 6 months followed by 5 to 8 ng/mL thereafter.
- Mycophenolate mofetil is the most commonly used antimetabolic maintenance immunosuppressive in the United States.
- Studies suggest that mycophenolate mofetil reduces the severity and incidence of acute rejection in simultaneous kidney-pancreas transplants regardless of the type of calcineurin inhibitor therapy.[8,9]
- Most centers use maintenance corticosteroids. A typical dose is 5 mg per day of prednisone by 1-month post transplantation.

Induction for Combined Transplantation—Liver/Kidney

- There is no consensus on the best approach to induction therapy in combined liver/kidney transplantation.
- At Washington University we use basiliximab induction with combined liver-kidney transplantation unless the patient is highly sensitized.
- It is thought that a newly transplanted liver can act as a "sink" for HLA antibodies and thus have an immunosuppressive effect.
- In highly sensitized patients, with high levels of donor-specific antibodies (DSA), there is still a risk of acute antibody-mediated rejection in the kidney.
- In highly sensitized patients, thymoglobulin should be used in an effort to reduce this risk.
- Another strategy to reduce the risk posed by preformed anti-HLA antibodies is to delay transplantation of the kidney after the liver transplantation for 10 to 24 hours (based on the cold ischemia time).
- In cases where the cross-match is positive pretransplant, a repeat cross-match can be performed after the liver transplant and before the kidney transplant.
- In these cases, the post liver cross-match can become negative reducing the immunologic risk to the kidney.

COMPLICATIONS

Pancreas Allograft Dysfunction

- The main causes of pancreas transplant dysfunction can be divided into surgical and medical causes.
- Surgical causes are most common in the early posttransplant period. Most pancreas transplants in the United States are enterically drained. See Table 31-2 and Figure 31-1.[10]

TABLE 31-2	MEDICAL AND SURGICAL COMPLICATIONS OF PANCREAS TRANSPLANT
Pancreas vascular thrombosis	Occurs in 3–10%. Manifests as pain and increase in pancreatic enzymes (lipase and amylase) and blood sugars. May occur early or late. Manifest as pain and increase in pancreatic enzymes. Of note, prolonged posttransplant hyperamylasemia is observed early posttransplant in up to 35% of all pancreas recipients.
Graft pancreatitis	Risk factors for early posttransplant graft pancreatitis include donor quality (age, obesity, history of prolonged resuscitation, excessive inotropic requirements), use of HTK (particularly when organ preservation time exceeds 12 hrs), prolonged preservation time, pancreatic duct outflow impairment, bladder drainage ("reflux pancreatitis").
Leaks of pancreatic enzymes	Anastomosis leak of enzymes into the intraperitoneal space causes less than 0.5% of all graft losses. Manifest by extreme abdominal pain and require urgent surgical exploration.
Abscess formation	Manifests as pain, fever, and sepsis in many cases. Requires urgent surgical exploration.

HTK, histidine-tryptophan-ketoglutarate.

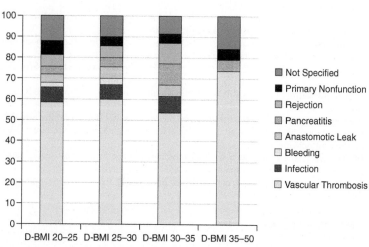

FIGURE 31-1. Causes of pancreas allograft failure within 3 months of transplantation according to donor body mass index based on United Network for Organ Sharing (UNOS) study. D-BMI, donor body mass index. (From Alhamad T, Malone A, Lentine KL, et al. Selected mildly obese donors can be used safely in simultaneous pancreas and kidney transplantation. *Transplantation.* 2017;101:1159–1166.)

- Medical complications include pancreas rejection and metabolic issues related to high blood sugars such as hyperkalemia, acidosis, and volume depletion due to osmotic diuresis when the kidney is functioning well.
- CMV pancreatitis can cause pancreas dysfunction.
- Suspicion for CMV pancreatitis is raised when CMV PCR levels in the blood are high in the setting of elevated lipase/amylase and/or hyperglycemia.
- The first signs of pancreas dysfunction are laboratory abnormalities on routine blood testing.
- Routine laboratory testing specific to pancreas transplant monitoring includes serum amylase, lipase for the assessment of exocrine function and blood sugars, HbA1c, and fasting C-peptide levels for the assessment of endocrine function.
- Tacrolimus or cyclosporine levels should be assessed as very high levels can cause elevations in enzyme levels.
- If pain is present with or without laboratory abnormalities, CT of the abdomen should be considered (usually noncontrast due to frequent kidney dysfunction in the setting of SPK).
- In recipient whose primary disease was type 1 diabetes, some transplant centers monitor anti-insulin, anti-islet cell, and/or anti-glutamic acid decarboxylase (GAD) autoantibodies to evaluate for recurrent disease.
- De novo antibodies have been associated with pancreas dysfunction.

Pancreas Allograft Rejection—Assessment

- Routine laboratory tests are important for monitoring pancreas function.
- Pancreas rejection should be suspected when any of the following occur:
  - Elevated serum lipase and/or amylase level
  - Elevated fasting plasma glucose level (could be a late marker for pancreas dysfunction)
  - Elevated hemoglobin A1c level (late marker)
  - De novo DSA or an increase in DSA titers
  - Unexplained fever or leukocytosis
  - New onset of graft tenderness
  - New onset of abdominal pain, discomfort
  - New onset of unexplained constipation
- For bladder-drained pancreas transplants the following can also suggest rejection:
  - Decrease in urinary amylase level in an 8- to 12-hour timed urine collection
  - Elevated serum creatinine level (in SPK transplant recipients)
  - New onset of hematuria
- There is relatively good concordance between kidney rejection and pancreas rejection in SPK, about 60%. Thus creatinine can be used to monitor for pancreas rejection.[11]
- In 20% of cases pancreas rejection can exist without kidney rejection and vice versa in SPK, thus care must be taken in the use of creatinine as a marker of pancreas rejection.[12]
- Definitive diagnosis of pancreas rejection requires a percutaneous needle biopsy of the pancreas.
- Before proceeding with biopsy, other intra-abdominal pathology should be ruled out by ultrasound and CT. This is of particular importance in the early posttransplant period (6 weeks). This is done to rule out thrombosis, leak, intra-abdominal abscess, pancreatic necrosis, ileus or bowel obstruction, or other abdominal pathology.

Pancreas Allograft Rejection—Acute Cellular Rejection

- Acute cellular rejection is classified into three grades according to the severity of inflammation and the degree of involvement of vascular endothelium.

- Grade I (mild)—active septal inflammation with evidence of inflammation in another component (septal veins, ducts, nerve branches, or focal acinar).
  - ○ Focal acinar inflammation is defined as a collection of ≥10 lymphocytes/eosinophils within an acinar area.
  - ○ Grade I includes one to two inflammatory foci per lobule with absent or minimal acinar injury.
- Grade II (moderate)—similar to grade I but includes mild intimal arteritis (<25% luminal compromise) or more than two inflammatory acinar foci per lobule with single-cell injury/dropout.
- Grade III (severe)—diffuse acinar inflammation with multiple-cell injury/dropout, moderate to severe intimal arteritis, or transmural/necrotizing arteritis.
- Borderline for cellular rejection: septal inflammation only.

Treatment
- Clinical trial evidence for treatment of pancreas rejection is lacking.
- At Washington University we target therapy according to the degree of inflammation per the Banff classification.
- Borderline acute cellular rejection:
  1. Augment maintenance immunosuppression with higher levels of tacrolimus (8 to 12 mcg/L) and full doses of mycophenolate mofetil (1000 mg twice daily) or mycophenolate sodium (720 mg twice daily) for 2 to 3 months.
  2. Pulse intravenous (IV) glucocorticoids (methylprednisolone 3 to 5 mg/kg daily for three doses, with a maximum daily dose of 500 mg), followed by a tapered dose of oral prednisone as follows: 60 mg daily for 2 days, then 40 mg daily for 2 days, then 20 mg daily for 2 weeks, then 10 mg daily for 2 weeks, then 5 mg daily indefinitely depending upon clinical response.
- Grades I, II, or III acute cellular rejection.
  1. Rabbit antithymocyte globulin (rATG)-Thymoglobulin at 6 to 10 mg/kg (1.5 to 2 mg/kg per dose in 5- to 7-daily or alternate-day doses, as tolerated).
     IV methylprednisolone, 125 to 250 mg, as premedication prior to the first two to three doses of rATG-Thymoglobulin, followed by a tapered dose of oral prednisone as detailed above for borderline acute cellular rejection.
  2. Augment maintenance immunosuppression (targeting a tacrolimus level of 10 to 12 mcg/L and full dosing of mycophenolate).
     Reduced doses of mycophenolate may be required during rATG therapy depending upon total white blood cell and platelet counts.

Pancreas Allograft Rejection—Antibody-Mediated Rejection
- The diagnosis of antibody-mediated rejection requires all three components:
  1. The presence of DSA
  2. C4d positivity in the interacinar capillaries
  3. Morphologic evidence of pancreas tissue injury
- Hyperacute antibody-mediated rejection is due to preformed DSAs and occurs within seconds to minutes of vascular anastomosis, leading to hemorrhagic necrosis in acini, islets, and ducts as well as graft thrombosis.
- Accelerated antibody-mediated rejection occurs within 24 to 48 hours after the anastomosis.
- Acute antibody-mediated rejection occurs within days, weeks, or months after transplantation.
- Approximately 75% of acute antibody-mediated rejection occurs within the first 6 months of transplantation.

Treatment
- Consists of:
  - Plasmapheresis: Minimum of three to five sessions of plasmapheresis. Plasmapheresis is performed daily or every other day as tolerated by the patient.
  - Intravenous immune globulin (IVIG): Doses of 100 mg/kg after each session of plasmapheresis, except after the final session, where a larger dose (500 to 1000 mg/kg, rounded to the nearest 10 g) is used.
  - Anti-B cell therapies such as rituximab: Given after the final session of plasmapheresis and IVIG. Single IV dose of 200 mg.
- Augment maintenance immunosuppression as we do in patients with acute cellular rejection and also administer oral prednisone as follows: 20 mg daily for 2 to 4 weeks, then 15 mg daily for 2 weeks, then 10 mg daily for 2 weeks, then 5 mg daily indefinitely.
- Monitoring the lipase and amylase levels assesses response to treatment of acute rejection. Blood sugar levels may remain high due to the use of high-dose corticosteroids for treatment of rejection.

SUMMARY

- The most common combined transplantations involving a kidney is simultaneous kidney-pancreas transplants.
- Pancreas allografts are more immunogenic than kidney allografts, therefore pancreas transplantation requires more induction and maintenance immunosuppression than kidneys alone or other combined kidney transplants (e.g., kidney-liver and heart-kidney).
- Maintenance immunosuppression of combined kidney-liver and heart-kidney transplants is usually similar to kidney transplant alone patients.
- SPK transplantation offers increased patient survival compared to deceased kidney transplants alone for type 1 diabetic patients once the initial postoperative course is successfully completed.
- Assessment of the need for kidney transplantation with liver transplantation in cirrhotic patients is difficult.
- Native kidney function frequently returns after successful liver transplantation in the setting of hepatorenal syndrome.

REFERENCES

1. Kandaswamy R, Stock PG, Gustafson SK, et al. OPTN/SRTR 2017 Annual data report: pancreas. *Am J Transplant.* 2019;19(S2):124–183.
2. *OPTN/SRTR 2017 Annual data report: liver.* 2017. Available at https://srtr.transplant.hrsa.gov/annual_reports/2017/Liver.aspx. Accessed June 14, 2019.
3. *OPTN/SRTR 2017 Annual data report: heart.* 2017. Available at https://srtr.transplant.hrsa.gov/annual_reports/2017/Heart.aspx. Accessed June 14, 2019.
4. Habib PJ, Patel PC, Hodge D, et al. Pre-orthotopic heart transplant estimated glomerular filtration rate predicts post-transplant mortality and renal outcomes: an analysis of the UNOS database. *J Heart Lung Transplant.* 2016;35(12):1471–1479.
5. Organ Procurement and Transplantation Network. *Policies.* Available at https://optn.transplant.hrsa.gov/governance/policies. Accessed June 19, 2019.
6. Robertson RP, Davis C, Larsen J, et al; American Diabetes Association. Pancreas and islet transplantation in type 1 diabetes. *Diabetes Care.* 2006;29(4):935.
7. Hart A, Smith JM, Skeans MA, et al. OPTN/SRTR 2017 Annual data report: kidney. *Am J Transplant.* 2019;19Suppl 2:19–123.

8. Merion RM, Henry ML, Melzer JS, et al. Randomized, prospective trial of mycophenolate mofetil versus azathioprine for prevention of acute renal allograft rejection after simultaneous kidney-pancreas transplantation. *Transplantation*. 2000;70(1):105–111.

9. Stegall MD, Simon M, Wachs ME, et al. Mycophenolate mofetil decreases rejection in simultaneous pancreas-kidney transplantation when combined with tacrolimus or cyclosporine. *Transplantation*. 1997;64(12):1695–1700.

10. Alhamad T, Malone AF, Lentine KL, et al. Selected mildly obese donors can be used safely in simultaneous pancreas and kidney transplantation. *Transplantation*. 2017;101:1159–1166.

11. Shapiro R, Jordan ML, Scantlebury VP, et al. Renal allograft rejection with normal renal function in simultaneous kidney/pancreas recipients: does dissynchronous rejection really exist? *Transplantation*. 2000;69(3):440–441.

12. Troxell ML, Koslin DB, Norman D, et al. Pancreas allograft rejection: analysis of concurrent renal allograft biopsies and posttherapy follow-up biopsies. *Transplantation*. 2010;90(1):75–84.

Index

Page numbers followed by f refer to figures; page numbers followed by t refer to tables.

A

Abdominal wall hernias, 152
ABMR. *See* Active antibody-mediated rejection
ABO blood typing, 303
ABO compatibility/incompatibility, 283
Abscess formation, 344t
Absolute contraindications, kidney transplant, 291, 291t, 294t
Absorption, in PD, 229
Acanthocytes, 18
Accelerated acute rejection, 325
ACE. *See* Angiotensin-converting enzyme
ACE inhibitor. *See* Angiotensin-converting enzyme inhibitor
Acetaminophen
  with active metabolites, 268t
  in renal impairment, 268
Acid-base
  balance, 158
  map, 53f
  regulation, 163
  status, 31, 34
Acid-base disorders, 52
  classification, 51
  definitions, 51
  electrolyte and, 130
  metabolic acidosis
    diagnostic testing, 54–55
    differential diagnosis, 55–57, 55t, 57t
    principles, 54
    treatment of, 57–58
  metabolic alkalosis
    diagnostic testing, 59
    differential diagnosis, 59
    principles, 58
    treatment, 60
    types of, 58t
  pathophysiology
    acid–base map, 53f
    acidosis, 52
    alkalosis, 53
    buffering, 51
    compensatory responses, 53, 54t
    excretion, 52
    physiologic response to acid load, 52f
    ventilatory response, 52
  respiratory acidosis
    diagnosis, 60–61
    principles, 60
    treatment of, 61
  respiratory alkalosis
    diagnosis, 61
    principles, 61
    treatment of, 61
Acidemia, defined, 51
Acid load, physiologic response to, 52f
Acidosis, 46, 52, 66, 130
Acquired renal cysts. *See also* Cystic disease of kidney
  clinical presentation, 155
  diagnostic criteria, 155
  differential diagnosis, 155
  epidemiology, 155
  outcome/prognosis, 156
  pathophysiology, 155
  treatment, 155
Activated clotting time (ACT), 258
Activated partial thromboplastin time (aPTT), 8, 259, 305t–306t
Active antibody-mediated rejection, 326–327, 327t. *See also* Immunologic complications after kidney transplantation
  chronic, 328, 328t
  donor-specific antibodies, 327, 327t
Active antibody-mediated rejection (ABMR)
  chronic, 328t
  diagnosis, 327t
  treatment of, 329
Active cancer, 300
Active T-cell-mediated rejection, chronic, 326
Active vitamin D, 137
Acute antihypertensive therapy, 164t
Acute cellular rejection, 326, 326t, 345–346
  grade I (mild), 346
  grade II (moderate), 346
  grade III (severe), 346
  treatment for, 328–329
Acute cellular rejection, Banff classification of, 326t
Acute fatty liver of pregnancy, 168, 169t
Acute hyperkalemia, 33

Acute hyperphosphatemia, 47
Acute hyponatremia
  defined, 20
  treatment for, 24–25
Acute interstitial nephritis (AIN). *See also*
    Acute kidney injury (AKI)
  causes of, 95t
  clinical presentation, 94–96
  definition, 94
  diagnostic testing, 96
  epidemiology, 94
  etiology, 94, 95t
  methicillin-induced, 97
  outcome, 97
  pathophysiology, 94
  prognosis for, 97
  treatment of, 96–97
Acute kidney injury (AKI), 10, 246. *See also*
    Renal diseases in pregnancy
  acute interstitial nephritis
    causes of, 95t
    clinical presentation, 94–96
    definition, 94
    diagnostic testing, 96
    epidemiology, 94
    etiology, 94, 95t
    outcome/prognosis, 97
    pathophysiology, 94
    treatment of, 96–97
  acute tubular injury
    causes of, 86t
    principles, 85–86
  atheroembolic renal disease
    about, 79–80
    diagnosis, 80–81, 81t
    epidemiology, 80
    outcome/prognosis, 82
    pathophysiology, 80
    prevention of, 80
    treatment, 81
  cardiorenal syndrome
    principles, 99
    treatment of, 99
  classification, 62, 63t
  clinical presentation, 63–64
  complications with DN and, 147–148
  contrast-induced nephropathy
    diagnostic testing, 87–88
    principles, 87
    treatment, 88
  crystalline nephropathies
    clinical presentation, 89, 90t–92t
    diagnostic testing, 89, 93
    ethylene glycol intoxication, 93–94
    outcome/prognosis, 94
    pathophysiology, 88–89

  prevention, 89
  treatment of, 93
  definition, 62
  diagnostic procedures
    biomarkers, 69–70
    serologic profile and special tests,
      69, 70t
    tissue diagnosis, 69
  diagnostic testing, 66–70
  dosing strategy of medications in, 261
  epidemiology, 62–63
  hepatorenal syndrome
    definition, 97
    diagnostic criteria for, 98t
    pathophysiology, 97–98
    treatment of, 98–99
  history, 64–65
    etiologies, 65
    infections, 65
    medications, 64
    risk factors, 65
    urine patterns and frequency, 64
    volume status, 64
  imaging
    point-of-care ultrasonography, 68, 69t
    renal ultrasound, 68
  intrinsic causes of, 79, 80t, 207
  ischemic, 86
  laboratories
    blood counts/coagulation screen, 68
    chemistry panel, 68
    urinary indices, 67, 68t
    urine examination, 66, 67t
  microvascular causes of, 79
    diagnosis, 82–85, 83t–84t
    principles, 82
    treatment, 85
  nephrotoxic, 86
  nondialytic management of, 70–71
  oliguric, 67
  physical examination, 65–66
    abdominal examination, 66
    cardiac examination, 66
    systemic signs, 66
    volume status, 65
  postrenal
    clinical presentation, 76
    definition, 73, 75t
    diagnostic testing, 76–77
    etiology, 74, 76
    management, 77–78
    pathophysiology, 76
  in pregnancy
    acute fatty liver of pregnancy, 168, 169t
    acute pyelonephritis, 167
    acute tubular necrosis, 167

HELLP syndrome, 168, 169t
HUS, 168, 169t
obstructive uropathy, 167
preeclampsia, 168
prerenal azotemia, 167
renal cortical necrosis, 168
treatment, 167
prerenal
definition, 72
etiology, 73, 74t
management, 73
prevention, 137
rhabdomyolysis, 86–87
RRT in, 71–72, 72t
Acute pancreatitis, 43
Acute phosphate nephropathy, 88
Acute pyelonephritis, 167
Acute renal failure trial network (ATN)
study, 246
Acute respiratory acidosis, causes of, 60
Acute respiratory alkalosis, 61
Acute tubular injury. See also Acute kidney
injury (AKI)
causes of, 86t
principles, 85–86
Acute tubular necrosis (ATN), 49, 81, 167
natural history of, 85–86
Acute uric acid nephropathy, 88
ADPKD. See Autosomal dominant polycystic
kidney disease; Autosomal dominant
polycystic kidney disease (ADPKD)
Adrenal vein sampling (AVS), 199
Adrogue–Madias equation, 24
Age
of living donor, 304
nonmodifiable risk factors in DN, 142
Aggressive medical therapy, 191
aHUS. See Atypical hemolytic uremic
syndrome (aHUS)
AIN. See Acute interstitial nephritis
AKI. See Acute kidney injury
Alanine-glyoxylate aminotransferase (AGT),
311
Albright hereditary osteodystrophy, 42
Albumin, 133, 254, 259t
Albumin excretion rate (AER), 309
Albumin-sensitive tests, 12
Albumin to creatinine ratio (ACR), 309
Albuminuria, 141, 143, 147
Albustix, 12
Albuterol, 35
Alcoholism, 48
Alcohol or starvation ketoacidosis, 56
Aldosterone, 28
resistance, 33
synthesis, 33

Alemtuzumab
lymphocyte-depleting antibody therapy,
343
monoclonal antibody, 314
Alkalemia, defined, 51
Alkali therapy, for concomitant acidosis, 148
Alkalosis, 29, 53
Allopurinol, 208
with active metabolites, 268t
for uric acid, 135
Alport syndrome, 15, 16t, 310
American Diabetic Association (ADA)
guidelines, 341
American Society of Nephrology, 207
Amikacin, dose calculation, 276
Amiloride, 32
Aminoglycoside
dosage adjustments, 272–277, 276t, 277t
loading dose calculation, 276t
maintenance dose calculation, 276t
therapeutic monitoring, 277t
therapy for PD patients and, 236
Amphotericin, and tubular damage, 30
Amyloidosis, 212
Analgesics, 268, 270. See also Drug dosing in
renal impairment
Anemia, 321–322
associated with CKD, 131, 133
and iron deficiency, 135
treatment of, 29
Angiography, 189
Angiotensin-converting enzyme (ACE)
inhibitor, 134, 164
related complications, 260
Angiotensin receptor blocker (ARB), 29,
134, 164, 270
Anion gap (AG) metabolic acidosis. See also
Metabolic acidosis
alcohol or starvation ketoacidosis, 56
diabetic ketoacidosis, 55
endogenous acid generation/accumulation,
57t
exogenous acid exposure/toxic
accumulation, 57t
lactic acidosis, 55
salicylate overdose, 56
toxic alcohol ingestions, 56
Antiangiogenic therapies, 208–209
Anti-B cell therapies, 347
Antibodies, donor-specific, 327, 327t
Antibody-mediated rejection, 346–347
Antibody therapies, induction and rejection,
315t. See also Kidney transplant
patient management
monoclonal, 314
polyclonal, 314

Anticoagulants. *See also* Drug dosing in renal impairment
  anti-Xa inhibitors, 263, 268
  direct thrombin inhibitors, 268
  heparins, 263
  vitamin K antagonists, 263
Anticoagulation, 257–258
  problems, 252
  related complications, 259
Antidiuretic hormone (ADH), 20
Antigen-presenting cells, 282
Antimetabolites, 317–318
Antimicrobials. *See also* Drug dosing in renal impairment
  aminoglycosides, 272–277, 276t, 277t
  antiretrovirals, 278
  dose adjustment for renal function, 272, 273t–275t
  vancomycin, 277–278, 277t
Antineutrophil cytoplasmic antibody (ANCA), 132
Antinuclear antibodies (ANA), 132, 310
Antiphospholipid syndrome (APS), 79, 82
Antiretrovirals, dosage adjustments, 278
Antiretroviral therapy (ART), 296
Antithymocyte globulin (ATGAM), 314
Anti-Xa inhibitors, dosage adjustments, 263, 268
Apixaban, direct oral anticoagulant agents (DOAC), 263
Apparatus
  for PD
    catheter and setup, 229–230, 230f
    dialysis solution, 230–231, 230t, 231t
    peritoneal membrane, 231–232, 232t
ARAS. *See* Atherosclerotic renal artery stenosis
ARB. *See* Angiotensin receptor blocker
Argatroban, 268
ARPKD. *See* Autosomal recessive inheritance pattern
Arrhythmias, 251
Arterial surgical complications, 332
Arteriovenous fistula (AVF), 9, 139
Arteriovenous graft (AVG), 139
Arthritis, 66
Asymptomatic hyponatremia, 24
Asymptomatic microscopic hematuria (AMH), 14, 15
Atheroembolic disease, 192
Atheroembolic renal disease. *See also* Acute kidney injury (AKI)
  about, 79–80
  diagnosis, 80–81, 81t
  epidemiology, 80
  outcome/prognosis, 82

pathophysiology, 80
prevention of, 80
treatment, 81
Atherosclerotic renal artery stenosis (ARAS), 184, 186
Atherosclerotic renovascular disease, 184–185
ATN. *See* Acute tubular necrosis
Atypical hemolytic uremic syndrome (aHUS), 128, 310
Auryxia, 137
Autoimmune diseases, 42
Automated cycler exchanges, 233
Automated PD, 233
Autosomal dominant hypophosphatemic rickets, 49
Autosomal dominant polycystic kidney disease (ADPKD), 149, 309–310
Autosomal recessive inheritance pattern (ARPKD), 149
Azathioprine, 118, 317, 318

B
Back pain, in PD, 239
Bacteria, 6
Bartter syndromes, 30
Basic metabolic profile (BMP), 305t–306t
Basiliximab
  monoclonal antibody, 314
  nondepleting antibody therapy, 342
Belatacept, dosing of, 317
Bicarbonate-based solutions, 249
Bicarbonate reabsorption, 52
Bicarbonate solutions, in rhabdomyolysis/hemolysis, 87
Bicarbonaturia, 32
Biguanides, 271, 271t
Biomarkers, diagnosis of AKI and, 69
Bisoprolol, β-blockers, 270
Bisphosphonates, 137
Bivalirudin, 268
BK virus. *See also* Nonimmunologic complications after kidney transplantation
  diagnosis, 336–337
  principles, 336, 336t
  risk factors for, 336t
  treatment of, 337
BK virus nephropathy (BKVN), 331
Blood
  coagulation parameters, 8
  loss, and transfusion, 9
  products, massive transfusion of, 59
  tests
    for hypernatremia, 26
    for hyponatremia, 23

Blood pressure (BP)
  control for renal biopsy, 8
  recordings
    in diagnosis of DN, 144
Blood urea nitrogen (BUN), 3t, 18
Body mass index (BMI), 300, 306
Bone
  disease in ESRD patients, 321
  resorption, increased, 39, 39t
Borderline acute cellular rejection, 346
Borderline rejection, 328
Bosniak renal cyst classification system,
    154t
Brincidofovir, 337
Buffering, 51
Bumetanide, diuretics in renal impairment,
    270
Busulfan, and hematuria, 15

C
Calcimimetics, 42
Calcineurin inhibitors (CNI), 103, 315,
    317
  during pregnancy, 171
  toxicity, 331
Calciphylaxis, 46
Calcitriol, 38, 44, 137
Calcium
  absorption, decreased, 42
  reabsorption of, 38
Calcium acetate, 47
Calcium balance, disorders of. *See also*
    Phosphorus metabolism, disorders of
  hypercalcemia
    causes of, 39t
    clinical presentation, 41
    diagnostic testing, 41
    malignancy-related, 40t
    principles, 39
    treatment, 41–42
  hypocalcemia
    clinical presentation, 43
    diagnostic testing, 44
    principles, 42–43
    treatment for, 44
  principles, 38–39
Calcium-based phosphate binders, 47
Calcium carbonate, 47
Calcium channel blockers, during pregnancy,
    171
Calcium oxalate, urinary crystal, 6t
Calcium phosphate, urinary crystal, 6t
Calculated PRA (cPRA), 288
Canada-USA (CANUSA) Study Group,
    232
Canagliflozin, 272

Cancer, and kidney transplant candidate
    evaluation, 299t, 300
Cancer-free waiting periods before
    transplant, 299t
Candida in urine, 6
Captopril challenge test, 199
Captopril radionuclide renogram, 187, 189
Cardiac examination, in AKI, 66
Cardiac risk assessment, 306, 307
Cardiac valvular disease, 152
Cardiorenal syndrome (CRS). *See also* Acute
    kidney injury (AKI)
  classification of, 99
  features of type 1, 99
  principles, 99
  treatment of, 99
Cardiovascular disease, hyperlipidemia and,
    131–132
Cardiovascular evaluation, of kidney
    transplant candidate, 294–295
Carotid imaging, 295
Cast nephropathy, 211–212
Casts, urinary
  defined, 6
  types of, 7t
Catastrophic APS, 82
Catheter and setup, 229–230, 230f
Catheter-site infections, in PD, 237
Cation-exchange resins, 36
Cefazolin, for PD patients, 236, 237t
Ceftazidime, for PD patients, 236, 237t
Centers for Medicare and Medicaid Services
    (CMS), 233
Central pontine myelinolysis, 22
Central venous catheter, 249, 251
Centrifugation, 254
Cerebral aneurysms, 152
Chelation, intravascular, 43
Chloride-resistant metabolic alkalosis
  about, 58t
  diagnostic testing, 59
  differential diagnosis, 59
  treatment for, 60
Chloride-responsive metabolic alkalosis
  about, 58t
  diagnostic testing, 59
  differential diagnosis, 59
  treatment for, 60
Chloride shunt, 33
Chlorthalidone, 270
Cholecalciferol (vitamin D3)
  for vitamin D replacement, 137
Chronic fungal infections, 296
Chronic hyperkalemia, 33, 37
Chronic hyperphosphatemia, 47
  treatment for, 47–48

Chronic hypertension, 163. *See also* Hypertensive disorders in pregnancy
  principles, 164
  treatment, 164, 164t
Chronic hyponatremia, 23
Chronic hypophosphatemia
  and osteomalacia in adults, 49
  and rickets in children, 49
Chronic kidney disease (CKD), 1, 42
  anemia, 131
  classification, 130, 132f
  definition, 130, 131f
  diagnosis, 132–133
  dialysis and renal transplant, preparation for
    immunizations, 138–139
    patient education, 138
  dosing of medications in, 261
  electrolyte/acid–base disorders, 130
  hyperlipidemia and cardiovascular disease, 131–132
  hypertension, 131
  medication errors in, 137
  mineral/bone disorders, 131
  and pregnancy, 169–171
  pregnancy in renal transplant recipients/ kidney donors
    after kidney donation, 171
    after renal transplant, 170–171
  referral for dialysis access/transplantation, 139
  RRT, initiation of, 139
  treatment
    AKI prevention, 137
    anemia and iron deficiency, 135–136
    CKD-MBD/SHPT, 136–137
    concomitant medications, 137–138
    edema and volume overload, 134
    hyperkalemia, 134–135
    hyperlipidemia, 135
    hypertension, 134
    hyperuricemia, 135
    metabolic acidosis, 135
    nephrology consultation, 134
Chronic kidney disease-mineral and bone disorder (CKD-MBD), 131, 133, 136
Chronic respiratory acidosis, causes of, 61
Chronic respiratory alkalosis, 61
Chvostek sign, 43
Cidofovir, 337
Cirrhosis with ascites, 98t
Cisplatin, and tubular damage, 30
Citrate anticoagulation, 249, 253
Citrate-containing blood products, 43
Citrate toxicity, 258
CKD. *See* Chronic kidney disease

Clearance calculation, 3
Clearance targets, defined, 233–234
Clotrimazole troche, oropharyngeal candidiasis prevention, 318
CMV. *See* Cytomegalovirus
CNI. *See* Calcineurin inhibitors
Cockcroft–Gault equation, 2, 3t, 261
Colchicine, 135
Colonic diverticulosis, 152
Compatibility testing
  serologic methods for, 284–286, 286f
  solid phase methods for, 286–288, 287f, 288f
Compensatory responses for primary acid–base disturbances, 53, 54t
Complement-dependent cytotoxicity (CDC) testing, 284, 284t, 285
Computed tomography angiography (CTA), 188
Computed tomography (CT) scans
  for ADPKD, 150
  for MCKD, 157
Computed tomography urography (CTU), 18
Concentric onion skin lesions, 85
Concomitant disorders, 130
Concomitant medications, 137
Congenital adrenal hyperplasia, 202
Connective tissue disorder, 65
Conn syndrome, 30
Constipation treatment, 239
Continuous ambulatory peritoneal dialysis (CAPD), 233
Continuous cycling peritoneal dialysis (CCPD), 233
Continuous renal replacement therapy (CRRT). *See also* Renal replacement therapy (RRT)
  anticoagulation in, 249
  complications of, 250–253
  drug dosing in CRRT, 250
  fluids in, 249
  principles of, 248–249, 248t
  regimen for CRRT, 250
Continuous venovenous hemodiafiltration, 247, 248, 249
Continuous venovenous hemodialysis (CVVHD), 248
Continuous venovenous hemofiltration, 248
Contrast-induced nephropathy. *See also* Acute kidney injury (AKI)
  diagnostic testing, 87–88
    diagnostic procedures, 88
    imaging, 88
    laboratories, 87–88
  principles, 87
  treatment, 88

Contrast-induced nephropathy (CIN), 87
Contrast nephropathy, 192
Convective elimination, 250
Corticosteroid, 96
  excess, 59
  therapy, 329
Costimulation inhibitors, 317
Creatine kinase, 47
Creatine phosphokinase (CPK), 31
Creatinine, 2, 3t
Creatinine clearance (CrCl), 3–4
Creatinine kinase (CK) elevation, 68
Crossmatch-positive transplants, 290
CRRT. *See* Continuous renal replacement
    therapy
CRS. *See* Cardiorenal syndrome
Crystalline nephropathies. *See also* Acute
    kidney injury (AKI)
  clinical presentation, 89, 90t–92t
  diagnostic testing, 89, 93
  ethylene glycol intoxication, 93–94
  outcome/prognosis, 94
  pathophysiology, 88–89
  prevention, 89
  treatment of, 93
Cushing syndrome, 30
Cyclic adenosine monophosphate (cAMP),
    149
Cyclophosphamide, 171
Cyclosporine
  calcineurin inhibitors (CNI), 315, 317
  decreasing response to aldosterone, 33
Cyst
  hemorrhage, 151
  infection, 151
Cystic disease of kidney
  acquired renal cysts
    clinical presentation, 155
    diagnostic criteria, 155
    differential diagnosis, 155
    epidemiology, 155
    outcome/prognosis, 156
    pathophysiology, 155
    treatment, 155
  medullary cystic kidney disease
    classification, 156
    clinical presentation, 156
    diagnostic criteria, 157
    differential diagnosis, 157
    epidemiology, 156
    outcome/prognosis, 157
    pathophysiology, 156
    treatment, 157
  medullary sponge kidney
    diagnosis, 158
    epidemiology, 157

    outcome/prognosis, 158
    pathophysiology, 157
    treatment, 158
  polycystic kidney disease
    classification, 149
    clinical presentation, 149–150
    complications, 151–152
    diagnostic criteria, 150, 150t
    differential diagnosis, 151
    epidemiology, 149
    outcome/prognosis, 153
    pathophysiology, 149
    patient education, 152–153
    treatment, 151
  simple renal cysts
    clinical presentation, 153
    diagnostic criteria, 153
    differential diagnosis, 154, 154t
    epidemiology, 153
    outcome/prognosis, 155
    pathophysiology, 153
    treatment, 154
  tuberous sclerosis
    diagnosis, 159
    epidemiology, 158–159
    pathophysiology, 159
    treatment, 159–160
  von Hippel-Lindau (VHL) syndrome
    diagnosis, 160
    epidemiology, 160
    pathophysiology, 160
    treatment, 161
Cystoscopy, 19, 309
Cytomegalovirus (CMV), 293. *See also*
    Nonimmunologic complications
    after kidney transplantation
  clinical presentation, 335
  principles, 332
  prophylaxis, 335
  treatment of, 335–336, 335t
Cytomegalovirus (CMV) IgG antibodies,
    296

D
Dabigatran, 268
Damage biomarkers, 70
Dapagliflozin, dosing of, 272
Delayed graft function (DGF), 302
Deoxycorticosterone-producing tumors,
    202
Deposition, extravascular, 43
Desirudin, 268
Dextrose, 228
Diabetes insipidus (DI), 163
Diabetes mellitus, post-transplant, 321
Diabetic ketoacidosis (DKA), 31, 55

Diabetic nephropathy (DN)
clinical presentation, 143–144
history, 144
physical examination, 144
complications
AKI, 147–148
hyperkalemia, 148
hypoglycemia, 147
definition, 141, 144
diagnostic testing
diagnostic procedures, 145
imagng, 145
laboratory testing, 145
differential diagnoses, 144
epidemiology, 141
modifiable risk factors
hyperglycemia, 142
hypertension, 142
obesity, 142
monitoring/follow-up, 148
nonmodifiable risk factors
age, 142
genetic factors, 142
race, 142
pathophysiology of, 141
prevention, 142
screening, 142–143, 143t
treatment
glycemic control, 145–146
hypertension, 146–147
Diabetic neuropathy, 341
Diabetic retinopathy, 341
Dialysate, 250
Dialysate flow rates, 253
Dialysis disequilibrium syndrome, 226
Dialysis patients
aminoglycosides for, 277
vancomycin for, 278
Dietary restriction of phosphate, 47
Diethylenetriamine-penta-acetic acid
(DTPA), 190
Diffusion
and convection, 249
in PD, 228
Diffusive elimination, 250
Dilutional hyponatremia, 98
Dipeptidyl peptidase-4 inhibitors, 271–272
Dipstick testing, 18
Direct oral anticoagulant agents (DOAC),
263, 269t
Direct thrombin inhibitors, dosage
adjustments, 268
Disorders of sodium, 20
Diuretics, 22, 30, 59, 71, 134. See also Drug
dosing in renal impairment
loop, 270

potassium-sparing, 271
thiazide, 270
Diuretic therapy, 99
DKA. See Diabetic ketoacidosis
DN. See Diabetic nephropathy
DOAC. See Direct oral anticoagulant agents
Donation after brain death (DBD), 290
Donation after cardiac death (DCD), 290,
324
Donor recipient mismatched antigens,
principle of, 284f
Donor-specific antibody (DSA), 324, 327,
327t
Dose. See also Drug dosing in renal
impairment
adjustment of medications
in AKI, 71
in renal insufficiency, 268
of TPE, 257
Drug activity, parameters of, 263,
264t–267t
Drug dosing in renal impairment
dosage adjustments of drugs
analgesics, 268, 270
anticoagulants, 263, 268, 269t
antihypertensives, 270
antimicrobials, 272–278, 273t–275t,
276t, 277t
diuretics, 270–271
hypoglycemic agents, 271–272
nephrotoxicity/alternatives to common
drugs, 262t
overview, 261
and pharmacokinetic principles, 261, 263,
264t–267t, 268t
during RRT, 278
Dual marginal kidneys, transplant of, 290
Dynamic contrast-enhanced CT, 189
Dysmorphic RBC, 18

E
EBV. See Epstein-Barr virus
Echogenicity, 8
Eculizumab, ABMR treatment, 329–330
Edema and volume overload, 134
Edoxaban
direct oral anticoagulant agents (DOAC),
263
and dose adjustments in renal
insufficiency, 268
EKG. See Electrocardiography
Electrocardiography (EKG), 32, 34–35
Electrolyte
and acid-base disorders, 130
disturbances, 210, 251–252
Electron microscopy, 337

ELISA. *See* Enzyme-linked immunosorbent assay
Empagliflozin, dosing of, 272
End diastolic velocity (EDV), 188
Endocrine complications. *See also* Kidney transplant patient management
 bone disease, 321
 hyperlipidemia, 320
 obesity, 321
 post-transplant diabetes mellitus, 321
Endogenous acid generation/accumulation, 57t
Endotoxic shock, 43
End-stage renal disease (ESRD), renal transplantation for, 280
Enzyme-linked immunosorbent assay (ELISA), 284, 284t
Eosinophiluria, 96
Epilepsy, 159
Epithelial cells
 renal tubular, 6
 squamous, 5
 transitional, 5
Eplerenone, aldosterone antagonists, 33
Epoetin alfa, 136
Epstein-Barr virus (EBV), 293. *See also* Nonimmunologic complications after kidney transplantation
 diagnosis, 338
 principles, 337–338
 treatment of, 338
Epstein-Barr virus (EBV), 296
Ergocalciferol (vitamin D2), 137
Erythrocytosis, post-transplant, 322
Erythropoiesis-stimulating agents (ESA), 136
Estimated glomerular filtration rate (eGFR), 271t, 280
Estimated post transplant survival (EPTS), 289
Estrogen exposure, 150
Ethacrynic acid, 270
Ethylene glycol
 ingestion, 56
 intoxication, 56
Euvolemic hyponatremia, 24
Exenatide, in severe renal impairment, 272
Exit-site and tunnel infection, in PD, 237
Exogenous acid exposure/toxic accumulation, 57t
Extended-interval (EI) dosing of aminoglycosides, 272
Extracellular fluid (ECF), 38

F
Fabry disease, 311
Familial hyperaldosteronism type I (FH-I), 196
Familial hypocalcemia, 42

Familial hypocalciuric hypercalcemia (FHH), 40, 41
Familial x-linked hypophosphatemic rickets (XLH), 49
Family history of hematuria, 5
Fanconi syndrome, 30, 49, 210
Febuxostat, 135,
Fentanyl, with active metabolites, 270
Ferric citrate, 137
Ferrous sulfate, for anemia/iron deficiency, 136
Fertility in women with CKD, 169
FFP. *See* Fresh frozen plasma
FHH. *See* Familial hypocalciuric hypercalcemia
Fibrates, 135
Fibrinoid necrosis, 85
Fibroblast growth factor 23 (FGF23), 39, 45
Fibromuscular dysplasia (FMD), 184
Flow crossmatch, 286
Fluconazole, oropharyngeal candidiasis prevention, 318
Fluid leakage, in PD, 239–240
Fludrocortisone suppression test, 199
Fluoroquinolones, 337
FMD. *See* Fibromuscular dysplasia
Focal segmental glomerulosclerosis (FSGS), 101–105, 144, 298
 C1q nephropathy and, 105
 primary, 102–103
  outcomes of, 103
  symptoms of, 103
  treatment of, 102–103
 secondary, 103–105
  genetic causes of, 103
  HIV infection and, 104
  sickle cell disease and, 104
  treatment of, 104
Fomepizole, 56
Fondaparinux, 263
Fractional excretion of sodium (FENa)
 calculation of, 67, 68t
Fresh frozen plasma (FFP), 254, 258, 259t
FSGS. *See* Focal segmental glomerulosclerosis
Fungal peritonitis, 237
Fungi, 6
Furosemide, 134
Furosemide stress test (FST), 71

G
Gadolinium, 189
Gadolinium-based contrast agents, 43, 138
Gastric drainage, vomiting or, 59
Gastric secretions, 29
Gastrointestinal (GI) symptoms, 41
Gene expression assays, 325
Genetic factors, nonmodifiable risk factors in DN, 142

Genetic testing
  for ADPKD, 150
  for VHL, 160
Genital edema, 240
Gentamicin
  dose calculation, 276
  and tubular damage, 30
Gestational hypertension, 163
Gestational hypertension and preeclampsia, 312
GFR. *See* Glomerular filtration rate
Gitelman syndromes, 30
Glipizide, with active metabolite, 271
Glomerular basement membrane (GBM), 328
Glomerular diseases in pregnancy, 171
Glomerular filtration rate (GFR), 42k, 71, 162
  defined, 1
  estimation, 2–4, 3t, 4t
    equation-based estimates of, 2, 4t
    serum markers, 2, 3t
    timed collections, 3–4
  proteinuria and, 10
Glomerular hyperfiltration, 141
Glomerular hypertrophy, 145
Glomerular proteinuria, 10
Glomerulonephritis, 15, 69
Glucagon-like peptide-1 receptor agonists, 272
Glucocorticoid, anti-inflammatory agents, 315
Glucocorticoid remediable hyperaldosteronism, 30
Glutathione S-transferase, 70
Glucocorticoid-remediable aldosteronism (GRA), 196
Glyburide, with active metabolite, 268t, 271
Glycemic control, treatment of DN, 145–146
Goldblatt model, 185–186
Goodpasture syndrome, 65
Gordon syndrome, 33, 202
Gout, 312
Graft pancreatitis, 344t
Gram-positive infections, 237
Granular casts, 7t
Granulocyte-macrophage colony-stimulating factor (GM-CSF), 29
Granulomatous disease, 40
Gross hematuria, 14

H
Hamartomas, 159
Head computed tomography, 23

Heavy chain deposition disease (HCDD), 212
HELLP syndrome. *See* Hemolysis, elevated liver enzymes, and low platelets syndrome
Hematologic complications. *See also* Kidney transplant patient management
  anemia, 321–322
  post-transplant erythrocytosis, 322
Hematuria, 9, 14–19, 76, 151. *See also* Proteinuria
  associated conditions, 15
  clinical presentation
    algorithm for microscopic hematuria, 17f
    history, 15, 17t
    physical examination, 17–18
  definition, 14
  diagnostic testing
    diagnostic procedures, 19
    imaging, 18–19
    laboratories, 18
  epidemiology, 14
  etiology, 14–15, 16t
  microscopic, 309
  monitoring, 19
Hemodialysis, 41, 48, 56
  access to, 219–220
  anticoagulation during, 224
    with heparin, 224
  complications of, 224
    access, 224–226
    dialyzer reactions as, 226–227
    from infections, 225
    recirculation, 225
    for urea clearance, 226
  initiation of, 217
  mechanisms for, 220, , 221t
    maintenance guidelines in, 221t
    prescriptions as part of, 220–222
  modalities, 218
  mortality rates with, 217
Hemoglobin A1c (HbA1c), 305t–306t
Hemoglobinuria, 66
Hemolysis, 46
Hemolysis, elevated liver enzymes, and low platelets (HELLP) syndrome, 79, 82, 168, 169t
Hemolytic uremic syndrome (HUS), 79, 82, 127–128, 168, 169t
Henderson–Hasselbalch equation, defined, 51
Heparin
  dosage adjustments, 263
  with HIT, 252
  intravenous, 249
  low-molecular-weight, 263
  reducing aldosterone synthesis, 33
  unfractionated, 258, 263

Heparin-induced thrombocytopenia (HIT), 249

Hepatic C virus (HCV), 296

Hepatitis
B virus (HBV), 293, 296
C virus (HCV), 293
kidney transplant candidate and, 296

Hepatitis B immunization, 138

Hepatitis C virus (HCV)-positive donor kidneys, 290

Hepatorenal syndrome (HRS). *See also* Acute kidney injury (AKI)
definition, 97
diagnostic criteria for, 98t
pathophysiology, 97–98
physiology, 341, 342
treatment of, 98–99

Herbal products, with aristolochic acid, 64

Hereditary kidney disease, living donor evaluation in
Alport syndrome, 310
atypical hemolytic uremic syndrome, 310
autosomal dominant polycystic kidney disease, 309–310
Fabry disease, 311
kidney stone, 310
primary hyperoxaluria, 311
systematic lupus erythematosus, 310
thin basement membrane disease, 310

Hernias, 239

Herpes simplex virus (HSV), 293

HHD. *See* Home hemodialysis

Histidine-tryptophan-ketoglutarate (HTK), 344t

Histocompatibility testing for kidney transplantation, 284, 284t

HIV-positive patients
kidney transplantation for, 290

HLA. *See* Human leukocyte antigen

Home hemodialysis (HHD), 241–244. *See also* Peritoneal dialysis (PD)
access training and care, 244
characteristics of, 243t
dialysis prescription, 242
patient selection, 242
water supply, 242

Hoodia gordonii, 64

Hormone replacement therapy (HRT), 305t–306t

Hospital-acquired hypernatremia, 25

24-hour urine protein collection, 13

HRHA. *See* Hyporeninemic hypoaldosteronism

HRS. *See* Hepatorenal syndrome

Human chorionic gonadotropin (HCG), 305t–306t

Human herpesvirus 5 (HHV-5), 332

Human immunodeficiency virus (HIV), 293
and kidney transplant candidate, 296, 298

Human leukocyte antigen (HLA), 293
donor and recipient matching, 283, 283f, 284f
and immunology of transplant, 281–282
molecules, antigen presentation by, 282
typing, 282–283, 303

Humoral hypercalcemia, 40t

Hungry bone syndrome, 43, 48

HUS. *See* Hemolytic uremic syndrome

Hyaline casts, 7t

Hydrochlorothiazide, 270

Hydromorphone, with active metabolites, 270

Hyperacute rejection, 325

Hypercalcemia. *See also* Calcium balance, disorders of
causes of, 39t
clinical presentation, 41
diagnostic testing, 41
malignancy-related, 40t
principles
decreased renal excretion, 40
familial hypocalciuric hypercalcemia (FHH), 40
granulomatous disease, 40
immobilization, 40
increased bone resorption, 39
increased intestinal absorption, 40
malignancy, 40
Milk-alkali syndrome, 40
primary hyperparathyroidism, 39
tertiary hyperparathyroidism, 40
treatment, 41–42
and tubular damage, 30
vitamin A intoxication, 40
vitamin D intoxication, 40

Hyperglycemia, 240
in development of DN, 141
modifiable risk factor in DN, 142

Hyperinsulinemia, 142

Hyperkalemia, 71, 134–135, 148. *See also* Potassium balance, disorders of
clinical presentation, 34
defined, 32
diagnostic testing
electrocardiography, 34–35
laboratories, 34, 34t
IV calcium for treatment of, 35
pathophysiology, 33–34
acute hyperkalemia, 33
chronic hyperkalemia, 33
renin and aldosterone in, 34t
treatment of, 35–37

Hyperkalemic periodic paralysis, 33

Hyperlipidemia, 135, 240–241, 320
and cardiovascular disease, 131–132
Hypernatremia, 25–27. *See also* Water
balance, disorders of
causes of, 25f
classification, 25
clinical presentation
history, 26
physical examination, 26
definition, 25
diagnostic testing
blood, 26
urine, 26
epidemiology, 25
etiology, 25, 25f
pathophysiology, 26
treatment, 27
Hyperparathyroidism, 49
Hyperphosphatemia, 43. *See also* Phosphorus
metabolism, disorders of
causes of, 46t
clinical presentation, 47
defined, 45
diagnostic testing, 47
pathophysiology
impaired renal excretion, 45–46
phosphate load, increased, 46
transcellular shift, 46
treatment for
acute hyperphosphatemia, 47
chronic hyperphosphatemia, 47–48
Hypertension, 131, 133, 152, 304, 312, 320
chronic
principles, 164
treatment, 164, 164t
modifiable risk factor in DN, 142
in pregnancy, 163
drug options, 164t
management, 166
renovascular, 185t
treatment, 146–147
Hypertensive disorders in pregnancy,
163–167. *See also* Renal diseases in
pregnancy
chronic hypertension
principles, 164
treatment, 164, 164t
preeclampsia
diagnosis, 165, 166t
principles, 165, 165t
treatment, 165–167
Hypertonic hyponatremia, 20, 21
Hypertonic saline, 24
Hypertriglyceridemia, 135
Hyperuricemia, 135
Hypervolemic hyponatremia, 24

Hypocalcemia, 89. *See also* Calcium balance,
disorders of
clinical presentation, 43
diagnostic testing, 44
principles
calcium absorption, decreased, 42
extravascular deposition/intravascular
chelation, 43
PTH level/effect, decreased, 42
septic shock, 43
treatment for, 44
Hypoglycemia, 147
Hypoglycemic agents. *See also* Drug dosing
in renal impairment
biguanides, 271, 271t
dipeptidyl peptidase-4 inhibitors,
271–272
glucagon-like peptide-1 receptor agonists,
272
insulin, 272
sodium-glucose cotransporter-2 inhibitors,
272
sulfonylureas, 271
Hypoinsulinemia, 46
Hypokalemia, 49, 241, 252. *See also*
Potassium balance, disorders of
clinical presentation, 30–31
history, 31
physical examination, 31
defined, 29
diagnostic testing
electrocardiography, 32
laboratories, 31, 31t
pathophysiology, 29–30
serum renin/aldosterone in, 31t
treatment for, 32
Hypokalemic periodic paralysis, 29
Hypomagnesemia, 30, 42, 49, 252
Hyponatremia, 20–25, 163. *See also* Water
balance, disorders of
causes of, 21f
classification
hypertonic hyponatremia, 20
hypotonic hyponatremia, 20
pseudohyponatremia, 20
clinical presentation
history, 23
physical examination, 23
defined, 20
diagnostic testing
blood, 23
imaging, 23
urine, 23
epidemiology, 20–21
etiology
hypertonic hyponatremia, 21

hypotonic hyponatremia, 21
isotonic hyponatremia, 21
pathophysiology, 22
risk factors, 22
SIADH, causes of, 22t
treatment
acute/symptomatic hyponatremia, 24–25
asymptomatic hyponatremia, 24
Hypoparathyroidism, 42
Hypophosphatemia, 252. *See also*
Phosphorus metabolism, disorders of
clinical presentation, 49
defined, 48
diagnostic testing, 49
moderate, treatment for, 50
pathophysiology
extracellular phosphate, redistribution
of, 48
intestinal absorption, decreased, 48
renal excretion, increased, 49
severe, treatment for, 50
Hyporeninemic hypoaldosteronism
(HRHA), 34
Hypotension, 250
after renal biopsy, 9
Hypothermia, 29, 252
Hypotonic hyponatremia, 20, 21
Hypovolemia, correction of, 41
Hypovolemic hyponatremia, 24

I
Iatrogenic after thyroidectomy, 42
IgA nephropathy, 298
ILDA. *See* Independent living donor advocate
Immobilization, 40
Immune checkpoint inhibitor (ICIs), 210
Immunizations, 318. *See also* Chronic kidney
disease (CKD)
to CKD patients
hepatitis B, 138
influenza vaccination, 138–139
pneumococcal vaccination, 138
Immunofluorescence (IF), 337
Immunoglobulin
depletion, 260
plasma half-life of, 256
removal of, 256–257
Immunohistochemistry (IH), 337
Immunologic complications after kidney
transplantation
diagnostic testing, 325
differential diagnosis, 324–325
principles, 324
rejection types
accelerated acute, 325
active antibody-mediated, 326, 327t

acute cellular, 326, 326t
borderline, 328
chronic, active antibody-mediated, 328,
328t
chronic active T-cell–mediated, 326
hyperacute, 325
subclinical, 328
treatment
acute cellular rejection, 328–329
antibody-mediated rejection, 329–330
Immunology of kidney transplant. *See also*
Kidney transplantation
antigen presentation by HLA molecules,
282
barriers to transplantation, 283
histocompatibility testing for
transplantation, 284, 284t
HLA donor/recipient matching, 283,
283f, 284f
HLA/MHC, 281–282
HLA typing, 282–283
serologic methods for compatibility
testing, 284–286, 286f
solid phase methods for compatibility
testing, 286–288, 287f, 288f
Immunosuppression, 314
Impaired insulin signaling in podocytes, 141
Independent living donor advocate (ILDA),
302, 303
Induction for combined transplantation
liver/kidney, 343
pancreas, 342–343
Induction immunotherapy, 342
Infection prophylaxis, 318
Infectious complications, in PD
exit-site and tunnel infection, 237
peritonitis, 234–237, 235t–236t, 237t,
238t
Influenza inactivated vaccine, 297t
Influenza vaccination, 138–139
Informed consent
and living donor evaluation, 302
Insulin, 45, 272
and hyperkalemia, 35
Insulin-like growth factor–binding protein 7
(IGFBP7), 70
Intermittent hemodialysis (IHD), 246, 247t
Interstitial fibrosis or tubular atrophy
(iIFTA), 326
Interventional radiology, 252
Intestinal absorption, increased, 40
Intracranial aneurysms, 295
Intraglomerular hypertension, 141
Intraperitoneal doses of antibiotics, 237t
Intravenous excretory pyelography, 158
Intravenous heparin, 249

Intravenous immunoglobulin (IVIG), 21,
    260, 347
Intravenous urography, 19
Inulin, 3
Ionized calcium, 41
Iron deficiency, 135
Ischemic acute kidney injury, 86
Ischemic nephropathy, defined, 185
Isotonic hyponatremia, 21

J
Juvenile nephronophthisis, 156

K
Kayexalate, 36
Kidney
    donation
        eligibility for, 304
        exclusion criteria for, 308t
    donor types, 290
    failure, 340
    function, 307
    stone, 310
Kidney allocation system (KAS), 288–290,
    289t
Kidney allograft survival, 283f
Kidney disease, recurrence of
    focal segmental glomerulosclerosis, 298
    IgA nephropathy, 298
    lupus nephritis, 298, 300
Kidney Disease Improving Global Outcomes
    (KDIGO), 246
    classification, 10
    guidelines, 62, 130
Kidney Disease Outcomes Quality Initiative
    (KDOQI)
    guidelines, 233
Kidney Donor Profile Index (KDPI), 288,
    289t
Kidney function, assessment of, 1–9
    diagnostic testing
        GFR estimation, 2–4, 3t, 4t
        imaging studies, 6, 8
        renal biopsy, 8–9
        urinary assessment, 4–6, 5t, 6t, 7t
    differential diagnosis, 1–2
    principles, 1
Kidney injury molecule-1 (KIM-1), 69
Kidney transplantation
    absolute/relative contraindications for,
        291, 291t
    immunology of transplant
        antigen presentation by HLA
            molecules, 282
        barriers to, 283
        histocompatibility testing for, 284, 284t

    HLA donor/recipient matching, 283,
        283f, 284f
    HLA/MHC, 281–282
    HLA typing, 282–283
    serologic methods for compatibility
        testing, 284–286, 286f
    solid phase methods for compatibility
        testing, 286–288, 287f, 288f
    kidney allocation system, 288–290, 289t
    kidney donor types, 290
    and outcomes, 281
    principles, 280
    recipient/donor evaluation for, 291
    referral for dialysis access, 139
    special populations for, 290
    transplant surgical procedure, 292
    waitlist management, 281
Kidney transplant candidate, evaluation of
    cancer, 299t, 300
    cardiovascular evaluation, 294–295
    infection
        about, 295–296
        hepatitis, 296
        human immunodeficiency virus, 296,
            298
        vaccinations for kidney transplant
            candidates, 297t
    obesity, 300
    peripheral arterial disease, 295
    principles, 293–294, 293t, 294t
    recurrence of kidney disease
        focal segmental glomerulosclerosis, 298
        IgA nephropathy, 298
        lupus nephritis, 298, 300
    waitlist management, 300
Kidney transplant patient management
    antibody therapies, induction and
        rejection, 315t
        monoclonal, 314
        polyclonal, 314
    endocrine/metabolic complications
        bone disease, 321
        hyperlipidemia, 320
        obesity, 321
        post-transplant diabetes mellitus, 321
    hematologic complications
        anemia, 321–322
        post-transplant erythrocytosis, 322
    hypertension, 320
    maintenance immunosuppression, 316f
        antimetabolites, 317–318
        calcineurin inhibitors, 315, 317
        costimulation inhibitors, 317
        glucocorticoid (prednisone,
            prednisolone), 315
        infection prophylaxis, 318

mammalian target of rapamycin
inhibitors, 317
pharmacology/drug–drug interactions,
318–320, 319t
malignancy, 322
pregnancy, 322–323
principles, 314
transplant-recipient outcomes, 320
Kimmelstiel–Wilson nodules, 145
K-Phos neutral
for moderate hypophosphatemia, 50

L
Labetalol, and dose adjustments, 270
Lactic acidosis, 55
Lanthanum carbonate, 48
Latent tuberculosis, 296
Leflunomide, 337
Left ventricular ejection fraction, 295
Left ventricular hypertrophy (LVH), 295
Liddle syndrome, 30, 201
Lifestyle modifications, 135
Light and heavy chain deposition disease
(LHCDD), 212
Light microscopy, 93, 337
Linagliptin, dosing in renal dysfunction, 272
Live-donor transplantation, 290
Liver cysts, 152
Liver/kidney transplantation
combined, 341–342, 342t
minimum criteria for, 342t
Liver-type fatty acid–binding protein
(L-FABP), 70
Live vaccines, 281
Living kidney donor candidate, evaluation of
ABO blood typing, 303
age, 304
cardiac risk assessment, 306, 307
in hereditary kidney disease
Alport syndrome, 310
atypical hemolytic uremic syndrome,
310
autosomal dominant polycystic kidney
disease, 309–310
Fabry disease, 311
kidney stone, 310
primary hyperoxaluria, 311
systematic lupus erythematosus, 310
thin basement membrane disease, 310
HLA typing, 303
hypertension, 304
independent living donor advocate, 303
informed consent, 302
medical evaluation, 304, 305t–306t, 307t,
308t
medical outcome of living kidney donation

long-term medical outcome after
donation, 311–312
perioperative complications, 311
obesity, 306
postdonation follow-up, 312
principle, 302
psychosocial evaluation, 303–304
renal assessment
kidney function, 307
microscopic hematuria, 309
proteinuria, 309
pyuria, 309
Lixisenatide
Loin pain hematuria syndrome, 16t
Loop diuretics, 24, 270
Low-density lipoprotein (LDL), 240
Lower extremity Doppler ultrasound, 295
Low–molecular-weight heparins, 263
Lupus nephritis, 298, 300
Lupus podocytopathy, 119

M
Macroalbuminuria, 143
Magnetic resonance angiography (MRA), 189
Magnetic resonance imaging (MRI), 150
Magnetic resonance urography (MRU), 19
Maintenance immunosuppression, 316f.
        See also Kidney transplant patient
        management
antimetabolites, 317–318
calcineurin inhibitors, 315, 317
for combined transplantation-pancreas, 343
costimulation inhibitors, 317
glucocorticoid (prednisone, prednisolone),
315
infection prophylaxis, 318
mammalian target of rapamycin
inhibitors, 317
pharmacology and drug-drug interactions,
318–320, 319t
Major histocompatibility complex (MHC),
and immunology of transplant,
281–282
Major histocompatibility complex class
I-related chain B (MICB), 327
Malabsorption syndromes, 48
Malignancy, 40, 40t
of kidney transplant patient, 322
Malignant tumors, for VHL, 160
Malnutrition, 48
protein loss and, 241
Mammalian target of rapamycin inhibitors
(mTORi), 317
Mannitol, 21
Manual exchanges, in PD, 233
Markers of hemolysis, 47

Maternal endothelial dysfunction, 165
MCKD. *See* Medullary cystic kidney
    disease
MDRD equation, 2, 3
Mean fluorescence intensity (MFI), 287
Measured GFR (mGFR), 307
Mechanical complications, in PD. *See also*
        Peritoneal dialysis (PD)
    back pain, 239
    fluid leakage, 239–240
    hernias, 239
    outflow failure, 239
    sclerosing encapsulating peritonitis,
        240
Medical outcome of living kidney donation
    long-term medical outcome after
        donation, 311–312
    perioperative complications, 311
Medications
    for AKI, 64
    errors in CKD, 137
    nephrotoxic, 261
    for RAS/RVHTN, 191
Medullary cystic kidney disease (MCKD).
        See also Cystic disease of kidney
    classification, 156
    clinical presentation, 156
    diagnostic criteria, 157
    differential diagnosis, 157
    epidemiology, 156
    outcome/prognosis, 157
    pathophysiology, 156
    treatment, 157
Medullary sponge kidney (MSK)
    diagnosis, 158
    epidemiology, 157
    outcome/prognosis, 158
    pathophysiology, 157
    treatment, 158
Medullary tissue, 337
Membrane plasma separation, 256
Meperidine, with active metabolites, 268t,
    270
Metabolic acidosis, 33, 71, 135. *See also*
        Acid-base disorders
    diagnostic testing, 54–55
    differential diagnosis, 55–57, 55t, 57t
    principles, 54
    treatment of, 57–58
Metabolic alkalosis. *See also* Acid-base
        disorders
    diagnostic testing, 59
    differential diagnosis, 59
    principles, 58
    treatment, 60
    types of, 58t

Metabolic complications. *See also* Kidney
        transplant patient management
    bone disease, 321
    hyperlipidemia, 320
    obesity, 321
    post-transplant diabetes mellitus, 321
Metabolic complications, in PD. *See also*
        Peritoneal dialysis (PD)
    hyperglycemia, 240
    hyperlipidemia, 240–241
    hypokalemia, 241
    protein loss and malnutrition, 241
Metformin
    for CKD patients, 137
    DN patients and, 146
    dosing of, 271
    Food and Drug Administration
        recommendations for, 271t
Methanol, 56
Methylprednisolone, for acute cellular
        rejection, 346
Metolazone, 270
Metoprolol, and dose adjustments, 270
MHC. *See* Major histocompatibility complex
Microalbuminuria, 142, 143, 143t
Microangiopathic hemolytic anemia, 85
Microscopic hematuria, 309
    causes of, 16t
    urologic pathology for, risk factors, 17t
Microvascular causes of AKI, 79. *See also*
        Acute kidney injury (AKI)
    diagnosis, 82–85, 83t–84t
    principles, 82
    treatment, 85
Midodrine, for HRS, 98
Mild hypercalcemia, 41
Milk-alkali syndrome, 40, 59
Mineral and bone disorders, 131
Mineralocorticoid excess, 200
    diagnosis, 202
    treatment, 202
Minoxidil, 171
Mircera, 136
Moderate hypophosphatemia, treatment
        for, 50
Modification of Diet in Renal Disease
        (MDRD) study, 261
Monoclonal immunoglobulin deposition
        disease (MIDD), 212, 314
Morphine, with active metabolites, 268t, 270
MSK. *See* Medullary sponge kidney
mTORi. *See* Mammalian target of
        rapamycin inhibitors
Multiphasic computed tomography
        urography, 18
Multiple myeloma, 65

Mycophenolate, 171, 318
Mycophenolate mofetil (MMF), 103, 317
Mycophenolic acid (MPA), 317
Myeloma kidney, 144
Myoglobinuria, 66

N
National Cholesterol Education Program
    Adult Treatment Program (NCEP
    ATP) III guidelines, 135
Native kidney biopsy, 8
Nephritic syndrome, 14, 15
Nephrogenic systemic fibrosis (NSF), 138
Nephrolithiasis, 41, 76, 89, 152
Nephrology consultation, 134
Nephrotic range proteinuria, 10
Nephrotoxic acute kidney injury, 86
Nephrotoxicity, and alternatives to common
    drugs, 262
Nephrotoxins, for AKI, 64
Neurologic symptoms, 41
Neuromuscular excitability symptoms, 43
Neuromuscular symptoms, 49
Neutra-Phos, for moderate
    hypophosphatemia, 50
Neutra-Phos K, for moderate
    hypophosphatemia, 50
Neutropenia, treatment of, 29
Neutrophil gelatinase–associated lipocalin
    (NGAL), 69, 70
Niacinamide, 47
Nitroprusside, with active metabolites, 268t
Nonalbumin proteins, 12
Nonanion gap acidosis, 34, 55
Non–calcium-based binders, 47
Nongap (hyperchloremic) metabolic acidosis,
    56. *See also* Metabolic acidosis
Nonglomerular hematuria, 15
Nonimmunologic complications after kidney
    transplantation
  BK virus
    diagnosis, 336–337
    principles, 336, 336t
    treatment of, 337
  cytomegalovirus
    clinical presentation, 335
    principles, 332
    prophylaxis, 335
    treatment of, 335–336, 335t
  Epstein-Barr virus
    diagnosis, 338
    principles, 337–338
    treatment of, 338
  infections, 332
  principles, 331, 331t
  surgical complications, 332, 333t–334t

Noninvasive cardiac stress testing, 295
Nonreabsorbable anion, 30
Nonsteroidal anti-inflammatory drugs
    (NSAID)
  for AIN, 95
  and hematuria, 15
  in renal injury, 268
Nonsteroidal anti-inflammatory medications,
    135
Norepinephrine, for HRS, 98
Normal anatomic renal changes in
    pregnancy, 162
Normal hemodynamic changes in pregnancy,
    162
Nuclear factor of activated T cells (NFAT),
    316f
Nutritional status, in CKD, 133
Nutritional support, in AKI, 71
NxStage, 253

O
Obesity, 321
  for kidney transplant candidate, 300
  and living donor evaluation, 306
  modifiable risk factor in DN, 142
Obstructive nephropathy, 74, 144
Obstructive sleep apnea (OSA), 194
Obstructive uropathy, 73, 74, 76, 167
  congenital causes of, 75t
  extrinsic causes of, 75t
  intrinsic causes of, 75t
Octreotide, for HRS, 98
Oliguric AKI, 67
Oncogenic osteomalacia, 49
Oral calcium supplements, 44
Oral cephalosporin, 237
Oral contraceptive pills (OCP),
    305t–306t
Oral contraceptives, and hematuria, 15
Oral phosphate binders, 48
Oral sodium loading test, 198
Organisms, in urinary assessment
  bacteria, 6
  fungi, 6
  parasites, 6
Organ Procurement and Transplantation
    Network (OPTN), 302, 342
Organ transplantation, combined
  combined liver/kidney transplantation,
    341–342, 342t
  complications
    pancreas allograft dysfunction,
      343–347, 344f, 344t
    pancreas transplantation, 340–341
    risks/benefits, 341
  principles, 340

Organ transplantation, combined (*Continued*)
treatment
liver/kidney, induction for, 343
maintenance immunosuppression for
combined transplantation—pancreas,
343
pancreas, induction for, 342–343
Orthostatic (postural) proteinuria, 11
Osmolar gap, 56
Osmotic demyelination, 22
Osmotic diuresis, 49
Osteolytic hypercalcemia, 40t
Outflow failure, defined, 239

P
Paired exchanged kidneys, 290
Pancreas allograft dysfunction, 343–347
causes of, 343, 344f
pancreas allograft rejection
acute cellular rejection, 345–346
antibody-mediated rejection, 346–347
assessment, 345
Pancreas transplantation, 146
indications for, 340–341
risks/benefits, 341
Pancreas vascular thrombosis, 344t
Pancreatic enzymes, leaks of, 344t
Panel-reactive antibody (PRA), 286, 293
Papillary necrosis, 144
Paraprotein
amyloidosis, 212
cast nephropathy, 211–212
classification of, 213t
electrolyte abnormalities, 214t, 215
Parasites, 6
Parathyroidectomy, 40, 42
Parathyroid hormone (PTH), 38, 133
decreased, 42
effect, decreased, 45
role of, 45
Patient education
for dialysis and renal transplant, 138
Patient selection
in HHD, 242
in PD, 229
Patiromer (Veltassa), 36
Pauci-immune GN, 120–123
PD. *See* Peritoneal dialysis
Peak systolic velocities (PSV), 188
Penicillinaseresistant antibiotic, 237
Percutaneous transluminal renal angioplasty
(PTRA), 190, 191
Peripheral arterial disease (PAD), 295
and kidney transplant candidate, 295
Peritoneal dialysis (PD), 36, 41, 246, 247t.
See also Home hemodialysis (HHD)

adequacy of
clearance targets, 233–234
ultrafiltration targets, 234
apparatus
catheter and setup, 229–230, 230f
dialysis solution, 230–231, 230t, 231t
peritoneal membrane, 231–232, 232t
catheter, 139
contraindications for PD, 229
indications for change to, 241
infectious complications
exit-site and tunnel infection, 237
peritonitis, 234–237, 235t–236t, 237t,
238t
mechanical complications
back pain, 239
fluid leakage, 239–240
hernias, 239
outflow failure, 239
sclerosing encapsulating peritonitis, 240
metabolic complications
hyperglycemia, 240
hyperlipidemia, 240–241
hypokalemia, 241
protein loss and malnutrition, 241
modalities and prescription
automated cycler exchanges, 233
manual exchanges, 233
prescriptions, 233
patient selection, 229
physiology
absorption, 229
diffusion, 228
ultrafiltration, 228–229
principles, 228
Peritoneal dialysis patients, signs/symptoms
in, 235t–236t
Peritoneal dialysis solution, 230–231, 230t,
231t
Peritoneal equilibration test (PET), 232
Peritoneal membrane, 231–232, 232t
Peritonitis, 234–237, 235t–236t, 237t,
238t
Persistent isolated microscopic hematuria,
309
Persistent pain, at renal biopsy, 9
Persistent proteinuria, 11
PHA. *See* Pseudohypoaldosteronism
Pharmacokinetic principles, dosing and, 261,
263, 264t–267t, 268t
Pharmacology and drug-drug interactions,
318–320, 319t
Pheochromocytomas
clinical presentation, 203–205
diagnostic testing, 204
medications associated with, 204t

principles, 202–203
treatment, 205
Phosphate
 binders, 137
 dietary restriction of, 47
 load, increased, 46
Phosphatonins, 45
Phosphorus
 enteric absorption of, 47
 fractional excretion of, 49
 in PD solutions, 231
Phosphorus metabolism, disorders of. *See also* Calcium balance, disorders of
 hyperphosphatemia
  causes of, 46t
  clinical presentation, 47
  defined, 45
  diagnostic testing, 47
  pathophysiology, 45–46
  treatment for, 47–48
 hypophosphatemia
  clinical presentation, 49
  defined, 48
  diagnostic testing, 49
  pathophysiology, 48–49
  treatment, 50
 principles, 44–45
Physiologic balance of acid–base status, defined, 51
PIRRT. *See* Prolonged intermittent renal replacement therapy
Plasma calcium, 49
Plasma creatinine, 47
Plasma exchange method, 254–256
 centrifugation, 254
 membrane plasma separation, 256
Plasma half-life of immunoglobulins, 256
Plasmapheresis, 347
Plasma phosphorus levels, 45
Plasma renin activity (PRA), 187
Pneumococcal conjugate vaccine (PCV13), 297t
Pneumococcal polysaccharide vaccine (PPSV23), 297t
Pneumococcal vaccination, 138
Pneumocystis jiroveci prevention, 318
Point-of-care ultrasonography (POCUS), 68, 69t
Polarized microscopy, 93
Polyclonal antibody, 314
Polycystic kidney disease. *See also* Cystic disease of kidney
 classification, 149
 clinical presentation, 149–150
  history, 150
  physical examination, 150

complications
  extrarenal manifestations, 152
  renal manifestations, 151–152
 diagnostic criteria, 150, 150t
 differential diagnosis, 151
 epidemiology, 149
 outcome/prognosis, 153
 pathophysiology, 149
 patient education, 152–153
 treatment, 151
Polydipsia, 26
Polyglandular autoimmune syndrome type I, 42
Polymerase chain reaction (PCR) amplification, 282
Polyuria, 26, 41
Posthypercapnic state, 59
Postrenal acute kidney injury. *See also* Acute kidney injury (AKI)
 clinical presentation, 76
 definition, 73, 75t
 diagnostic testing, 76–77
 etiology, 74, 76
 management, 77–78
 pathophysiology, 76
Poststreptococcal glomerulonephritis, 65
Post-transplant diabetes mellitus (PTDM), 315
Post-transplant lymphoproliferative disorders (PTLD), 314
Potassium
 in PD solutions, 231
 replacement, 32
Potassium balance, disorders of
 hyperkalemia
  clinical presentation, 34
  defined, 32
  diagnostic testing, 34–35, 34t
  pathophysiology, 33–34
  treatment of, 35–37
 hypokalemia
  clinical presentation, 30–31
  defined, 29
  diagnostic testing, 31–32, 31t
  pathophysiology, 29–30
  treatment of, 32
 principles, 28–29, 28t
Potassium phosphate, for severe hypophosphatemia, 50
Potassium-sparing diuretics, 271
Preangioplasty, 188
Preeclampsia, 82, 164, 168. *See also* Hypertensive disorders in pregnancy
 diagnosis, 165, 166t
 principles, 165, 165t
 treatment, 165–167
Preemptive transplants, 280

Pregnancy
  kidney transplantation and, 322–323
  in renal transplant recipients/kidney donors
    after kidney donation, 171
    after renal transplant, 170–171
Prerenal acute kidney injury. *See also* Acute
    kidney injury (AKI)
  causes of, 74t
  definition, 72
  etiology, 73, 74t
  management, 73
Prerenal azotemia, 167
  pathophysiology of, 73f
Prescription, 233
  TPE (*See also* Therapeutic plasma
    exchange (TPE))
    anticoagulation, 257–258
    dose of TPE, 257
    replacement solution, 258, 259t
    vascular access, 257
Primary aldosteronism, 195
  bilateral disease, 196
  causes of, 196
  clinical presentation, 196–197
  evaluation for, 197–199
  treatment, 199–200
  unilateral disease, 196
Primary hyperaldosteronism, 30, 59
Primary hyperoxaluria, 311
Primary hyperparathyroidism, 39
Primidone, with active metabolites, 268t
Procainamide, with active metabolites, 268t
Prolonged intermittent renal replacement
    therapy (PIRRT), 252–253. *See also*
    Renal replacement therapy (RRT)
Prophylactic therapy, 335
Prophylaxis, treatment of rejection, 318
Propranolol, and dose adjustments, 270
Protein loss and malnutrition, 241
Proteinuria, 10–14, 96, 309, 312. *See also*
    Hematuria
  classification
    glomerular proteinuria, 10
    overflow proteinuria, 10
    tubular proteinuria, 10
  classification of, 143t
  clinical approach to, 13–14
  definition, 10
  diagnosis
    quantitative methods, 12–13, 13t
    semiquantitative methods, 11–12, 12t
  etiology
    orthostatic (postural) proteinuria, 11
    persistent proteinuria, 11
    transient (functional) proteinuria, 11
  quantification of, 18

Proteinuric kidney diseases, 144
Prothrombin time (PT), 8, 259
Prothrombin time/international normalized
    ratio (PT/INR), 305t–306t
Proton loss, 30
Proximal tubule reabsorption, 45
Pseudohyperkalemia, 33, 34
Pseudohypoaldosteronism (PHA), type I, 33
Pseudohyponatremia, 20
Pseudohypoparathyroidism, 42
Pseudomonas aeruginosa, 237
Psychosocial evaluation of living donor,
    303–304
PTH. *See* Parathyroid hormone
PTRA. *See* Percutaneous transluminal renal
    angioplasty
Pulmonary hemorrhage, 66
Pulse intravenous (IV) glucocorticoids, 346
Pyuria, 309

Q

Quantitative methods. *See also* Proteinuria
  24-hour urine protein collection, 13
  spot urine ACR, 12–13, 13t
  spot urine PCR, 12

R

Rabbit antithymocyte globulin (rATG)-
    Thymoglobulin, 314
Race, nonmodifiable risk factors in DN,
    142
Radix tripterygii, 64
Randomized evaluation of normal *vs.*
    augmented level replacement therapy
    (RENAL) study, 247
Rapid plasma regain (RPR), 293
Rasburicase, 208
Rash, 66
RBC. *See* Red blood cells
Recurrent flash pulmonary edema, 187
Recurrent glomerular disease, 298
Red blood cells (RBC)
  casts, 7t, 18
  for urinary assessment, 4
Refeeding syndrome, 48
Referral for dialysis access/transplantation,
    139. *See also* Chronic kidney disease
    (CKD)
Refractory hypertension, 191
Regional citrate, 258
Rejection types. *See also* Immunologic
    complications after kidney
    transplantation
  accelerated acute rejection, 325
  active antibody-mediated rejection, 326,
    327t

acute cellular rejection, 326, 326t
borderline rejection, 328
chronic, active antibody-mediated rejection, 328, 328t
chronic active T-cell-mediated rejection, 326
hyperacute rejection, 325
subclinical rejection, 328
Relative contraindications to kidney transplant, 291, 291t
Renal allograft dysfunction, differential diagnosis of, 331t
Renal angiography, 189
Renal angiomyolipomas, 159
Renal artery stenosis (RAS), 194
    clinical presentation, 186–187, 186t
    diagnostic testing, 187, 187t
        imaging, 188–190
        laboratories, 187–188
    epidemiology
        atherosclerotic renovascular disease, 184–185
        FMD, 185
    pathophysiology
        ARAS, 186
        Goldblatt model, 185–186
    principles, 184
    treatment, 190, 191t
        medications, 191
        nonpharmacologic therapies, 191–192
Renal assessment. See also Living kidney donor candidate, evaluation of
    kidney function, 307
    microscopic hematuria, 309
    proteinuria, 309
    pyuria, 309
Renal biopsy, 69, 93, 96. See also Kidney function, assessment of
    complications, 8–9
    indications, 8
    preprocedural evaluation, 8
Renal calcium excretion, 42
Renal cortical necrosis, 168
Renal cysts, 160
Renal diseases in pregnancy
    AKI in pregnancy
        principles, 167–168, 169t
        treatment, 167
    CKD and
        about, 169–170
        pregnancy in renal transplant recipients/kidney donors, 170–171
    glomerular diseases in pregnancy, 171
    hypertensive disorders, 163–167
        chronic hypertension, 164, 164t
        preeclampsia, 165–167, 165t, 166t

principles, 162–163, 163t
SLE and pregnancy, 171
Renal elimination, 35
Renal excretion, decreased, 39t, 40
Renal failure, 45
Renal function, dose adjustment for, 272, 273t–275t
Renal hemodynamics, 162
Renal imaging, 8
Renal injury, localization of, 1
Renal losses, 30
Renal parenchymal disease, 194
Renal phosphate wasting, 49
Reninoma, 202
Renin-secreting tumors, 202
Renal potassium regulation, 28
Renal replacement therapy (RRT)
    advantages/disadvantages of, 247t
    in AKI, 71–72, 72t
    continuous RRT (CRRT)
        anticoagulation in, 249
        complications of, 250–253
        drug dosing in CRRT, 250
        fluids in, 249
        principles of, 248–249, 248t
        regimen for CRRT, 250
    dosage adjustments during, 278
    dosing of, 246–248
    initiation of, 139
    modalities of, 246
    prolonged intermittent RRT, 253
Renal to aortic ratio (RAR), 188
Renal tuberculosis, 144
Renal tubular acidosis (RTA), 31, 56, 57t
Renal tubular epithelial cells, 6
Renal ultrasound, 6, 68, 93
Renal vascular disease, 144
Renal vascular hypertension (RVHTN).
        See also Renal artery stenosis (RAS)/Renal vascular hypertension (RVHTN)
    angiotensin II-dependent, 185
    angiotensin-independent/volume-dependent, 185
Renin-angiotensin-aldosterone (RAAS) system, 33, 162, 185
Renin inhibitors (Aliskiren), 147
Renovascular hypertension, 185t
Replacement solution, 248, 250, 258
    complications related to, 259
    pros and cons of, 259t
Resistive index (RI), defined, 188
Respiratory acidosis. See also Acid-base disorders
    diagnosis, 60–61
    principles, 60
    treatment of, 61

Respiratory alkalosis, 48. *See also* Acid-base disorders
  diagnosis, 61
  principles, 61
  treatment of, 61
Restenosis, 192
Retrograde pyelogram (RPG), 19
Rhabdomyolysis, 43, 46, 65, 86–87. *See also* Acute kidney injury (AKI)
Rituximab, 118, 171
Rivaroxaban, direct oral anticoagulant agents (DOAC), 263
Routine urine dipstick, 11–12, 12t
RRT. *See* Renal replacement therapy
RTA. *See* Renal tubular acidosis
RVHTN. *See* Renal vascular hypertension

S

Salicylate overdose, 56
Saline infusion test, 198
Salt tablets, 24
Salt-sensitive hypertension, 201
Saxagliptin, dosing in renal impairment, 271
Scleroderma renal crisis, 82
Sclerosing encapsulating peritonitis, 240
Secondary hyperaldosteronism, 30
Secondary hyperparathyroidism (SHPT), 131, 136
Seizure prophylaxis, with magnesium sulfate, 167
Selective serotonin reuptake inhibitors (SSRI), 22
Semiquantitative methods. *See also* Proteinuria
  albumin-sensitive tests, 12
  positive dipstick, implications of, 12
  routine urine dipstick, 11–12, 12t
Sepsis, 65
Septic shock, 43
Sequence-specific oligonucleotide (SSO), 282
Sequence-specific primers (SSP), 283
Serologic methods for compatibility testing, 284–286, 286f
Serologic testing, 18
Serum albumin, 133
Serum creatinine, 18, 87
Serum free light chain (FLC) ratios, 133
Serum markers, 2, 3t. *See also* Glomerular filtration rate (GFR)
Serum osmolality calculation, 56
Serum protein electrophoresis (SPEP), 211
Sevelamer carbonate, 48
Severe hypercalcemia, 41
Severe hypophosphatemia, treatment for, 50
SIADH. *See* Syndrome of inappropriate antidiuretic hormone

Simple renal cysts. *See also* Cystic disease of kidney
  clinical presentation, 153
  diagnostic criteria, 153
  differential diagnosis, 154, 154t
  epidemiology, 153
  prognosis, 155
  pathophysiology, 153
  treatment, 154
Simultaneous kidney and pancreas (SPK) transplantation, 340
Sirolimus, 171
Sitagliptin, dosing in renal impairment, 271
SLE. *See* Systemic lupus erythematosus
Slow continuous ultrafiltration (SCUF), 249
Sodium, distal delivery of, 35
Sodium-glucose cotransporter-2 inhibitors, 272
Sodium-glucose cotransporter-2 (SGLT-2) inhibitors, 146
Sodium polystyrene sulfonate (SPS), 36
Sodium restriction, 134
Solid phase methods for compatibility testing, 286–288, 287f, 288f
Solid phase testing, 287
Solitary native kidney, renal biopsy of, 8
Spiral computed tomography scan, 188
Spironolactone, 32
  aldosterone antagonists, 33
  for severe HF, 271
Spot urine ACR. *See* Spot urine albumin to creatinine ratio
Spot urine albumin to creatinine ratio, 12–13, 13t
Spot urine PCR. *See* Spot urine protein to creatinine ratio
Spot urine protein to creatinine ratio, 12
Squamous epithelial cells, 5
Staphylococcus aureus, 237
Steal syndrome, 226
Sterile precautions, 251
Sterile technique, 244
Stress biomarkers, 70
Struvite stones, 310
Subacute antihypertensive therapy, 164t
Subclinical rejection, 328
Sucroferric oxyhydroxide, 137
Sulfamethoxazole, 318
Sulfonylureas, 146, 271
Supraventricular arrhythmias, 251
Sustained low efficiency dialysis (SLED), 246
Symptomatic hyponatremia, 24–25
Syndrome of inappropriate antidiuretic hormone (SIADH), 22t
Syndromes of mineralocorticoid excess, 30

Systemic hemodynamics, 162
Systemic lupus erythematosus (SLE), 115, 310
  and pregnancy, 171
  complication, 119
  renal pathology for, 115–116
  treatment for, 116–118

T
Tacrolimus, calcineurin inhibitors (CNI), 315, 317
Tamm–Horsfall protein, 156
TBMD. *See* Thin basement membrane disease
T-cell reactivity assays, 325
T cells, 282
Temporizing measures, for liver transplantation, 98
Terlipressin, for HRS, 98
Tertiary hyperparathyroidism, 40
Therapeutic plasma exchange (TPE)
  complications
    ACE inhibitor-related, 260
    anticoagulation-related, 259
    replacement solution-related, 259
    TPE procedure–related, 259–260
    vascular access–related, 259
  current renal indications for, 254, 255t
  kinetics of substance removal in
    plasma half-life of immunoglobulins, 256
    removal of immunoglobulin, 256–257
    volume of distribution, 256
  plasma exchange method, 254–256
    centrifugation, 254
    membrane plasma separation, 256
  principles, 254
  rationale for, 254
  TPE prescription
    anticoagulation, 257–258
    dose of TPE, 257
    replacement solution, 258, 259t
    vascular access, 257
Thiazide diuretics, 22, 99, 270
Thiazolidinediones (rosiglitazone, pioglitazone), 146
Thin basement membrane disease (TBMD), 310
Three-pore model, 232
Thrombi, 85
Thrombocytopenia, 260
Thrombotic microangiopathy (TMA)
  clinical presentation, 128
  definitions, 127
  pathophysiology, 127
  treatment, 129

Thrombotic thrombocytopenic purpura (TTP), 127, 129, 79, 254
Thyroid-stimulating hormone, in hyponatremia, 23
Thyrotoxicosis, 40
Tissue inhibitor of metalloproteinases-2 (TIMP-2), 70
TLS. *See* Tumor lysis syndrome
Tobramycin, dose calculation, 276
Tocilizumab, ABMR treatment, 329
Torsemide, diuretics in renal impairment, 270
Total body potassium, 28
Toxic alcohol ingestions, 56
TPE. *See* Therapeutic plasma exchange
Traditional dosing, of aminoglycosides, 272
Tramadol, with active metabolites, 268t, 270
Transcellular shift, 46
Transient (functional) proteinuria, 11
Transitional epithelial cells, 5
Transjugular intrahepatic portosystemic shunt (TIPS), 98
Translesional pressure gradient, 189
Transplant glomerulopathy, 328
Triamterene, 32
Trimethoprim, 318
Triple phosphate, urinary crystal, 6t
Trousseau sign, 43
Tuberous sclerosis. *See also* Cystic disease of kidney
  diagnosis, 159
  epidemiology, 158–159
  pathophysiology, 159
  treatment, 159–160
Tubular proteinuria, 10
Tubular toxins, and tubular damage, 30
Tubulointerstitial fibrosis, 145
Tumoral calcitriol production, 40t
Tumor lysis syndrome (TLS), 43, 46, 88
Tunneled presternal catheters, 229
Tunnel infections, in PD, 237
Type 4 RTA, 148

U
Ultrafiltration, 249
  failure, 234
  in PD, 228–229
  targets, defined, 234
Ultrasonography
  for AKI in patients, 68
  for MCKD, 157
  for simple renal cysts, 153
Ultrasound diagnostic criteria, 150, 150t
Unclassified metabolic alkalosis
  massive transfusion of blood products, 59
  Milk-alkali syndrome, 59
Unfractionated heparin, 258, 263

United Kingdom Prospective Diabetes Study (UKPDS), 142
United Network for Organ Sharing (UNOS), 287, 340
Urea reduction ratio (URR), 246, 248
Urea tablets, 24
Ureteral surgical complications, 332
Ureterorenoscopy, 19
Uric acid
  in hyponatremia, 23
  levels, 47
  urinary crystal, 6t
Urinalysis, 4, 96
Urinary assessment, 4–6, 5t, 6t, 7t
Urinary calcium, 41
Urinary casts. See Casts, urinary
Urinary crystals, 6, 6t
Urinary indices, 67, 68t
Urinary tract infection, prevention, 318
Urine
  alkalinization, 208
  anion gap, 55
  chemokine measurements, 325
  culture, 8, 18
  cytology, 18
  electrophoresis, 211
  examination, in AKI, 66
  excretion, 132
  patterns and frequency, 64
  phosphorus, 24-hour, 49
  potassium excretion, 31
  sediment findings, 89
  tests
    for hypernatremia, 26
    for hyponatremia, 23

V
Valganciclovir (VGCV), 335, 335t
Valvular heart disease, 295
Vancomycin
  dosage adjustments, 277–278, 277t
  for PD patients, 236, 237t
Varicella (Varivax), 297t
Varicella zoster virus (VZV), 293
Vascular access, 257
  complications related to, 259
Vasoconstriction, 87
Vasopressin antagonists, in SIADH, 24
Velphoro, 137
Venous surgical complications, 332
Viral blips, 296
Vitamin A intoxication, 40
Vitamin D, 38, 45, 137
  deficiency, 42, 48, 49
  intoxication, 40

replacement, 137
rickets dependent on, 42
Vitamin K antagonists, dosage adjustments, 263
Vomiting or gastric drainage, 59
von Hippel-Lindau (VHL) syndrome.
    See also Cystic disease of kidney
  diagnosis, 160
  epidemiology, 160
  pathophysiology, 160
  treatment, 161

W
Waitlist management
  in kidney transplantation, 281
  for kidney transplant candidate, 300
Warfarin, 263
  direct oral anticoagulant agents, 263
  and hematuria, 15
Water balance, disorders of
  hypernatremia
    classification, 25
    clinical presentation, 26
    definition, 25
    diagnostic testing, 26
    epidemiology, 25
    etiology, 25, 25f
    pathophysiology, 26
    treatment, 27
  hyponatremia
    causes of, 21f
    classification, 20
    clinical presentation, 23
    defined, 20
    diagnostic testing, 23
    epidemiology, 20–21
    etiology, 21
    pathophysiology, 22
    risk factors, 22
    SIADH, causes of, 22t
    treatment, 24–25
  principles, 20
Water homeostasis, changes in, 163
WBC. See White blood cells
Wegener granulomatosis, 65
White blood cells (WBC)
  casts, 7t
  for urinary assessment, 4

X
Xanthine oxidase inhibitors, 135

Z
Zoster (Shingrix), 297t